D1610927

FROM DEVELOPMENT TO DEGENERATION AND REGENERATION OF THE NERVOUS SYSTEM

FROM DEVELOPMENT TO DEGENERATION AND REGENERATION OF THE NERVOUS SYSTEM

Edited by:

CHARLES E. RIBAK, PhD
Professor of Anatomy & Neurobiology
Department of Anatomy & Neurobiology
University of California at Irvine
  School of Medicine
Irvine, CA

CARLOS ARÁMBURO DE LA HOZ, PhD
Associate Professor
Department of Cellular & Molecular
  Neurobiology
Instituto de Neurobiología
Campus UNAM-UAQ Juriquilla
Universidad Nacional Autónoma de México
Querétaro, Qro. México

EDWARD G. JONES, MD, PhD
Director, Center for Neuroscience
University of California, Davis
Davis, CA

JORGE A. LARRIVA SAHD, MD, PhD
Professor, Department of Developmental
  Neurobiology & Neurophysiology
Instituto de Neurobiología
Campus UNAM-UAQ Juriquilla
Universidad Nacional Autónoma de México
Querétaro, Qro. México

LARRY W. SWANSON, PhD
Appleman Professor of Biological Sciences
Neuroscience Program
University of Southern California
Los Angeles, CA

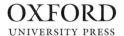

OXFORD
UNIVERSITY PRESS

2009

OXFORD
UNIVERSITY PRESS

Oxford University Press, Inc., publishes works that further
Oxford University's objective of excellence
in research, scholarship, and education.

Oxford   New York
Auckland   Cape Town   Dar es Salaam   Hong Kong   Karachi
Kuala Lumpur   Madrid   Melbourne   Mexico City   Nairobi
New Delhi   Shanghai   Taipei   Toronto

With offices in
Argentina   Austria   Brazil   Chile   Czech Republic   France   Greece
Guatemala   Hungary   Italy   Japan   Poland   Portugal   Singapore
South Korea   Switzerland   Thailand   Turkey   Ukraine   Vietnam

Published by Oxford University Press, Inc.
198 Madison Avenue, New York, New York 10016
www.oup.com

Oxford is a registered trademark of Oxford University Press

Library of Congress Cataloging-in-Publication Data

From development to degeneration and regeneration of the nervous system / Charles E. Ribak ... [et al.].
    p. ; cm.
Includes bibliographical references and index.
ISBN 978-0-19-536900-7
1. Central nervous system—Physiology. 2. Nervous system—Degeneration. 3. Nervous system—Regeneration.
4. Neuroplasticity. I. Ribak, Charles E.
[DNLM: 1. Central Nervous System—physiology. 2. Nerve Regeneration. 3. Neurodegenerative
Diseases—physiopathology. 4. Neuronal Plasticity. WL 300 F931 2009]
    QP370.F76 2009
    612.8'2—dc22
ISBN 978-0-19-536900-7

                                                                                                    2008022057

1 3 5 7 9 8 6 4 2

Printed in the United States of America
on acid-free paper

To the memory of Santiago Ramón y Cajal

FOREWORD

Lawrence Kruger

This volume celebrates the emergence of the twenty-first century Cajal Club as a welcome component of the scientific attempt to advance the understanding of the organizational principles of the nervous system and the passion of Santiago Ramón y Cajal, who devoted most of his life to advance this poorly understood subject before his entry onto the scene. The first Nobel prize in the field now called "neuroscience" was presented in 1906, and it also was the first shared Nobel award, thus acknowledging the principle of international interaction and cooperation that has served the glorious development of all fields of science for the past century. The centenary of the formal acceptance of the evidence Cajal adduced in support of the "neuron doctrine" was widely feted across the world over the past year, and in keeping with a recent trend of becoming a global organization, the Cajal Club aptly met in Mexico for the first time. Quite frankly, the scientific content and tenor of the meeting set a new standard of excellence and a broadly felt sense of camaraderie.

Half a century ago the Cajal Club was a rather jejune social club for neuroanatomists seeking a future for their subject with limited tools, and still heavily immersed in the long tradition of descriptive anatomy from which Cajal had attempted to revolutionize the field with experimental approaches establishing the rules of neural connectivity. The highlight of the meetings in that era was the dinner banquet, with emphasis on libations and an air of hi-jinks presided over with some regularity by either the jovial Pinckney J. Harman or the flamboyant, energetic Wendell J.S. Krieg. Its attachment to the American Association of Anatomists in the United States (AAA) and to the Federation of American Societies of Experimental Biology (FASEB) meetings limited its breadth. The Cajal Club's eventual transfer to status as a "social" at the annual Society for Neuroscience meetings largely continued its prior tradition, although serious theme discussions and formal presentations gradually emerged, adding stimulating content to the fun of the occasion.

The propitious decision to organize a Cajal Club meeting in Querétaro, Mexico, adds the next logical step in the evolution of what Cajal probably would have hoped for—the club's firm internationalization. Following on the special first meetings abroad in the previous century in Madrid and Stockholm, arranging a meeting in the beautiful historic colonial portion of the Mexican highlands and the seat of the revolution from Spanish colonial rule enabled emphasizing the impact of the Spanish roots of modern trends in neuroscience deriving from Cajal's life work. It should be remembered that, in the latter part of his career, Don Santiago served with some vigor in the Senate of Spain, soon to be dominated by the dictatorship of Generalissimo Franco and a brutal civil war that led to the flight of many of his disciples to the Western hemisphere. The development of neuroscience in Mexico, and especially as it has recently flowered in the beautiful new university campus and laboratories in Querétaro, would surely have delighted Cajal, for it embodies his heritage in exemplary fashion and reveals the recent spread of advanced research in the neurosciences beyond the Federal District of Mexico City into modern new centers of excellence and enlightened leadership. The poignant essay in this volume by José Luis Díaz of the émigrés from the world of Cajal to the new world of Latin America (including the Caribbean), and initially to the rapidly expanding and generously supported labs in the United States, by distinguished students of Cajal, provides a luminous historical account of the global importance of the Spanish school in modern neuroscience.

The meeting also provided an opportunity to host an exhibit devoted to materials from the career of Cajal's final surviving student, Rafael Lorente de Nó, presented lovingly by his estimable devoted disciple in Querétaro, Jorge Larriva Sahd. It was also a most suitable occasion to bestow the Krieg Lifetime Achievement Award to honor Ricardo Miledi, who continues to work productively at the University of California, Irvine, and increasingly at the splendid UNAM facilities in Mexico, employing cutting-edge techniques of molecular biology in expanding his high-impact, profoundly important contributions to fundamental neurobiology. It is of particular interest to note the changing concepts of the synapse deriving from the recent understanding of extra-synaptic neurotransmitter receptors pioneered by Miledi in two of his important contributions from his youth that have attracted recent special attention (Eusebi, F. 2007. Ricardo Miledi and the foundation of synaptic and extra-synaptic neurotransmitter receptor physiology. *J Physiol* 581:890–2)—precisely the sort of work that we imagine would have conceptually delighted Cajal, if he had survived into modern times. Let us hope that Miledi's dual appointment (UCI-UNAM) serves to acknowledge that there are no meaningful borders to cross between the national scientific communities and that this first meeting of the Cajal Club in Mexico will be the first of many future exchanges among the brotherhood (and sisterhood) of neuroscientists.

The organization of a Cajal Club meeting in Mexico for the first time formally recognizes the link of Mexican neuroscientists to Cajal and to Spain; several of the excellent articles in this book reveal both the truly international character of neuroscience research in Mexico as well as the vigorous growth of the field as a leading component of Mexican science today. On a personal note, having devoted much of my career to studying the somatosensory system, the scientific highlight of the meeting for me was the presentation made by Ranulfo Romo, the annual Pinckney J. Harman Memorial Lecturer. His essay in this volume provides a masterful conceptual advance in the power of quantitative neurobiology in addressing the mysteries of sensory perception. Other chapters contained in this volume were presented in English by our españolophonic colleagues—a courtesy much appreciated by their many monolingual friends from the United States.

The meeting also provided a propitious occasion for the inauguration of the newly built, technologically advanced, and acoustically superb auditorium in the new, elegant, and modern laboratory setting together with new clinical diagnostic facilities at the recently developed Juriquilla University campus in Querétaro, imaginatively set in a handsome indigenous landscape. The warm hospitality of Professor Carlos Arámburo and the ability of the staff, faculty, and organizing multinational committee to organize a diverse sophisticated scientific program was appreciably enhanced by arranging a special evening museum event and dinner in downtown Querétaro, as well as tours of the extraordinary captivatingly beautiful remnants of colonial times in the cathedral and the charming provincial cities of San Miguel de Allende and Guanajuato. How they diverted a severe coastal storm from interfering with the scientific and social programs shall remain an admired and much-appreciated mystery.

Having attended numerous previous meetings of the Cajal Club over the past 50 years and serving a traditional presidential stint as Nucleolus and Nissl Body of this venerable organization, I am moved to declare with alacrity that this extraordinarily successful first meeting of the Cajal Club in Mexico portends a productive future for this organization and the expectation that it shall thrive beyond national boundaries. The diversity of subjects in this volume and the quality and originality of their content testify to the growth and sophistication of the exhilarating field so remarkably fostered by the singular efforts of Cajal and his ever-expanding scientific progeny. Viva nuestra revolución científica.

PREFACE

This book arose from the idea of two of the editors to have an international meeting of the Cajal Club in Mexico for the very first time in the club's 60-year history. Most of the officers and board members of the Cajal Club had collaborated with or mentored scientists from Mexico, and so it seemed like a logical idea to meet with them and exchange information on the nervous system. The topic chosen by the Mexican and American organizers was similar to the title of one of Cajal's great books, "Degeneration and Regeneration of the Nervous System." The co-organizers decided that it was time to address this topic with a current perspective. Neural development was included because many of the processes involving neurons in development are re-engaged in the types of processes that neurons must undergo following a brain injury or other insult.

As indicated in the Foreword by Dr. Lawrence Kruger, the meeting was held in Querétaro, Mexico, from the 19th to the 21st of August, 2007, and was a great success. This meeting was truly an international one, with about 50 worldwide neuroscience leaders and over 350 attendees, including many graduate students from Latin America and the United States. Not only did the meeting provide the opportunity for renewing old friendships, but it also built new scientific bridges between neuroscientists in the United States of America and Mexico. For the Instituto de Neurobiología of the Universidad Nacional Autónoma de México (UNAM), the opportunity to host this meeting was a great platform to increase its international profile. This meeting also provided an occasion to render homage again to Don Santiago Ramón y Cajal, whose heritage can be traced to several academic "grandsons" at the Instituto de Neurobiología and whose contributions have formed and enriched what is now known as the Mexican School of Research on Integrative Neurobiology.

The chapters in this volume fall into four categories: Cajal's Legacy, Neuronal Migration and Development, Degenerative Brain Diseases, and Neural Plasticity and Regeneration. In the first section of the book, an introductory chapter, Chapter 1, provides insight into the scientists exiled from the School of Cajal in Madrid and where these scientists migrated, especially those who came to Mexico and established productive careers.

The chapters in Part 2 address important issues about brain development. Chapters 2 and 3 examine the cellular and molecular mechanisms by which neurons are generated from the ventricular zone in the forebrain and migrate to their destinations in the cerebral cortex. Both of these chapters on cortical development also discuss the critical role of the Cajal–Retzius cell, the only neuronal type in the central nervous system named after Cajal. Chapter 4 provides insight into a special region of the forebrain, the hypothalamus (specifically its paraventricular nucleus), and its development from the wall of the third ventricle. This first section of the book ends with two chapters that examine the clinical relevance of brain development in certain disease states in humans. Chapter 5 provides insight into the nature and cause of neural tube defects, whereas Chapter 6 gives an overview of the normal and abnormal development of human electroencephalographic recordings during the first year of age.

Part 3 provides comprehensive information about several degenerative disorders of the brain. Chapter 7 is written by one of the discoverers of the morphology of catecholamine-containing neurons in the brain, and his details about the dopaminergic neurons in the substantia nigra and their loss in Parkinson's disease is a current account of degenerative mechanisms operating in this disorder. The world's expert on the structure of myelinated axons has authored Chapter 8, and the studies that he describes illustrate the severe loss of these important communicating cables in the aged brain. Chapter 9 provides insight into brain aging mechanisms in a canine model, whereas Chapter 10 describes important cellular and molecular mechanisms involving human cortical neurons in Alzheimer's disease. The last chapter in this section, Chapter 11, describes the cellular pathology found in human epilepsy. Together, these chapters summarize much of our current knowledge about the major molecular and cellular changes found in several degenerative diseases of the brain.

The last section of the book addresses the issues of brain plasticity and regeneration in the adult brain. According to Cajal, neurons in the adult brain did not exhibit the properties of regrowth to connect damaged circuits. As stated by Cajal (p. 738, *Degeneration and Regeneration of the Nervous System*), "if experimental neurology is some day to supply artificially the deficiencies in question, it must accomplish these two objects: it must give to the sprouts, by means of adequate alimentation, a vigorous capacity for growth; and place in front of the disoriented nerve cones and in the thickness of the tracts of the white matter and neuronic (neurogenic) foci specific orienting substances." The promise of stem cells obtained from the inner cell mass of embryos for the cure of degenerative disorders of not only the brain, but also other parts of the body, is the major medical challenge of the twenty-first century. The first of the chapters in Part 4, Chapter 12, describes how the brain's own stem cells provide newly generated neurons to the hippocampal dentate gyrus and how these neurons extend their dendrites into an established neuropil to become integrated into neural circuitry. The following two chapters, Chapters 13 and 14, examine some of the neuroplastic changes that take place in motor and sensory cortices of awake behaving primates. The final two chapters of the volume address the issue of regeneration in the injured spinal cord and the factors that may contribute to its success. These chapters highlight the importance of the need for axonal guidance for regeneration as stated in the quote from Cajal above.

Several people contributed substantially to this endeavor. The editors would like to acknowledge the help provided at the Cajal Club meeting in Mexico by Lee A. Shapiro, Richard H. Thompson, Manuel Corona, Diego Prieto, Paola Méndez-Probst, Manuel Salas Alvarado, Alfredo Varela-Echavarría, Alfredo Feria Velasco, Gonzalo Martínez, and Hugo Merchant. We also appreciate the support of the Instituto de Neurobiología, the Coordinación de la Investigación Científica (Dr. René Drucker-Colín), the Graduate Programs in Neurobiology and Biomedical Sciences, and the Facultad de Medicina, UNAM (Dr. José Narro Robles), Cajal Club, IBRO, Society for Neuroscience, CONCyTEQ, COCIBA, SA de CV, Carl Zeiss, Mexico, and the Government of Querétaro. Last, and certainly not least, we gratefully acknowledge the help and support provided by Oxford University Press, specifically Craig Panner and David D'Addona.

CONTRIBUTORS

LUIGI F. AGNATI, MD, PhD
Department of Biomedical
  Sciences
Section of Physiology
University of Modena
Modena, Italy

ALFONSO ALBA, PhD
Universidad Autónoma de San Luis
  Potosí
S.L.P., México

MANUEL ALVAREZ, PhD
Instituto de Fisiología
  Celular
Universidad Nacional Autónoma de
  México
México, D.F., México

AILEEN J. ANDERSON, PhD
Reeve-Irvine Research Center
Departments of Physical Medicine &
  Rehabilitation and Anatomy &
  Neurobiology
Christopher Reeve Paralysis
  Foundation Core Director
University of California-Irvine,
Irvine, CA

VÉRONIQUE M. ANDRÉ, PhD
Mental Retardation Research
  Center
David Geffen School of
  Medicine
University of California
  Los Angeles
Los Angeles, CA

TIZIANA ANTONELLI, MD, PhD
Department of Clinical and
  Experimental Medicine
Section of Pharmacology
University of Ferrara
Ferrara, Italy

GLORIA AVECILLA, MSc
Unidad de Investigación en
  Neurodesarrollo
Instituto de Neurobiología
Universidad Nacional Autónoma de
  México
Campus Juriquilla
Querétaro, México

RAMÓN BARTOLO
Department of Neuroscience
Instituto de Neurobiología UNAM
Campus Juriquilla
Querétaro Qro., México

NATALE BELLUARDO, PhD
Department of Experimental
  Medicine
Section of Human Physiology
University of Palermo
Palermo, Italy

JORGE BUSCIGLIO, PhD
Department of Neurobiology & Behavior
Institute for Brain Aging and
  Dementia
University of California-Irvine
Irvine, CA

LILIANA CAMARILLO, PhD
Instituto de Fisiología Celular
Universidad Nacional Autónoma de
  México
México, D.F., México

CARLOS CEPEDA, PhD
Mental Retardation Research
  Center
David Geffen School of Medicine
University of California Los Angeles
Los Angeles, CA

SILVIA CORDERO, PhD
Instituto de Fisiología Celular
Universidad Nacional Autónoma de
  México
México, D.F., México

BRIAN J. CUMMINGS, PhD
Physical Medicine and
  Rehabilitation
University of California-Irvine
Irvine, CA

JUAN A. DE CARLOS, PhD
Instituto Cajal (CSIC)
Department of Molecular,
  Cellular and Developmental
  Neurobiology
Madrid, Spain

CARLOS ARÁMBURO DE LA HOZ, PhD
Instituto de Neurobiología
Campus UNAM-UAQ
  Juriquilla
Universidad Nacional Autónoma de
  México
Querétaro, Qro. México

ATUL DESHPANDE, PhD
Department of Neurobiology &
  Behavior
Institute for Brain Aging and
  Dementia
University of California-Irvine
Irvine, CA

José Luis Díaz, MD
Department of History and Philosophy
   of Medicine
Faculty of Medicine
National Autonomous University of
   Mexico (UNAM)
México, D.F., México

Antonio Fernández-Bouzas,
   MD, PhD
Unidad de Investigación en
   Neurodesarrollo
Instituto de Neurobiología
Universidad Nacional Autónoma de
   México
Campus Juriquilla
Querétaro, México

Thalía Fernández, PhD
Unidad de Investigación en
   Neurodesarrollo
Instituto de Neurobiología
Universidad Nacional Autónoma de
   México
Campus Juriquilla
Querétaro, México

Luca Ferraro, PhD
Department of Clinical and
   Experimental Medicine
Section of Pharmacology
University of Ferrara
Ferrara, Italy

Robin S. Fisher, PhD
Mental Retardation Research
   Center
David Geffen School of Medicine
University of California Los
   Angeles
Los Angeles, CA

Kjell Fuxe, MD
Department of Neuroscience
Karolinska Institutet
Stockholm, Sweden

Fernando García-Moreno, PhD
Instituto Cajal (CSIC)
Department of Molecular,
   Cellular and Developmental
   Neurobiology
Madrid, Spain

Susanna Genedani, PhD
Department of Biomedical
   Sciences
Section of Physiology
University of Modena
Modena, Italy

Thalía Harmony, MD, PhD
Unidad de Investigación en
   Neurodesarrollo
Instituto de Neurobiología
Universidad Nacional Autónoma de
   México
Campus Juriquilla
Querétaro, México

Elizabeth Head, PhD
Department of Neurology
Institute for Brain Aging &
   Dementia
University of California,
   Irvine
Irvine, CA

Adrián Hernández, PhD
Instituto de Fisiología Celular
Universidad Nacional Autónoma de
   México
México, D.F., México

MITRA J. HOOSHMAND
Reeve-Irvine Research Center
Anatomy & Neurobiology
University of California, Irvine
Irvine, CA

EDWARD G. JONES, MD, PhD
Director, Center for Neuroscience
University of California, Davis
Davis, CA

HANS S. KEIRSTEAD, PhD
Co-Director of the Sue and
    Bill Gross Stem Cell
    Research Center
Reeve-Irvine Research Center
Department of Anatomy &
    Neurobiology School of Medicine
    University of California at Irvine
Irvine, CA

MAX KLEIMAN-WEINER
Mental Retardation Research Center
David Geffen School of
    Medicine
University of California
    Los Angeles
Los Angeles, CA

LUIS LEMUS, PhD
Instituto de Fisiología Celular
Universidad Nacional Autónoma de
    México
México, D.F., México

MICHAEL S. LEVINE, PhD
Mental Retardation Research
    Center
David Geffen School of Medicine
University of California
    Los Angeles
Los Angeles, CA

ROGELIO LUNA, PhD
Instituto de Fisiología Celular
Universidad Nacional Autónoma de
    México
México, D.F., México

PAUL MANGER, PhD
School of Anatomical Sciences
Faculty of Health Sciences
University of Witwatersrand
Johannesburg, Republic of South Africa

DANIEL MARCELLINO, PhD
Department of Neuroscience
Karolinska Institutet
Stockholm, Sweden

JOSÉ LUIS MARROQUÍN, PhD
Centro de Investigación en
    Matemáticas
Guanajuato, México

GARY W. MATHERN, MD
Mental Retardation Research Center
Department of Neurosurgery
David Geffen School of Medicine
University of California Los
    Angeles
Los Angeles, CA

CARMEN MÉNDEZ, BIOL, PhD
Departamento de Embriología
Facultad de Medicina
Universidad Nacional Autónoma de
    México
México, D.F., México

JUAN CARLOS MÉNDEZ
Department of Neuroscience
Instituto de Neurobiología UNAM
Campus Juriquilla
Querétaro Qro., México

HUGO MERCHANT, PhD
Instituto de Neurobiología UNAM
Campus Juriquilla
Querétaro Qro., México

AMAYA MIQUELAJÁUREGUI, PhD
Instituto de Neurobiología
Universidad Nacional Autónoma de
    México
Querétaro, Qro. México

GIUSEPPA MUDÓ, PhD
Department of Experimental
    Medicine
Section of Human Physiology
University of Palermo
Palermo, Italy

VERÓNICA NÁCHER, PhD
Instituto de Fisiología Celular
Universidad Nacional Autónoma de
    México
México, D.F., México

THOMAS NASELARIS, PhD
Helen Lewis Neuroscience
    Institute
University of California,
    Berkeley
Berkeley, CA

RODRIGO NÚÑEZ VIDALES
Departamento de Embriología
Facultad de Medicina
Universidad Nacional Autónoma de
    México
México, D.F., México

GLORIA OTERO, MD, PhD
Facultad de Medicina
Universidad Autónoma
del Estado de México, México

ENRIQUE PEDERNERA, MD, PhD
Departamento de Embriología
Facultad de Medicina
Universidad Nacional Autónoma de
    México
México, D.F., México

OSWALDO PÉREZ
Department of Computational
    Neuroscience
Instituto de Neurobiología UNAM
Campus Juriquilla
Querétaro Qro., México

ZACHARY D. PEREZ
Department of Anatomy &
    Neurobiology
University of California at Irvine
    School of Medicine
Irvine, CA

ALAN PETERS, PhD
Department of Anatomy and
    Neurobiology
Boston University School of
    Medicine
Boston, MA

ENEIDA PORRAS-KATTZ, MD
Unidad de Investigación en
    Neurodesarrollo
Instituto de Neurobiología
Universidad Nacional Autónoma
    de México
Campus Juriquilla
Querétaro, México

LUIS PRADO
Department of Neuroscience
Instituto de Neurobiología UNAM
Campus Juriquilla
Querétaro Qro., México

CHARLES E. RIBAK, PhD
Department of Anatomy &
  Neurobiology
University of California at Irvine
  School of Medicine
Irvine, CA

JOSEFINA RICARDO-GARCELL, MD,
  PhD
Unidad de Investigación en
  Neurodesarrollo
Instituto de Neurobiología
Universidad Nacional Autónoma de
  México
Campus Juriquilla
Querétaro, México

RANULFO ROMO, MD, DSc
Department of Neuroscience
Instituto de Fisiología Celular
Universidad Nacional Autónoma de
  México
México, D.F., México

JORGE A. LARRIVA SAHD, MD,
  PhD
Department of Developmental
  Neurobiology &
  Neurophysiology
Instituto de Neurobiología
Campus UNAM-UAQ
  Juriquilla
Universidad Nacional Autónoma
  de México
Querétaro, Qro. México

DESIRÉE L. SALAZAR
Reeve-Irvine Research Center
Anatomy & Neurobiology
University of California, Irvine
Irvine, CA

EFRAÍN SANTIAGO-RODRÍGUEZ, MD,
  PhD
Unidad de Investigación en
  Neurodesarrollo
Instituto de Neurobiología
Universidad Nacional Autónoma de
  México
Campus Juriquilla
Querétaro, México

LEE A. SHAPIRO, PhD
Department of Surgery and
  Neurosurgery
Texas A&M University College of
  Medicine
Teague Veterans Medical Center
  and Scott & White Hospital
Temple, TX

MONICA M. SIEGENTHALER, PhD
Reeve-Irvine Research Center
Sue and Bill Gross Stem Cell
  Research Center Department
  of Anatomy & Neurobiology
School of Medicine
University of California
  at Irvine
Irvine, CA

LARRY W. SWANSON, PhD
Neuroscience Program
University of Southern
  California
Los Angeles, CA

SERGIO TANGANELLI, PhD
Department of Clinical and
  Experimental Medicine
Section of Pharmacology
University of Ferrara
Ferrara, Italy

ALFREDO VARELA-ECHAVARRÍA, PhD
Instituto de Neurobiología
Universidad Nacional Autónoma de
   México
Querétaro, México

YURIRIA VÁZQUEZ, PhD
Instituto de Fisiología Celular
Universidad Nacional Autónoma de
   México
México, D.F., México

HARRY V. VINTERS, MD
Mental Retardation Research
   Center
Department of Neuropathology
David Geffen School of Medicine
University of California Los Angeles
Los Angeles, CA

IRENE YAMAZAKI, MD
Mental Retardation Research
   Center
David Geffen School of Medicine
University of California
   Los Angeles
Los Angeles, CA

ANTONIO ZAINOS, PhD
Instituto de Fisiología Celular
Universidad Nacional Autónoma de
   México
México, D.F., México

WILBERT ZARCO
Department of Neuroscience
Instituto de Neurobiología UNAM
Campus Juriquilla
Querétaro Qro., México

CONTENTS

FROM DEVELOPMENT TO DEGENERATION AND REGENERATION OF THE NERVOUS SYSTEM

Part 1

Cajal's Legacy

Chapter One

The Legacy of Cajal in Mexico

José Luis Díaz

> Spaniards,
> Spaniards of the exodus and of weeping:
> lift up your heads
> and do not look frowning upon me,
> for I am not he who sings of destruction
> but of hope.
>
> Léon Felipe
> *Spaniard of the Exodus and of Weeping*
> La Casa de España en México, 1939

THE SECOND SPANISH REPUBLIC AND THE REFUGEE TEACHERS

Many Mexican neuroscientists consider themselves to some extent to be descendants or at least beneficiaries of the School of Santiago Ramón y Cajal, whom we consider our patron saint. In this chapter I will attempt to outline the genealogy that links us to this great Spanish master not only scientifically, but culturally, linguistically, and philosophically—beyond a strictly academic affiliation to one that is social and political in nature. I therefore offer this as a tribute to our mentors, the disciples of the great Cajal, who were expelled from their homeland to make a home in Mexico. Their exodus was as dreadful for them as their settling in Mexico was auspicious for us. Indeed, to begin to examine the Mexican influence of the scientific work and thought of Santiago Ramón y Cajal, it is necessary to consider the exile of his students and colleagues to the Americas. This exile occurred as another tragic result of the devastating Spanish Civil War, which cut short the tenure of the Second Republic, an ideal that had the firm support of the vast majority of Spanish intellectuals, and in particular of those researchers close to the renowned neurohistologist in his last years.

   The academic, cultural, and political education of the émigrés was sponsored by a progressive social and cultural movement during the "Silver Age," which,

3

beginning at the end of the nineteenth century, reached its historical apex under the Second Spanish Republic (1931–36). This Republic was established on April 18, 1931, by a popular plebiscite that was acknowledged by King Alfonso XIII. The political direction and the objectives of the Republic were laid down in the Constitution of 1931, a document that defined Spain as a democratic republic of workers—including intellectuals and scientists. The Constitution decreed a series of reforms that were very advanced for its time, such as the autonomy of the municipalities and regions, women's right to vote, indirect elections, freedom of worship, civil marriages, and numerous measures of social and cultural protection. Research and education took a dominant role, as under the Republican-Socialist coalition led by Manuel Azaña, when the famous pedagogue Fernando de los Ríos implemented his educational policy. As a consequence of the immediate and efficient application of this policy, the number of schools was doubled; pedagogical missions were initiated; and an intense expansion of universities, the press, and the book publishing market took place. Madrid became a cultural and scientific center, and education and scientific research took on increasing importance.

The Republic's educational and scientific program made use of and revived an organization created in 1876 by professors who had been dismissed from the Central University of Madrid for defending academic freedom and refusing to bring their teaching into line with official religious, political, or moral dogmas. The organization was the *Institución Libre de Enseñanza* (Free Teaching Institution). During the half-century from its foundation to the establishment of the Republic, this institution had the support of liberal intellectuals committed to educational, cultural, and social reform. Through this body, the most advanced pedagogical and scientific theories on the European continent were introduced in Spain, making the publication *Boletín de la Institución Libre de Enseñanza* a powerful vehicle for the dissemination of its ideology, and the famous "Generation of '27" of poets, writers, painters, and other artists actually emerged out of its ranks, a product of its progressive ideas.

The *Junta para la Ampliación de Estudios* (Board for Advanced Studies), chaired by Santiago Ramón y Cajal himself, was created to support the training of highly qualified professionals in the humanities and sciences. Between 1907 and 1939, nearly all Spanish intellectuals and scientists furthered their studies with the help of scholarships or grants from this board, including Cajal's own students, who initially trained in its laboratories and subsequently at the best European universities, particularly in Germany, France, and the United Kingdom. In addition, as if it were a government department of research and culture, the Board created numerous centers and laboratories for studies in the humanities and sciences, such as the Centro de Estudios Históricos (Historical Studies Center), Instituto Nacional de Ciencias Físico-Naturales (National Institute of

Physico-Natural Sciences), and the famous Residencia de Estudiantes (Student Residence Hall).

The *Residencia de Estudiantes* stands among the most legendary creations of the Board, as it was a hotbed of extraordinary talent at a crucial moment in Spanish history. Indeed, in addition to creators as deservedly famous as the poet Federico García Lorca, filmmaker Luis Buñuel, painter Salvador Dali and biochemist Severo Ochoa, virtually all of Cajal's students and protégés lived together in the Residence. In fact, one of the laboratories that made up the Cajal Institute was located within its walls. Notable among its foreign visitors was the Mexican writer and scholar Alfonso Reyes, who would be a crucial figure in the Mexican reception of the exiles of the Spanish Republic.

THE CAJAL INSTITUTE: BREEDING GROUND FOR NEUROSCIENTIFIC RESEARCHERS

Within this historical and cultural context, we find the great Cajal, his school, his laboratories, and his teaching in those final years of his long, highly significant, and productive academic career (see Álvarez Leefmans 1994). At the time the Second Republic was established, the 79-year-old Nobel laureate was one of the most respected intellectuals in Spain and among the most celebrated neuroscientists in the world. In 1932 he delegated upon his closest and most favored protégé, Francisco Tello, the administration of his Institute, the activities of which had all but ended after a long period of difficulties. Two years later, in 1934, Cajal died in Madrid. It was merciful timing, as Cajal probably would not have been able to bear the devastation of the civil war that would break out two years later and result in the establishment of a dictatorial regime that would repress or expel virtually all of his colleagues and students.

At the time of his death, Cajal and his team were engaged in intense scientific research at all three locations of the Institute: the *Laboratorio de Investigaciones Biológicas* (Biological Research Laboratory), located in Cerro de San Blas and directed by Tello; the *Laboratorio de Fisiología Cerebral* (Cerebral Physiology Laboratory), initially directed by Juan Negrín and later by Gonzalo R. Lafora; and a *Laboratorio de Histología Normal y Patológica* (Normal and Pathological Histology Laboratory), located in the *Residencia de Estudiantes* and directed by Pío del Río Hortega.

It is worth noting Cajal's main direct protégés in those days. In age order, they were:

- José Francisco Tello (1880–1958)
- Gonzalo Rodríguez Lafora (1886–1971)

- Fernando de Castro (1896–1967)
- Rafael Lorente de Nó (1902–90)

As will be discussed below, with the end of the war these and Cajal's other direct protégés suffered an intense repression campaign within Spain, where they faced an extremely uncertain future. This was not the case for the Aragonese scientist Lorente de Nó, who left Spain prior to the war in 1931 and developed a remarkable career in the field of neuroscience. Working at the Rockefeller Institute until 1972, and from that time on at UCLA, Lorente de Nó retired to Tucson, where he lived until his death in 1990. During his retirement he was visited regularly by the young Mexican student Jorge Larriva, who without doubt could be considered his disciple in the broad sense of the term that I suggested in the first paragraph of this chapter. As proof of his affiliation, Larriva (2002) recently delivered an account and reminiscence of his mentor, which offers an erudite, sensible, and opportune depiction of the figure of one of the most outstanding of Cajal's direct protégés, heir both to his histological talent and his visionary theoretical capacity. An example of the first of these abilities was his contribution to the description of the arrangement of the cerebral cortex in columns; an example of the second was his inference of reverberating circuits in servomechanisms of neural networks, considered a pioneering development for the cybernetic model of the nervous function.

In addition to these students, who were largely trained in his laboratories and under his personal supervision, Cajal brought together three highly notable figures with training in the latest developments in the anatomical, physiological, and clinical sciences of the nervous system. It is important to mention these three researchers because they were responsible, in different ways, for the training of several students who would be called upon to import the teachings of the Cajal School to the Americas. In age order, they were:

- Nicolás Achúcarro (1880–1918)
- Pío del Río Hortega (1882–1945)
- Juan Negrín (1892–1956)

Nicolás Achúcarro was born in Bilbao in 1880 and died prematurely in Neguri (Vizcaya) in 1918. In addition to being an outstanding scientist, Achúcarro maintained links with prominent intellectuals and creators of his period: He was from the same region as the philosopher Miguel de Unamuno and was his disciple in Bilbao, and he shared a home with the notable poet and eventual Nobel laureate Juan Ramón Jiménez, another eventual exile of the war. As were many Spanish intellectuals of his time, he was exposed to progressive influences through Giner de los Ríos. Achúcarro engaged in preuniversity scientific studies in Wiesbaden before going on to study medicine in Madrid. Like many other students, he was a histology student of Cajal at the time. He completed his training with two famous European psychiatrists: Pierre Marie in the Salpetriere in Paris and Emil Kraepelin in Munich. Achúcarro's basic goal was to study the anatomopathological bases of neuropsychiatric illnesses, the same study that would be taken up again years later by Dionisio Nieto, particularly during his exile in Mexico, as is discussed in more detail below. Achúcarro brought together an extensive anatomopathological collection of mental illnesses and, through his ingenious methods of dyeing nerve tissue with tannin and ammoniacal silver oxide, he made highly significant contributions to the neuropathology of rabies, Alzheimer's dementia, and alcoholism. In 1908 he was appointed Director of the Pathological Anatomy Laboratory at the Psychiatric Hospital of Washington, but he returned to Spain in 1911 to direct the *Laboratorio de Histopatología del Sistema Nervioso* (Nervous System Histopathology Laboratory) in the Cajal Institute with a grant from the *Junta para la Ampliación de Estudios*. Shortly after receiving an honorary doctorate from Yale University, Achúcarro fell seriously ill. In distress and with tragic precision, he diagnosed himself in 1915 with a recently defined serious condition: Hodgkin's disease. And so, after a significant scientific career, he died at home in Neguri in 1918 . . . at only 37 years of age.

Pío del Río Hortega was born in Valladolid in 1882 and died in exile in Buenos Aires in 1945. On a grant from the *Junta para la Ampliación de Estudios*, he worked in Paris, London, and Berlin, although his principal training was at the Nervous System Histopathology Laboratory directed by Nicolás Achúcarro. After Achúcarro's death in 1918, Cajal named del Río Hortega the laboratory director, and he maintained a close relationship with the intellectuals of the *Residencia de Estudiantes*. del Río Hortega made his main contribution to science shortly before Achúcarro's death, when he modified the dye used by his mentor and colleague to a triple-silver impregnation with ammoniacal silver carbonate. This dyeing method was one of the most important contributions to neurohistology not only in Spain but throughout the world, as it enabled the observation of glial cells and the first descriptions of the microglia and oligodendroglia; in fact, for a time microglial cells were known as "Hortega cells." There occurred at this point a distancing between Cajal and del Río Hortega. It is said that this discovery, which Cajal had not believed, was the cause of the rift, although it has also been posited that it was a matter of a personal difference between them. Cajal and del Río Hortega reconciled around 1926.

In 1940, at the end of the Civil War, del Río Hortega was granted refuge in Argentina as an associate professor at the University of La Plata. He developed an outstanding career in Buenos Aires, where he founded what was named the Ibero-American Neurohistology School and categorized cerebral tumors from a histopathological perspective. Two outstanding students of his in Madrid—Isaac Costero and Dionisio Nieto—were political refugees in Mexico, as is discussed below.

Juan Negrín, one of the most outstanding personalities in the history of the Spanish Republic, was born in Las Palmas in 1892 and died in Paris in 1956. It is necessary to distinguish two separate facets of Negrin's life: the physiologist and the politician. As a physiologist, he was a PhD and *Privatdozent* at the University of Leipzig and Professor of Physiology in the Faculty of Medicine at the University of Madrid. In 1916 he was named Director of the Department of Cerebral Physiology at Cajal's Laboratory of Biological Research, and Director of the Physiology Laboratory located in the *Residencia de Estudiantes*. Negrín engaged in intense scientific research there, and in 1928 he introduced biochemistry in Spain as a branch of physiology.

Several of Negrín's students emigrated during the war. Outstanding among these are Severo Ochoa (who immigrated to the United States, where he would go on to receive the Nobel Prize), Francisco Grande Covián, José García Valdecasas, Rafael Méndez, Ramón Pérez Cirera, and José Puche Alvarez. These last three became outstanding professors in exile at the National Autonomous University of Mexico, and many of the current generation of Mexican neuroscientists had the good fortune either to be their students or to know them personally.

Negrín the politician is better known and is even more fascinating than Negrín the physiologist. He was a member of parliament for the Spanish Socialist Workers' Party (PSOE) and a member of the Constitutional Assembly of the Republic. He had the crucial role of Finance Minister in the Cabinet of Prime Minister Largo Caballero. At that time, Spain transferred gold to the Soviet Union in exchange for weapons for the Republic. This transaction turned Negrín into an extremely controversial figure in the Republican struggle. The most sober opinion suggests that Negrín, who was not a member of the Communist Party, considered in good faith that it was necessary for the Republic to arm itself to put down Franco's fascist uprising, even if it meant dealing with Stalin's totalitarian regime. Negrín was handed the difficult task of President of the Government from 1937 until the war was lost, when he was forced to flee the country. He maintained the honorary role of President of the Republic in exile in the United Kingdom until 1945, when he travelled briefly to Mexico. He died in Paris in 1956.

THE FALL OF THE REPUBLIC AND THE DOUBLE EXILE OF THE CAJAL INSTITUTE

Having outlined the characteristics of the Cajal Institute following the death of its founding director and the personalities of its most outstanding members, I now return to the fateful year of 1936, when the Spanish Civil War began. The most immediate antecedent to the war was the victory of Manuel Azaña's Popular Front in February of that year over the *Confederación Española de Derechas Autónomas*

(Spanish Confederation of the Autonomous Right; CEDA), an ultraconservative party that had been in power in the Republic for two years. Azaña claimed victory through a coalition of leftist parties. The victors held power by a narrow margin, though, and they were unable to directly satisfy the demands of radical worker groups for more and speedier reforms, and much less the reactionary sectors that resisted any changes. Spain was divided into two main factions that were becoming increasingly polarized: one conservative, monarchic, and Catholic; and the other socialist, radical, and anticlerical.

In this context of mutual contempt and hatred, and as a result of Azaña's victory, a large-scale mobilization of workers took place, with numerous strikes instigated by the communist and anarchist unions, calling for immediate and dramatic reforms. At the same time, on the opposite end of the political spectrum, another mobilization was taking place: that of the extreme right, led by the Spanish Falange and the so-called National Block, movements sympathetic to Italian Fascism and German Nazism. In July 1936 the assassination of the right-wing parliamentary Calvo Sotelo hastened the military uprising of Generals Mola and Franco, and the Civil War began. After three tragic and bloody years, the war ended in 1939 with the victory of the Nationalists, Francisco Franco's assumption of power, and the establishment of his cruel dictatorship that would last until the death of the "Caudillo" in 1976. The mass repression of opposition resulted in the exile of a large number of republicans from every walk of life, particularly intellectuals and scientists. The Cajal Institute was not unaffected by this deconstruction, or to the diaspora of its greatest exponents.

A distinction needs to be made between internal and external exile. Following is a brief and difficult review of the internal exile of the Institute within Spain as a consequence of the repression. In 1939 its director, Cajal's successor Jorge Francisco Tello, faced a trial before the Tribunal of Political Responsibilities and a purging trial by the Tribunal of the Medical Association. As a result, he was stripped of his position as the Cajal Institute's director, expelled from the Royal Academy, and dismissed from his faculty position, which was given back to him in 1949, six months before his retirement. Lorenzo Ruíz de Arcaute died in the bombing of Madrid. Fernando de Castro was purged and subsequently tolerated. Joaquín Alonso was stripped of his positions as professor and prosector. Juan Miguel Herrera was sentenced and imprisoned, then fled into exile in Panama, where he introduced the study and practice of pathology. Something similar happened to Rodríguez Pérez, who after being imprisoned went into exile in Colombia, where he worked as a professor in pathology. Rodríguez Puchol was imprisoned and forbidden to return to the academy until he managed to establish a professional relationship with Gregorio Marañón. Luis Calandre Ibáñez faced two summary war trials and was subsequently restricted to private practice. Antonio de Zulueta was sentenced and prohibited from practicing his profession.

Other members and students of the Cajal Institute fled into exile outside Spain, in many cases risking their lives. The list of Institute members in external exile is as follows:

* Pío del Río Hortega, in Argentina
* Students of del Río Hortega: Gonzalo R. Lafora, Isaac Costero, and Dionisio Nieto, in Mexico
* Juan Negrín, in France and the United Kingdom
* Students of Negrín: Rafael Méndez, Ramón Pérez Cirera, and José Puche, in México; Severo Ochoa, in the USA

The welcoming of Spanish exiles in Mexico is one of the noblest and most celebrated chapters in the history of Mexican foreign policy. Much has been written on the subject (see Fresco 1950; Various 1982), but in the context of this discussion of exiles from the Cajal Institute, it is worth recalling briefly the role of Mexican president Lázaro Cárdenas's vigorous policy to welcome Spanish exiles, through which he not only saved their lives but also fostered a renascent and flourishing science, the development of which had been interrupted between 1910 and 1920 due to the devastation of the Mexican Revolution. To provide a productive environment, particularly for academics and intellectuals, Alfonso Reyes, one of the most outstanding Mexican intellectuals of the period and indeed of the whole twentieth century, instigated the creation of *La Casa de España en México* (The House of Spain in Mexico), the seed for what has become the renowned *Colegio de México*.

At the same time, the *Universidad Nacional Autónoma de México* (National Autonomous University of Mexico; UNAM) provided researchers in the humanities and sciences with teaching and research positions, and in doing so benefited greatly from the injection of a stream of creative, disciplined, honest, and bold thinkers. Cajal's students were the promoters of several laboratories that in time would come to be prominent institutions in biomedical research, particularly in Mexican neurosciences. Indeed, Lafora, Costero, and Nieto used a grant from the Rockefeller Foundation to establish the *Laboratorio de Estudios Médicos y Biológicos* (Medical and Biological Studies Laboratory), set up by these disciples of Cajal in Mexico near the former School of Medicine in 1941. The researchers' salaries were paid by *La Casa de España*. This laboratory was conceived in the image and likeness of its alma mater, the Cajal Institute, as a center for basic clinical research into the anatomo-functional aspects of the nervous system. In time, this laboratory would become the *Instituto de Estudios Médicos y Biológicos* (Medical and Biological Studies Institute) and finally the *Instituto de Investigaciones Biomédicas* (Institute of Biomedical Research). From 1993, the majority of neuroscientists at this Institute formed a *Centro de Neurobiología* (Neurobiology Center), located in Juriquilla in the state of Querétaro, and later converted into an institute in 2002. Meanwhile, at the National Cardiology Institute, under the direction and management of its founder, Ignacio Chávez, a pathology department was opened with Isaac Costero as its director, followed by a pharmacology department headed by Rafael Méndez.

CAJAL INSTITUTE EXILES TEACH AND CONDUCT RESEARCH IN MEXICO

To better understand the influence of the Cajal School in Mexico, more detailed sketches of the scientific profiles of Lafora, Puche, Méndez, Costero, and Nieto are necessary. Gonzalo Rodríguez Lafora (see biography by Valenciano, 1977) was born in Madrid in 1886. His fields of expertise were clinical neuropsychiatry and neurohistological research. He was a direct disciple of Cajal and, in his time, was responsible for one of the laboratories of the Cajal Institute. In 1925 he founded the Medical-Pedagogical Institute and Carabanchel Sanatorium, as well as the seminal magazine *Archivos de Neurobiología*, which brought together interests in histology, physiology, and pathology of the nervous system in its two aspects—the neurological and the psychiatric, before they became distinct specialist fields of study. He performed a series of pioneering works into sexuality, which led to his interest, although critical, in the psychoanalytical theory of Freud. His adherence to the Republic was firm, expressed in his promotion of psychiatric reform within the framework of the new regime. Before the end of the war, in 1938, he fled from Spain, whose republic was on the verge of defeat, and came to Mexico, where he received a warm welcome and came to be a veritable celebrity as a prototype of the erudite scientific psychiatrist in the nine years of his exile there. By 1939, the National Academy of Medicine in Mexico had already named him an honorary member and the Mexican Society of Neurology and Psychiatry accepted him with open arms. Lafora's celebrity grew when he diagnosed Gregorio "Goyo" Cárdenas, a serial killer of women, as suffering from "crepuscular" crises of an epileptic nature. His diagnosis sparked conflict with the Mexican psychiatric institution, as some of its members considered this unlawful meddling. The conflict subsequently subsided, although the distancing it caused with the Mexican psychiatric profession was notable. Lafora began to explore the possibility of returning to Spain, and in 1947, when he considered the invitation to return to be genuine and safe, he made the journey to Madrid, where a long "purging" process awaited him, and he was reincorporated into the Cajal Institute and the Spanish psychiatric profession until his death in 1971. Unlike those discussed below, Lafora had a relatively provisional stay in Mexico, marked by his notable and controversial personality as a neuropsychiatrist. He left much less of a mark as a professor and researcher in his host country, apart from his participation in the foundation of the Medical and Biological Studies Laboratory.

José Puche was born in Valencia in 1895. He studied medicine in Catalonia and came to be the Dean of the University of Valencia and the Director of Military Health during the Civil War. Even though he originally belonged to the physiology group of Pi Suñer in Barcelona, he went to Madrid for his graduate thesis in the laboratory of Juan Negrín, where he was exposed to the school of Cajal. Exiled after the war to France and Mexico, he was absorbed initially by the *Instituto Politécnico* until 1958, when he became a professor of the Physiology Department in the School of Medicine at the National University and remained there until his death in 1979. In this position he undertook tireless research and teaching projects. In the last years of his life he could be seen delivering impeccable papers in the National Congress of Physiological Sciences as if he were only a graduate student and not a marvellous teacher of more than 80 years of age. A sweet man of exquisite manners and impeccable expression in Spanish, Puche introduced many students to physiological research and in his later years embarked on a study of feeding and glucose regulation in the crayfish, whereby he initiated the study of circadian rhythm physiology in Mexico. Among his many students it is worth remembering the figure of the brilliant and internationally reputed neurophysiologist Hugo Aréchiga, recently and prematurely deceased.

Rafael Méndez, born in Lorca in the Murcia region in 1906, was also a disciple of Juan Negrín and, in addition, was mentored by the pharmacologist Teófilo Hernando. The poet Federico García Lorca, one of Méndez's several artist friends from the *Residencia de Estudiantes*, dedicated his poem "*Reyerta*" ("Quarrel") to him. In 1928 Méndez left Spain for Edinburgh, together with Severo Ochoa, to study pharmacology and biochemistry. During the period of the Republic, and particularly during the presidency of his mentor Negrín, Méndez was involved in some incredible adventures that he himself related (subsequently recorded by Fernández Guardiola, 1997), and he was given the post of Undersecretary of Internal Affairs. With the fall of the Republic, Rafael Méndez went first to the University of Loyola in Chicago, then to Harvard, and finally, at the request of Ignacio Chávez, to Mexico, where he joined the Institute of Cardiology as a pharmacologist in 1947. This same group featured other great teachers of Mexican neuroscience, including Arturo Rosenblueth. During his time in the Institute of Cardiology, Méndez became a world-renowned expert in the mechanism of action of digitalis. After retiring from the Institute he worked as the Health Institutes Coordinator, where he displayed a characteristic bonhomie that helped earn him the respect of all of his colleagues. A teacher to generations of cardiologists trained in the Institute, it is worth noting among his disciples in the laboratory pharmacologists such as Gustavo Pastelín and Emilio Kabela. He returned to Spain on a few occasions toward the end of Franco's rule and played an important advisory role in the restitution of Spanish science and the return of several exiled scientists to the Iberian peninsula. He died in Mexico in 1991.

Isaac Costero was born in Burgos in 1903 and died in Mexico City in 1979. He was probably Pío del Río Hortega's closest protégé and colleague at the

Cajal Institute. Around 1930, he went to the Erlich Institute in Frankfurt on a grant from the *Junta para la Ampliación de Estudios*. He learned del Río Hortega's techniques and used them to analyze the behavior of human brain microglia in culture to study the functions of microglia and oligodendroglia in glial tumors such as gliomas and pragliomas. In 1932 he studied in Berlin at the Albert Fischer Institute of Biology, where he learned autopsy techniques that would eventually become the basis for Mexican pathology. In exile in Mexico, Costero founded the Department of Pathological Anatomy at the National Cardiology Institute. There he studied the cerebral alterations of rheumatic fever, the normal and pathological states of the carotid body, the evolution of heart attacks, and the physiopathology of arteriosclerosis. He also carried out studies on cerebral cysticercosis and hepatic cirrhosis caused by alcoholism. Costero received huge recognition in Mexico. In 1968 he was made President of the National Academy of Medicine, in 1972 he was awarded the National Prize for Sciences, and in 1979 he received an honorary doctorate from the UNAM. Upon leaving the Cardiology Institute in 1977, he joined the National Neurology Institute's Cerebral Research Unit, where he remained until his death in 1979. It was there that I had the opportunity to interact with him. Two of Costero's outstanding students were Ruy Pérez Tamayo, the pathologist, scientist, and professor to generations of medical practitioners and researchers in biomedicine, who has also made a prolific and indispensable contribution to the philosophy of science; and Adolfo Martínez Palomo, also a biomedical researcher and promoter of science, who has recently written about the Spanish doctors in exile, particularly his teacher Costero (Martínez Palomo 2006). Another of Costero's students, Rosario Barroso, was at his side to the end.

Dionisio Nieto is possibly the member of the Cajal School who continued to develop Cajal's teaching in Mexico in the most specific and prolonged manner, particularly because he devoted himself to neuropsychiatric research in the tradition established by Achúcarro, whom he never met but whom he admired deeply. Nieto arrived in Mexico with a very solid education in two fields: German psychiatry and Spanish neurohistology, two traditions he successfully joined together in his research and teaching work. He acquired a high level of competence in both of these fields, and it was Cajal himself who encouraged him to take up the analysis of psychiatric pathological principles using neurohistological techniques. This mission, approved by Cajal, would be fully developed by Nieto while in exile in Mexico. He was given positions at the UNAM and the *La Castañeda* Public Mental Hospital. In both places, his work was scrupulous and productive. As mentioned previously, he was the central figure behind the establishment of the Medical and Biological Studies Laboratory, and after Lafora and Costero departed, Nieto remained in his position there for the rest of his life. In the mental hospital he established the Pabellón Piloto wing, a model of efficiency, research, and hygiene in an institution whose resources were overstretched and in many ways deficient.

At the mental hospital, Nieto soon confronted numerous cases of neurocysti-cercosis—a cerebral parasitosis that often led to neurological and psychiatric complications. He made significant efforts to diagnose neurocysticercosis using a cerebrospinal fluid reaction. However, his best-known studies were those involv-ing the application of the del Río Hortega and Golgi techniques in the study of neuropsychiatric illnesses, the pathology of which was still quite undefined in the 1940s and 1950s. Nieto analyzed the neuropathology of epilepsy and schizo-phrenia in pioneering studies that were not successfully replicated until decades later. Nieto was also the first psychiatrist in Mexico to introduce the analysis and use of various psychoactive drugs, particularly antipsychotics, antidepressants, antimanics, and hallucinogens. He studied and published biological and especially biochemical hypotheses on psychoses at a time when the prevailing paradigm was psychoanalysis and skepticism about the value of cerebral research in psychiatry. In this way, Nieto was an underappreciated, inadequately recognized figure in Mexi-can psychiatry, even though he enjoyed the respect of most specialists for his eru-dition and his honest and open attitude (Sacristán 2007).

Nieto's influence and, through him, that of the Cajal School, was perhaps more significant and less controversial in Mexican neurosciences than in psychia-try, particularly given his work as a researcher for the *Instituto de Investigaciones Biomédicas* (Biomedical Research Institute) for more than 40 years, where I had the privilege of being his student between 1965 and 1972 and to continue a close association with him until his death on January 5, 1985 (Díaz 1987). He had an enormous influence on all the nervous system researchers who trained at that institute and on two direct students who became highly prominent in Mexican neuroscience: Alfonso Escobar in the fields of neuroanatomy and neuropathology, and Augusto Fernández Guardiola (1927–2004), considered the founder of psy-chophysiology in Mexico. Fernández Guardiola was another Spanish refugee who, arriving in Mexico at a young age, completed a degree in medicine and worked tirelessly on the neurophysiological bases of sleep, epilepsy, pain, and consciousness. Fernández Guardiola was another outstanding figure among the Spanish exiles, a teacher of many researchers currently working in neuroscience in Mexico (Díaz 2004). In his last years, he published a delightful tribute to those exiles who were students of Cajal (Fernández Guardiola 1997) and whom he knew and worked with personally, both in the realm of physiological sciences in Mexico and as a fellow exile. This book is, of course, of supreme importance for the subject herein discussed.

THE SCHOOL EXILED, TRAVELLING, TRANSPLANTED

The Mexican school of neurosciences in the tradition established by Cajal has several attributes that have endured and are still evident today. First, it takes an anatomo-functional and integrative approach to the nervous system. This approach is faithful to the tradition of meticulous observation of the great Spanish thinker and to the functional inferences that characterized his thought, as reflected in the original Cajal Institute and in the one that has been gradually rebuilt in Madrid following the restoration of democracy, and particularly since 1986 when it was established in its current location. The school is also defined by an empirical approach based on evidence gained through observation. This does not mean philosophical empiricism, but rather an empirical foundation for all theories. There is in this sense a greater emphasis on hands-on methodology and on observation, and less on statistical approaches, made possible by a rigorous scientific ethical framework and a commitment to veracity. For example, Nieto based his psychopharmacological studies in the sensitivity of the clinical interview, and his meticulous observations of the mental effects of the medications under study have been corroborated in subsequent double-blind studies. Cajal's students in Mexico always maintained a monistic approach with regard to the mind–body relationship and a critical and tenacious opposition to any dualist or purely mentalist approach that might attempt to separate mental faculties and pathologies from their necessary cerebral basis.

In addition to these methodological features, there is among Cajal's heirs— particularly among the Spanish refugees—a notable degree of scholarly and political independence, humble expression, and unwavering intellectual honesty. It was rare for them to occupy executive academic positions, as they preferred research and teaching work. They almost always remained above personal or group interests, and by doing so often constituted reference points of balance and dignity in the institutions where they worked and for which they displayed admirable loyalty and dedication. These rigorous and demanding teachers demonstrated notable intellectual generosity in their teaching and training of students, although always within the framework of a strict tutorship and a theoretical commitment that Cajal himself had been known for in his recommendations for scientific research. And like the founder of the school himself, they had no shortage of gruffness, insistence on creativity, and no-nonsense reserve.

Spaniards by origin and temperament, the exiles of the Cajal Institute, like many other refugees of the Second Republic, gratefully and lovingly chose to take Mexican citizenship. On the memorable occasion of the tribute given by the UNAM to their Spanish exile professors, the respected and temperate philosopher Eduardo Nicol declared with his eyes full of tears: "We were born Mexican in 1939." Similarly, and no less unforgettably, Rafael Méndez made the following remark:

> It is not the date of arrival or the number of generations one has here that indicates one's love for Mexico. When it comes to a genuine love and respect for Mexico, a person of pure indigenous blood should not be seen as any more Mexican than a person descended from an Asturian or Andalusian grandfather. And those of us who were not born in Mexico but have bound our bodies and souls to your land feel as Mexican as they do. (Pastelín 1984)

ACKNOWLEDGMENTS

I thank Martin Boyd for the speedy translation of this essay. I would also like to thank Dr. Juan de Carlos of the Cajal Institute of Madrid for the talk we had during the meeting of the Cajal Club in the UNAM's Institute of Neurobiology, and further interviews in which he not only provided me with invaluable information on the history of the Institute and of its first members, but also corrected some mistakes of the present manuscript.

REFERENCES

Álvarez Leefmans, F.J. 1994. *Las neuronas de Don Santiago*. Mexico City: Pangea.

Aréchiga, H. 1991. *Cincuenta años del exilio español en la UNAM*. Mexico City: UNAM.

Campos, R., O. Villasante, and R. Huertas, eds. 2007. *De la "edad de plata" al exilio: Construcción y reconstrucción de la psiquiatría española*. Madrid: Frena.

Díaz, J.L. 1987. Su aportación al problema cerebro-mente. In *Homenaje a Dionisio Nieto*. Mexico: Department of Psychiatry and Mental Health, Faculty of Medicine, UNAM. In Nieto 1990, 37–39.

Díaz, J.L. 1991. La enseñanza de los Científicos. In Aréchiga 1991, *Cincuenta años del exilio español en la UNAM*, 125–33.

Díaz, J.L. 2004. Obituary: Augusto Fernández Guardiola. *Humanidades* (UNAM) 272: 24–5.

Fernández Guardiola, A. 1997. *Las neurociencias en el exilio español en México*. Mexico City: Fondo de Cultura Económica, Colección La Ciencia para Todos, 153.

Fresco, M. 1950. *La emigración Republicana Española: Una victoria para México*. Mexico City: Editores Asociados.

Martínez Palomo, A. 2006. Médicos. In *Científicos y humanistas del exilio español en México*, 127–41. México City: Academia Mexicana de Ciencias.

Nieto, A. 1990. *La obra científica de Dionisio Nieto*. Mexico City: UNAM.

Pastelín, G. 1994. Semblanza del Doctor Rafael Méndez. In *Rafael Méndez, imagen y obra escogida*. Mexico City: UNAM, Dirección General de Proyectos Académicos.

Sacristán, C. 2007. En defensa del paradigma científico: El doble exilio de Dionisio Nieto en México. In Campos, Villasante, and Huertas 2007, 327–46.

Valenciano Gayá, L. 1977. *El Doctor Lafora y su época*. Madrid: Ediciones Morata.

Various. 1982. *El exilio español en México*. Mexico City: Fondo de Cultura Económica, 1939–82.

Part 2

Neuronal Migration and Development

Chapter Two

Tangential Cell Movements During Early Telencephalic Development

Juan A. De Carlos and Fernando García-Moreno

INTRODUCTION

The telencephalon is a structure that appears early in embryonic development due to a bilateral evagination (protrusion) of the neural tube in the cephalic region. The paired structures that are generated are known as telencephalic vesicles, and they give rise to the cerebral hemispheres that contain the pallium (cerebral cortex and hippocampus) and the subpallium (striatum and rhinencephalon).

   At the time of the formation of the telencephalon, the pallium wall is extremely thin as compared to the neighboring subpallium. Indeed, its cortical neuroepithelium is considered to be a pseudo-stratified epithelium containing densely packed cells in a columnar disposition. As in the subpallium, the germinative area of the pallium is the ventricular zone, which is the area lining the embryonic ventricles. Here, neurons are generated intermittently, in successive waves during precise developmental time windows, to establish the appropriate structures. As a rule, the cells generated in a given location do not remain close to their origin for long. They embark on a journey that may be extremely long at times to reach the specific area where they will reside. For a long time it has been known that newborn neurons use two different mechanisms to reach their desired destination, radial and tangential migration, two classes of migration that were clearly demonstrated by nineteenth-century classical histology. Indeed, at the Cajal Institute, we have

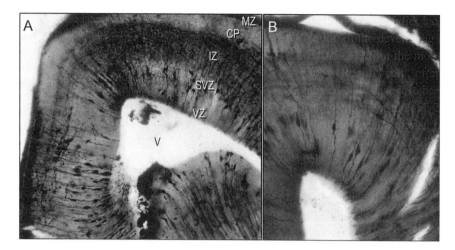

Figure 2.1. Coronal sections through the telencephalon of a rodent embryo impregnated using the Golgi method and showing the two types of cell displacement, radial and tangential. Microphotographs taken from some original histological preparations made by Cajal more than 100 years ago and conserved at the Cajal Institute. In picture **(A)** we have labelled the different layers of the developing neuroepithelium as we know them today: marginal zone (MZ), cortical plate (CP), intermediate zone (IZ) with many impregnated fibers and the germinative areas, the subventricular and ventricular zones (SVZ, VZ). The ventricle (V) is also labeled above the ganglionic eminence. Medial is left, and dorsal is up. Picture **(B)** shows several labeled cells undergoing radial migration and two cells migrating tangentially through the lower intermediate zone, at higher magnification. (See color Figure 2.1)

preserved some fine preparations made by Cajal with the Golgi method that display both types of migration in the telencephalon of rodent embryos (Figure 2.1). In these, it is clear that cells undergoing radial movement are oriented perpendicular to the pial surface and those that migrate tangentially (orthogonally) lie parallel to the piamater.

RADIAL MIGRATION

In radial migration, newborn cells move from their site of origin in the ventricular zone towards the pial surface following an inside-out sequence (Angevine and Sidman 1961). However, these cells can stop at diverse levels along their path to colonize different strata, that is, different layers of the cerebral cortex. Using light and electron microscopy (1972), Pasko Rakic demonstrated that newborn cells attach to the radial glia and use it as a scaffold to ascend to the desired cortical level. This type of migration is gliophilic because the radial glia are needed for embryonic migration. It is now known that radial glia disappear in newborn animals because they are generally transformed to astrocytes (Hunter and Hatten 1995). However, there are certain exceptions in the cerebellum and retina, where specific radial glia persist throughout adult life, such as the Bergman and Müller cells, respectively (Pinto and Götz 2007).

During embryonic stages, the radial glia fulfill two important functions. First, they serve as a scaffold for newly generated cells to migrate (Rakic 1972) and second, they divide to produce new radial glia, as well as true neurons (Noctor et al. 2001; Tamamaki et al. 2001). This type of radial migration implies that cells remain relatively close to the brain area in which they are generated. By contrast, tangential migration allows the cells to move over long distances and colonize other brain regions, sometimes very far from their site of origin.

TANGENTIAL MIGRATION

Although tangential movements of cells have been known since the time of Cajal (see Fig. 2.1), radial migration was usually considered the main mechanism used by newborn cells to reach their adult destinations. Perhaps this is because tangential migration occurs mainly at very early developmental stages (García-Moreno et al. 2007a, 2007b).

The first dynamic demonstration of tangential cell displacements was obtained by retroviral labeling (Walsh and Cepko 1988; Price and Thurlow 1988), mainly in the cerebral cortex, although the interpretation of such movements was uncertain and poorly understood. Using novel methods, such as time-lapse video imaging of cortical slices in culture, the great majority of migrating cells in the intermediate zone (adjacent to the germinative ventricular zone and the future white matter) followed a radial course. However, a minority (about 12%) ceased to migrate radially and instead moved perpendicular to the glial fibers within this cortical stratum (O'Rourke et al. 1992).

Perhaps the most studied and best understood tangential migration is that which occurs from the adult subventricular zone toward the olfactory bulbs. This migration provides the olfactory bulbs with new cells, even during the adult period, and it constitutes the so-called rostral migratory stream (RMS) (Lois and Alvarez-Buylla 1994). This type of tangential migration does not occur very early in telencephalic development, because the olfactory bulbs begin to appear in mice at E13. However, it has the peculiarity that it is maintained throughout the life of the animal.

For several years we have been interested in the early stages of telencephalic development, studying the initial stages in the development of the cerebral cortex and the olfactory structures. Thus, in the last 15 years our understanding of how the cortical neuroepithelium transforms into a complex 6-layered structure has changed enormously. In this chapter, we are going to review our contributions to the current understanding of cortical development and of the migratory patterning in the early stages of telencephalic development.

At the beginning of the 1990s there were two important theories regarding the development of the cerebral cortex. The first of these posited that some corticopetal fibers arrive at the upper part of the telencephalic neuroepithelium, coming from certain deep mesencephalic nuclei. These fibers initiate the formation of the primordial plexiform layer, an external and primitive white matter that arises in amphibians and reptiles (Marín-Padilla 1971, 1978, 1990). As such, the arrival of these afferent fibers induces the onset of cortical development, which was described as having a dual origin. Indeed, this primitive layer is split so that the cortical plate cells that accumulate within it form a superficial marginal zone (future layer 1) and a deep subplate. The newly generated cortical plate forms layers 2–6 of the cerebral cortex, because the site of generation of the cells that populate these layers in the ventricular zone differs from that which form layer 1 and from that of the subplate cells that are derived from the upper part of the neuroepithelium (Marín-Padilla 1978).

In addition, it was believed that all the cells that form part of the cerebral cortex (at least the cells that occupy layers 2–6) are generated in the germinative areas (ventricular and subventricular zones) of the cortical neuroepithelium itself (Bayer and Altman 1991). Furthermore, the majority of cortical cells migrate away from their site of generation along the processes of radial glial to form the cortical layers, following a deep to superficial sequence (Rakic 1972). Finally, a small neuronal population was thought to move randomly by tangential displacement throughout the lower part of the cortical neuroepithelium (ventricular, subventricular, and intermediate zones), extending from the hippocampus to the temporal cortex (Fishell et al. 1993). This distribution might be supported by the sharp boundaries formed by differential gene expression across the developing telencephalon (Rubenstein et al. 1994).

NEW TECHNIQUES: NEW DISCOVERIES

Over the past 15 years, the classical histological methods of silver impregnation in fixed tissue have given way to new, more selective labeling techniques. This advance was due to the use of a selection of novel compounds that do not damage the cells and that are suitable inject in living animals, as well as in whole isolated culture or fixed brains. Among the most popular dyes is the family of the carbocyanine lipophilic fluorescent tracers, of which DiI has been the most commonly used (Honig and Hume 1986, 1989).

Using DiI to label the neuroepithelium of E13–E15 rat embryos (before the generation of the cortical plate and when there is only one superficial stratum, the preplate), we studied the early development of the major cortical efferent and afferent projections through the internal capsule, the axonal pathway between the cortical and subcortical structures (De Carlos and O'Leary 1992). We initially found that subplate axons are the first fibers to exit the developing cortex and extend into the nascent internal capsule. Subsequently, we demonstrated that thalamic axons extend through the internal capsule toward the cortex, concurrent with the extension of preplate axons from the cortex. In this way, these two axonal populations co-establish the internal capsule. We also showed that the subcortical distribution of subplate axons is very limited because they extend through the internal capsule into the thalamus, preceding the definitive cortico-thalamic projection that arises from layer 6 neurons (De Carlos and O'Leary 1992). Because our experiments showed that the thalamocortical axons were the first afferents to extend into the cortex, these findings indicated that the preplate layer cannot contain early fibers originating from beyond the cortex, although they do not challenge the theory of the dual origin of the mammalian neocortex (Marín-Padilla 1978). Thalamic axons do not arrive until E16 in the rat, at which time the cortical plate is beginning to emerge. This is also some days after preplate neurons have extended axons long distances within the cortex, as well as into the internal capsule. Therefore, the early fibers in the upper part of the neuroepithelium (preplate) are not afferent to the cortex; rather, they must arise from preplate cells, that is Cajal–Retzius and subplate cells. Because the thalamic axons do not invade the cortical plate until E18 (Catalano et al. 1991; De Carlos et al. 1995a), our findings (De Carlos and O'Leary 1992) suggest that the early differentiation of the preplate and the initial development of the cortical plate—in other words, the beginning of cerebral cortex development—occur independently of afferent fibers.

Once the suggestion that afferent fibers are required to induce the development of the cerebral cortex was excluded, we looked for other possibilities that might induce distant cells and/or fibers to interact with the cortical neuroepithelium at early developmental stages. Two different possibilities were tentatively studied, and both turned out to be involved in the entry of cells and fibers into the developing cortex. First, we studied the growth of the olfactory placodes in the rat, describing all the cellular elements generated in these structures during their development. Among these, we described the existence of a novel cell population that originates in the olfactory placode and that migrates to the rostral part of the telencephalon, mainly spreading over its dorsal surface at early stages of embryonic development (De Carlos et al. 1995b; 1996a). The neuronal nature of these novel migrating cells was established with an antibody directed against the neuron specific class III beta-tubulin (TuJ1, gift from Dr. Frankfurter), which labels all neuronal cells after their last mitosis (Lee et al. 1990). This neural population migrates very early in development, before other placode-derived cells, following a tangential pathway in the dorsal mesenchymal tissue. In this way, it reaches the dorsal part of the telencephalic vesicles, apparently without associating with any fiber. Despite their origin, these cells do not express olfactory markers and, at present, their function is unknown. However, because these cells introduce their axons into the preplate (De Carlos et al. 1995b, 1996a), it is likely that they interact with preplate cells just when this layer begins to form, suggesting a possible involvement in the earliest stages of cortical development.

Another site considered as a possible entry point to the cortical neuroepithelium for cells and fibers was the limit between the dorsal and basal telencephalon (pallial–subpallial boundary). This possibility has been studied using a new method that we set up in our laboratory: whole embryo culture in roller bottles, combined with injecting embryos from E12 to E14 (at the preplate stage or the beginning of cortical development). Briefly, embryos were individually dissected from pregnant dams in a petri dish containing Hank's balanced solution at 37°C. Under the dissecting microscope, the muscular uterine wall and the decidua were removed, and the Reichert's membrane was opened and dissected to reveal the vascularized visceral yolk sac and the embryo within it. The yolk sac was partially broken at its avascular site, maintaining the integrity of the vitelline arteries and veins but exposing the embryo attached by the umbilical vessels, taking care not to cut into the chorioallantoic placenta. The amnion was removed and the vessels of the viteline stalk were tucked under the tail of the embryo. Once the embryo had been exposed, a small amount of carbocyanine dye (DiI and/or DiA) was injected into the basal telencephalon, either in the germinative area of the lateral ganglionic eminence (LGE) or in the area of the cortico-striatal boundary. These dyes help trace the migratory behavior of the newly generated LGE cells, and/or they serve to detect any cell or fiber entering the dorsal telencephalon. Finally, the injected embryos were transferred to glass bottles containing heat-inactivated rat serum as the culture medium, and placed in a roller drum housed in an incubator chamber at 37°C subjected to continuous gassing with a mix containing 95% oxygen (see more details in De Carlos et al. 1996b). Embryos were incubated for 24–48 hours, fixed, vibratome sectioned, and studied with the aid of a fluorescent microscope equipped with the appropriate filter cubes.

Using this methodology, we were able to define two important anatomical relationships. First, some cells generated in the LGE reach the lateral and basolateral telencephalic area, including the olfactory cortex, using the radial glia of the eminence as a migratory substrate. Second, some cells generated in the LGE migrate toward the cortical neuroepithelium, transgress the cortico-striatal boundary, and then move long distances tangentially into the preplate/marginal zone of the neocortical primordium (Figure 2.2A). This finding is extremely important because it demonstrates that not all cells that form part of the cerebral cortex are generated within the neocortical neuroepithelium, reaching their appropriate position by radial migration along the cortical radial glia. Instead, we must acknowledge the dual origin of the cerebral cortex. Thus, whereas some cortical cells are generated inside the pallium and use radial displacement to

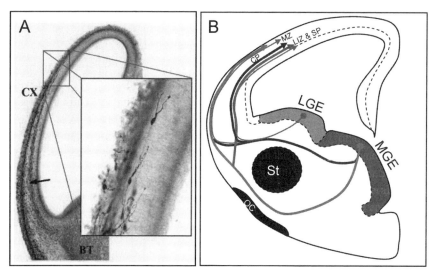

Figure 2.2. Tangential migration of cortical interneurons. **(A)** Microphotograph taken of a coronal section from the telencephalon of an E15 rat embryo immunostained with an antibody against the neurotransmitter GABA. The migratory GABAergic cells coming from the basal telencephalon (BT) enter the cortex (CX) through the marginal and intermediate zone (arrow). The box in the dorsal telencephalon shows a higher magnification of the leading tangential migrating cells as they progress toward the hippocampal anlage, bearing a fine trailing process and a robust and sometimes bifurcated leading process. **(B)** Cartoon representation of a coronal section from the left hemisphere of a mouse embryo at E14–E15 of development. Green arrows trace the migratory routes taken by the cortical cells generated in the medial ganglionic eminence (MGE; blue) and bordering the developing dorsal and ventral striatum (St). Both dorsal and ventral routes bifurcate at the level of the pallial–subpallial boundary to reach the cortex through the marginal zone (MZ) or the lower intermediate zone (LIZ). Red arrows trace the migratory routes following by the cortical interneurons generated in the lateral ganglionic eminence (LGE; orange), which also bifurcate as they enter the cortex. The striatum (St) and the olfactory cortex (OC) are chemorepellent areas for cortical interneurons generated in the basal telencephalon (see Marín and Rubenstein, 2001). CP, cortical plate; SP, subplate. (See color Figure 2.2)

reach their appropriate stratum, other cortical cells are generated in the subpallium and reach the cortex by tangential migration (De Carlos et al. 1996b, Figure 5C).

These discoveries constituted a breakthrough and led to a rapid change in the concept of cortical development. One year after our first description of the possible basal telencephalic origin and tangential migration of cortical cells, two different laboratories working separately with slice culture preparations from mice (Anderson et al. 1997) and rats (Tamamaki et al. 1997) confirmed our first description and extended it by demonstrating the GABAergic nature of these tangentially migrating cells. The GABAergic character is very interesting because it indicates that these cells are exclusively cortical interneurons (inhibitory cells with short axons). At present, numerous laboratories worldwide are still working on different aspects of their genesis and mechanisms of migration, as well as the routes and fate of these tangentially migrating cortical cells. Subsequently, it has been accepted that all cortical projection (pyramidal) neurons are exclusively generated in the germinative area (ventricular zone/VZ and subventricular zone/ SVZ) of the cortical neuroepithelium and most, if not all, of the cortical interneurons are generated in the basal telencephalon, specifically in the three subdivisions of the ganglionic eminence (the lateral/LGE-, medial/MGE- and caudal/ CGE-regions).

As a rule, cortical pyramidal cells reach their appropriate stratum by means of radial migration, using the cortical radial glial. Meanwhile, cortical interneurons reach the developing cortex by tangential migration (a non-glia dependent mechanism) using two different strata for their displacement. These strata are the upper part of the neuroepithelium, or marginal zone (MZ), and the lower intermediate zone (IZ), essentially a fibrillar stratum (future white matter) localized above the SVZ (Figures 2.3, 2.4). Genetic studies have shown that the *Dlx1* and *Dlx2* transcription factors are selectively expressed at early developmental stages in the three ganglionic eminences, and that they are necessary for tangential migration. Indeed, if *Dlx1/2* are ablated, most interneurons in the developing cortex and hippocampus are lost (Anderson et al. 1997; Pleasure et al. 2000). However, these experiments do not discriminate whether the three subdivisions of the ganglionic eminence are able to generate cortical interneurons or they do

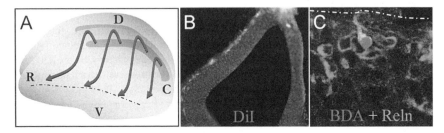

Figure 2.3. Origin of Cajal–Retzius cells and their tangential migration. **(A)** Cartoon representing a view of the telencephalon of an E11 mouse embryo from the left side. Cajal–Retzius cells originate in the cortical hem (purple band). The blue arrows indicate the migratory routes taken by Cajal–Retzius cells to cover the entire telencephalic surface. The migration is in an oblique caudal to rostral direction. **(B)** Coronal section from the telencephalon of an E10 mouse embryo injected with DiI in the cortical hem and cultured in toto for 24 hours. Cells generated in the cortical hem (injection site) migrate toward the basal telencephalon through the upper part of the preplate (red). The section was counterstained with DAPI (blue nuclei). **(C)** Migrating cell labelled with BDA injected in the cortical hem (red). The section was immunostained for *Reelin,* which labels the Cajal–Retzius cells (green) in the cortical preplate. Migrating cells express *Reelin.* (See color Figure 2.3)

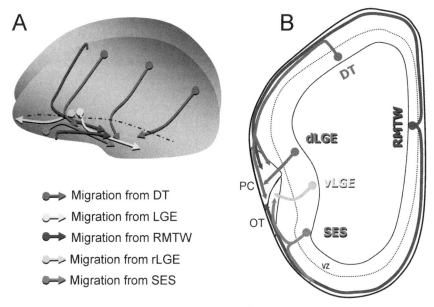

A

●→ Migration from DT
○→ Migration from LGE
●→ Migration from RMTW
○→ Migration from rLGE
●→ Migration from SES

B

DT

RMTW

dLGE

PC   vLGE

OT

SES

VZ

Figure 2.4. Early tangential migrations in the telencephalon converging in the olfactory cortex. **(A)** Cartoon of the telencephalon of an E11 mouse embryo, a lateral view of the left hemisphere. The different migratory routes identified in our studies are represented with a color code. Each cell population generated at E11 that was studied converges in the area of the developing olfactory cortex. Migration from the dorsal telencephalon (DT) and the ros-tromedial telencephalic wall (RMTW; red and blue arrows, respectively) crosses the cortical preplate initially following a rostral course. When the cells reach the pallial–subpallial bound-ary (dashed line), they change their migratory direction toward the caudal pole, together with some cell populations that originated in the lateral ganglionic eminence (LGE; yellow arrow) and in the septo-eminential sulcus (SES; orange arrow). In turn, a cell population emerges from the rostral area of the lateral ganglionic eminence (LGE; light blue arrow) that migrates rostrally, below the pallial–subpallial boundary, to the area of the prospective olfactory bulb (pOB). **(B)** Drawing representing a coronal section through the telencepha-lon of an E11 embryo. Diverse cell populations emerge from all proliferative telencephalic regions that use tangential displacement through the superficial preplate to reach the two main areas of the olfactory cortex, the piriform cortex (PC), and/or the olfactory tubercle (OT). VZ, ventricular zone. (See color Figure 2.4)

so to the same extent. Subsequent genetic studies have suggested that the MGE was the source of most neocortical interneurons (Sussel et al. 1999; Lavdas et al. 1999; Anderson et al. 2001). However, some authors refused to accept that the LGE generates any cortical cells, proposing instead that the cells generated in this structure run tangentially toward the olfactory bulbs through the rostral migratory stream (Wichterle et al. 2001). Studies have now revealed that the same genes are not expressed throughout the ganglionic eminence. For instance, whereas *Dlx1/2* are expressed in both the LGE and MGE (Anderson et al. 1997;

Stenman et al. 2003), *Nkx2.1* and *Mash1* are only expressed in the MGE (Sussel et al. 1999; Wichterle et al. 2001; Butt et al. 2005; Xu et al. 2005), such that the derivatives of this structure can be more readily defined. Likewise, *Gsh2* and *Er81* are expressed in the CGE (Corbin et al. 2003; López-Bendito et al. 2004).

A large amount of information has been generated on this subject over the years, but the source and diversity of the cells that undergo tangential migration are still not well understood. Thus, we have attempted to shed more light on all of these questions. It should be noted that in our initial experiments, embryos were removed from the uterus and exposed while attached by the umbilical veins to their membranes. Then, they were injected under the dissecting microscope and cultured in toto in roller bottles for 1 or 2 days (De Carlos et al. 1996b). However, most laboratories have studied tangential migrations of cortical interneurons generated in the basal telencephalon using cultured tissue slices. Our approach prevents the disruption of some putative rostro-caudal migratory routes that are lost in slice cultures, thereby forcing the newly generated cells to migrate erroneously through the intact piece of tissue in the experimental slice. We have compared the results obtained using our whole-embryo culture method with those we obtained in tissue slices, as used by other authors.

We first generated a three-dimensional computer reconstruction, from a coronal-sectioned E14 rat brain to study the macroscopic formation of the ganglionic eminences (Jiménez et al. 2002a). The first structure that emerges in the rat is the MGE at E12, whereas the LGE emerges at E12.5. Indeed, the MGE expands until E14, at which point it begins to decrease in size until E17. By contrast, the LGE grows progressively until the MGE fades away. Furthermore, it is significant that the LGE extends along the entire rostro-caudal axis, whereas the MGE emerges rostrally in the second third of the axis. Moreover, the interganglionic sulcus lies very deep in the rostral levels, separating both eminences and making the migration between both structures difficult at this point. For this reason, more migrating cells come from the medial to caudal levels of the rostro-caudal axis. We also demonstrated that both involved ganglionic eminences (LGE and MGE) give rise to a substantial number of cells that migrate tangentially, following several different routes to reach distinct layers of the mature cerebral cortex. In addition, we used different antibodies to study the tangentially migrating cells and demonstrated that they express mainly GABA, calbindin, and calretinin in a sequential fashion. Thus, they constitute a heterogeneous cell population that bears different markers and that probably fulfills different roles in the early development of the cortex (Jiménez et al. 2002a).

It is also important when studying tangential migration to understand the mechanisms used by the cells to move without the aid of any glial support. In 1892 Cajal formulated the neurotropic theory, suggesting that growth cones are provided with chemotactic sensitivity capable of recognizing attracting substances secreted by target cells. He hypothesized that the same mechanisms could also be involved in neuronal migration. To date, it is known that several molecules do indeed play such a role in axonal guidance and/or cell migration, including netrins, semaphorins, ephrins, and slits, as well as their corresponding receptors (Chisholm and Tessier-Lavigne 1999; Marín and Rubenstein 2001; Marín et al. 2001). For example, the Slit and Semaphorin families act as repulsive cues for axons in the mouse central nervous system. In the embryo, Slit1 is highly expressed in the VZ of the LGE and MGE (Yuan et al. 1999) and consequently, it has been suggested that Slit1 might repel LGE neurons, keeping them out of the VZ (Zhu et al. 1999). Combining both gain and loss of function approaches, it has also been suggested that Semaphorin 3A and 3F are repulsive and inhibit the passage of subsets of migrating MGE cells that express Neuropilin (Npn) 1/2, preventing them from entering the striatum as they migrate to the cerebral cortex (Marín et al. 2001).

In contrast, there are also positive or permissive factors that regulate tangential migration. For example, a couple of Neuroregulin 1 (Nrg1) isoforms exist that are expressed along the cortical migratory path of interneurons in the embryo. These Nrg1 isoforms act as long- and short-range attractants for tangentially migrating cells due to the expression of the ErbB4 receptor (Flames et al. 2004). The glial cell line–derived neurotrophic factor (GDNF) also serves as a potent chemoattractant of GABAergic cells via the glycosylphosphatydilinositol (GPI)-anchored receptor GFRalfa1 (Pozas and Ibañez 2005). Other factors, such as the brain-derived neurotrophic factor (BDNF) and neurotrophin 4 (NT4), were shown to stimulate tangential migration of MGE cells toward the cortex through TrkB signaling and PI3-kinase activation (Polleux et al. 2002). Hepatocyte growth factor/scatter factor (HGF/SF) also acts as a motogen for tangentially migrating interneurons via its mesenchymal-epithelial transition factor (MET) receptor (Powell et al. 2001).

In summary, data have been accumulated in the last five years that begin to shed light on the mechanisms that operate in tangential migration (see reviews in Marín and Rubenstein 2001; Corbin et al. 2001; Nakajima 2007). Modestly, our laboratory has contributed to elucidating the mechanisms behind tangential migration by describing the expression of the Slit receptor Robo-2 in the mantle zone of the LGE and in a band within the cortical mantle, which includes the upper part of the IZ and the cortical plate (CP). This receptor is not found in the lower part of the IZ and the PP/MZ, which correspond closely to the migratory routes used by tangential migrating cells. In addition, the band of Robo-2 expression in the LGE appears to be continuous with the expression in the cortex, although there is actually a gap between both bands that forms a free channel that is used by migrating cells to reach the cortex (Jiménez et al. 2002b). Likewise, we have data indicating that the cell adhesion molecule PSA-NCAM plays an important role in tangential migration. In this case, PSA-NCAM is expressed in the MZ, subplate (SP), and the lower IZ areas in the cortical neuroepithelium used by tangentially migrating cells (Jiménez et al. 2002b).

THE CAJAL–RETZIUS CELLS

Since their first description by Santiago Ramón y Cajal (1890) and Gustav Retzius (1893), the so-called Cajal–Retzius cells have turned out to be an attractive and enigmatic cellular population. They are the first neurons generated in the developing cortex, and they are located in layer 1 of the mammalian cerebral cortex. However, their sites of origin, molecular characteristics, and even their morphology remain under debate and are yet to be fully established. Morphologically, the Cajal–Retzius cells are the only neurons in the central nervous system with two or more axons (Cajal 1890). Despite being considered local circuit neurons, they express glutamate and not GABA (Hevner et al., 2003). During the mature life of the animal, the density of these neurons decreases, leading to the suggestion that they die after accomplishing their function during the initial stages of cortical development (Parnavelas and Edmunds 1983; Del Río et al. 1995; König et al. 1981). However, it is plausible that the cells generated at the initial stages of development would be diluted by the enormous increase in the tissue volume that occurs during brain maturation.

Cajal–Retzius cells are situated in the upper part of the neuroepithelium before the generation of the cortical plate. For this reason, they are thought to fulfill a relevant role in the development and establishment of the layered structure of the cerebral cortex. Accordingly, these cells are said to promote and direct the radial migration of neurons by means of the secretion of a large extracellular matrix protein, *Reelin* (Caviness 1982; Magdaleno et al. 2002). Mutant mice in which *Reelin* expression is suppressed (denominated as *reeler*) or where the *Reelin* receptors are inactivated, generate an aberrant cerebral cortex in which the layers are formed in the inverse order, with only layer 1 remaining in the appropriate position (Ogawa et al. 1995). This observation has been substantiated in various studies (Howell et al. 1997; Hiesberger et al. 1999; Trommsdorff et al. 1999; Herms et al. 2004), although several experiments performed in other mutant mice have raised doubts about this issue (Meyer et al. 2002, 2004). For example, mutant mice in which practically all of the Cajal–Retzius cells were eliminated, removing the source of *Reelin*, possess a correctly laminated cerebral cortex (Yoshida et al. 2006). Therefore, the function of Cajal–Retzius cells and the *Reelin* protein does not seem to be as clear or simple as it was believed some years ago. Furthermore, despite being a cell population that was described more than a hundred years ago, the sites in the brain where these cells are generated has remained unclear until recently. Thus, the mystery surrounding the Cajal–Retzius cells involves their origin, their function, and the compounds they express (reviewed in Soriano and Del Río 2005).

By means of BrdU injection, it was thought that 80% of the Cajal–Retzius cells in the developing mouse are generated at E10, and the remaining 20% at E11 (Hevner et al. 2003). However, the site of generation has remained an object of controversy among the scientific community. Whereas it was originally thought that these cells were generated in the underlying cortical neuroepithelium (Gorski et al. 2002; Alcántara et al. 1998), several authors have recently studied alternative origins, especially after the surprising discovery of the tangential migration of cortical GABAergic interneurons. Nevertheless, despite these efforts no consensus has been reached. Studies with genetic markers situate their origin in the neopallium, due to the widespread expression of the Tbr1 and Emx2 transcription factors (characteristic of the dorsal pallium) and the absence of Dlx expression (typical of the subpallium) (Hevner et al. 2003). Despite this evidence, other extracortical origins are still being considered, such as the MGE or the retrobulbar area (Meyer et al. 2002). Though many scientists still argue in favor of multiple origins for this unique population (Meyer et al. 2004), the medial telencephalic wall is the most likely site of their origin and may resolve this question. This structure includes the cortical hem (Meyer et al. 2002; Takiguchi-Hayashi et al. 2004), a region defined by the expression of different genes, such as *Wnt* and *Bmp* (Grove et al. 1998; Abu-Khalil et al. 2004; Shimogori et al. 2004). Indeed, the latest studies in the field seem to confirm the origin of the Cajal–Retzius cells in the cortical hem (Yoshida et al. 2006; García-Moreno et al. 2007a). Thus, in genetic lineage tracer experiments (Yoshida et al. 2006) cells that express the *Wnt3a* gene (a gene exclusively expressed in the cortical hem) populate the preplate at the correct stages, they express the protein *Reelin*, and they remain in the marginal cortical area, at least until the end of gestation.

In our laboratory, we demonstrated in whole embryo cultures that the main origin (if not the only one) of the Cajal–Retzius cells is the cortical hem, and we defined the tangential migratory routes that they take to reach the more distal point of the pallium (García-Moreno et al. 2007a). The injection of tracers in different areas of the cortical hem of mouse embryos and their observation after 24 hours in culture demonstrated a characteristic cellular migration. The cells emerge from the cortical hem and move tangentially through the incipient preplate very superficially, almost in contact with the pial membrane. In addition, the tangential migratory routes describe an oblique trajectory, in a rostral direction, from all levels of the cortical hem (rostral, medial, and caudal). It should be highlighted that the migration of the Cajal–Retzius cell population is different from the pattern described for neocortical development. The Cajal–Retzius cells have their origin in a dorsal, caudal, and medial area of the telencephalon, whereas the development of the preplate initiates in a ventral, rostral, and lateral area of the telencephalon (De Carlos and O'Leary 1992). Prior to the arrival of the cortical plate cells, the Cajal–Retzius cells must occupy the whole cortical extension, settling down and commencing their activities to promote and to facilitate radial neuronal migration.

Another issue surrounding this cell population is how their tangential displacement is controlled, and why neighboring populations respond in different ways to the similar assortment of molecular signals. To date, the only molecule suggested to participate in directing the migration and positioning of these cells is the chemokine CXCL12 (Stromal derived factor 1, SDF1), acting by means of its receptor CXCR4 expressed in the Cajal–Retzius cells (Stumm et al. 2003; Tissir et al. 2004). Although, there is evidence that the meninges and their expression of CXCL12 are necessary for the final and correct location of the Cajal–Retzius cells, it remains unclear whether this molecule acts during the migration of neuroblasts (Borrell and Marín 2006) or it affects the maintenance of the final position of Cajal–Retzius cells, next to the piamater (Paredes et al. 2006).

As we have seen, the preplate is generated with the arrival of an external cell population to the cortical neuroepithelium, the Cajal–Retzius cells. However, several cell populations inhabit the preplate before the arrival of the cortical plate cells (Jiménez et al. 2003). To further complicate the situation, recent studies in our laboratory have demonstrated that this cellular stratum is also used as a crowded highway by cell populations generated in different telencephalic areas that migrate tangentially to occupy other distant regions (García-Moreno et al. 2007b).

THE OLFACTORY CORTEX

The first sensory system to develop in the brain is the olfactory system. There-fore, the neurons that constitute this structure should be the first cells generated in the telencephalon (Valverde and Santacana 1994). More or less simultaneous to the generation of the Cajal–Retzius cells in the cortical hem, an important number of neuroblasts accumulate in the ventrolateral part of the telencephalon. This cell population is known by some authors as the piriform preplate, and it is thought to be comprised of several cell types. The early migration of radial glia from the cortico-striatal sulcus toward the piriform preplate suggests that some neuroblasts reach this telencephalic area by means of radial migration, as demon-strated by the experimental injection of tracers in this area (De Carlos et al. 1996b). In addition to this early contribution of the basal telencephalon to the primary olfactory regions, a separate cell population generated in the dorsal pallium has been reported to migrate ventrally through the preplate to colonize the piriform cortex surrounding the lateral olfactory tract (Tomioka et al. 2000; Jiménez et al. 2002a; Kawasaki et al. 2006).

The olfactory system consists of the olfactory bulbs (OB) and the primary olfactory cortex (OC). Though the piriform preplate still exists, the OB has not yet formed as an external, evaginated structure. Instead, the first olfactory neu-rons that are generated accumulate in the rostral telencephalic pole, in a region that we call the prospective olfactory bulb (pOB). Before OB evagination occurs, the OB projection neurons (the mitral and tufted cells) have already sent their axons toward the caudal pole, through the ventrolateral part of the telencephalon, forming the lateral olfactory tract (LOT) (López-Mascaraque et al. 1996). The piriform cortex (PC) is the area through which this tract passes. The region below the lot and PC is the olfactory tubercle (OT). Finally, the olfactory cortex is completed by the entorhinal cortex (EC), which is located in a caudal telencephalic area just where the LOT ends. The origin of the projecting cells that populate the OB is currently unknown, although it has been suggested that they reach the pOB by means of tangential migration (Nomura and Osumi 2004). However, it is well established that some olfactory interneurons (granular and periglomerular cells) are generated in a region surrounding the lateral ventricles, the subventricular zone, both during embryonic development and throughout adult life. From this area, the olfactory cells migrate rostrally to reach and enter the OB. Although these cells use tangential migration, they do not migrate superficially using the cortical preplate. Rather, they follow a deep pathway that is known as the rostral migratory stream (RMS) (Alvarez-Buylla et al. 1994). It has also been shown that these olfactory interneurons are generated during embryonic stages (from E13.5 in mice) in the subpallial LGE (Wichterle et al. 2001). Nevertheless, both the time of origin and the precise regions where the different cell populations that populate the olfactory cortex are generated remain largely unknown.

Studies from our laboratory using in toto mouse embryo culture, injections of several tracers, and immunohistochemistry, show that there are many cell populations from different proliferative regions of the telencephalon that migrate tangentially in the preplate stage (E10–E12), preferentially converging in the olfactory cortex (Figure 2.5) (García-Moreno et al. 2007b). In this way, tangential migration has been rediscovered as a general mechanism employed in embryonic development, especially in stages prior to the arrival of the cortical plate. Thus, cell populations follow different migratory routes that pass through the entire cortical preplate, from the dorsal and lateral pallium, and from the rostro-medial telencephalic wall (medial pallium). These cell populations coexist with the Cajal–Retzius cells in the preplate and they share common features, such as their tangential and oblique direction toward rostral levels. However, their migration through the preplate occurs at a deeper level rather than in apposition to the pial surface. It is interesting to note that there is orthogonal migration at the same time, throughout the piriform cortex toward the caudal pole. Caudally directed tangential migration is repeated by several cell populations but always in regions ventral to the pallial–subpallial boundary. Some of the neuronal migratory paths from the dorsal telencephalon have been described, as well as the molecular mechanisms that direct migration along these paths (Nomura et al. 2006). As such, ephrin A5 directs the ventral migration of these neurons, under the control of Pax6. Accordingly, the mutant mouse for Pax6 has reduced levels of ephrin A5

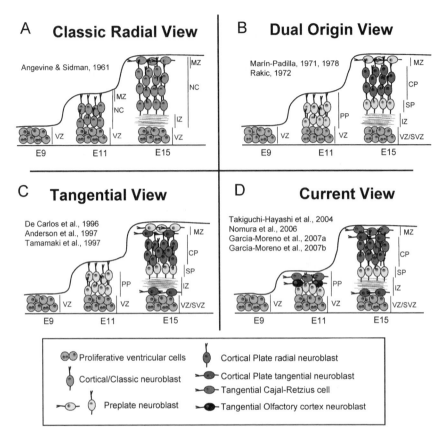

A **Classic Radial View**

Angevine & Sidman, 1961

MZ
NC
IZ
VZ

E9   E11   E15

B **Dual Origin View**

Marín-Padilla, 1971, 1978
Rakic, 1972

MZ
CP
SP
PP
IZ
VZ/SVZ

E9   E11   E15

C **Tangential View**

De Carlos et al., 1996
Anderson et al., 1997
Tamamaki et al., 1997

MZ
CP
SP
PP
IZ
VZ/SVZ

E9   E11   E15

D **Current View**

Takiguchi-Hayashi et al., 2004
Nomura et al., 2006
Garcia-Moreno et al., 2007a
Garcia-Moreno et al., 2007b

MZ
CP
SP
PP
IZ
VZ/SVZ

E9   E11   E15

Proliferative ventricular cells
Cortical/Classic neuroblast
Preplate neuroblast

Cortical Plate radial neuroblast
Cortical Plate tangential neuroblast
Tangential Cajal-Retzius cell
Tangential Olfactory cortex neuroblast

Figure 2.5. Evolution of our understanding of cerebral cortex development through different models. **(A)** Model validated up to 1970. All the cortical cells are generated in the germinative area of the neocortical (NC) epithelium, the ventricular zone (VZ). The first layer to develop, the marginal zone (MZ), and the inside-out gradient (radial migration) of the different waves of cell generations, are indicated. **(B)** Model validated from 1970 to 1996. Following the revised nomenclature of the Boulder Committee, this model establish the *dual origin theory*, whereby the cortical plate (CP; source of cortical layers 2–6) originated in the ventricular and subventricular zones (VZ, SVZ), and ascended using the radial glia to colonize the preplate (PP), which is considered of different origin. The PP is divided into an upper marginal zone (MZ; future layer 1) and a lower subplate zone (SP). **(C)** Model validated from 1996 to 2007. Introducing the arrival of different GABAergic cell populations that come from the basal telencephalon and reach the neuroepithelium by tangential migration. **(D)** The current view incorporates the latest discoveries on the early tangential migrations at preplate stages into the previous model; these cells converge at the olfactory cortex. The intermediate zone (IZ) is a fibrous layer present in all the models that will be the white matter in the adult. The lower bar in each model represents different embryonic ages (E9, E11, E15). (See color Figure 2.5)

and displays aberrant tangential migration that surpasses the ventral limits of the olfactory cortex. This population that migrates tangentially to reach the early olfactory cortex is the only one for which the molecular correlates are partially understood.

The LGE is a subpallial structure that gives rise mainly to the striatum (Puelles et al. 2000; Wichterle et al. 2001). The studies that first identified the origin of the cortical interneurons (De Carlos et al. 1996) also showed that cells generated in the LGE descended toward the olfactory cortex with the aid of radial glia. Recent work in our laboratory (Garcia-Moreno et al. 2007b) has revealed that the migratory itineraries that drive these neurons to the olfactory cortex subdivide the LGE into three regions based on the migratory pattern of their neurons (Puelles et al. 2000; Marín and Rubenstein 2002):

> The dorsal portion of the LGE (dLGE). Defined by the expression of Gsh2 but not of Gsh1 (Corbin et al. 2000; Toresson and Campbell 2001), this area probably corresponds to the pLGE1 and pLGE2 regions described by Flames et al. (2007). Cells generated in this area descend to the piriform cortex, as previously described (De Carlos et al. 1996) and immunohistochemically, they resemble the cell population that reaches the embryonic piriform cortex from pallial regions.

> The ventral portion of the LGE (vLGE). This area expresses both Gsh1 and Gsh2 (Yun et al. 2003). This area probably corresponds to the pLGE3 and pLGE4 regions, described by Flames et al. (2007). Cells generated in this area reach the olfactory cortex radially and colonize the olfactory tubercle, a region ventral to the piriform cortex. This population is clearly subpallial and differs greatly from those areas mentioned previously because it does not express Tbr1, a pallial transcription factor.

> The rostral tip of the LGE (rLGE). Cells generated in this area migrate radially to the olfactory cortex and then turn forward to begin a new tangential migration. This tangential migration runs parallel to the horizontal brain axis, taking them to the pOB, where the olfactory bulb will appear (García-Moreno et al. 2007b). This cell population is probably the first exogenous cell population to arrive at the olfactory bulb, at developmental stages prior to the appearance of the RMS, which is the main exogenous source of neurons in the olfactory bulb (Pencea and Luskin 2003; Tucker et al. 2006). At present, it is not known what type of cell migrates from the rLGE (interneurons or projection neurons).

The rostro-medial telencephalic wall (RMTW) generates a cell population that reaches the olfactory cortex following a dorsal route through the preplate. However, there is also another route in the same area generated by cells that move tangentially in the opposite direction. These cells move ventrally, crossing the surface of the medial pallium and the septum to reach and settle in the olfactory tubercle. The neurons that follow this route share the trajectory with those generated in another subpallial and rostral territory that divides the LGE and the septum, the septo-eminencial sulcus (SES). The neurons generated in this region also populate the olfactory bulb, and they are characterized by their Calbindin expression.

We found that all the tangential migrations during early telencephalic development that converge in the olfactory cortex run with a given direction, depending on their site of origin (García-Moreno et al. 2007b). As a general rule, cells generated in the pallium migrate tangentially along both the dorso-ventral and caudo-rostral axis. By contrast, those generated in the subpallium mainly migrate along the rostro-caudal axis, using the olfactory cortex as a substratum. As an exception, most cells generated in rLGE and some in the SES migrate rostrally through the subpallium to reach the pOB. Finally, cells generated in the pallium migrate caudally just when they cross the cortico-striatal boundary.

In summary, the telencephalon behaves differently in the stages prior to and after the arrival of the cortical plate. Tangential migration is a very well-established mechanism of cell movement in different neuronal types that share the same destination but differ in their origins. Therefore, we must consider tangential migration as a general strategy used in normal nervous system development, not an exception.

FINAL CONSIDERATIONS

Studying the generation and distribution of early cell populations in telencephalic development, we found that different coincident cell populations move using different migratory routes to reach distinct final destinations. However, all of these cells share a general mechanism as they use tangential migration for their displacements. Although the study of each population separately can isolate us from the behavior of the others, it is evident that each one will decisively influence the rest because they share the substratum over which they pass at the same developmental stages, and probably the factors that guide them. Therefore, although the developing telencephalon in the preplate stage is probably the best model by which to study the underlying mechanisms of tangential migration, it is necessary to study the telencephalon as a whole to see that the behavior of each cell type depends on that of the others.

Thus, when we consider all the cell movements that occur at a given developmental stage and in a given brain structure (e.g., the cerebral cortex), we can recognize the existence of a well-established telencephalic pattern of tangential migrations from the neocortical primordium to the olfactory cortex. This implies several changes to the model initially conceived to explain the development of the cerebral cortex (see Fig. 2.5). Although the development of this structure has been studied for a long time now, the most popular model was proposed in 1970, when a committee of scientists met in Boulder, Colorado, to unify the terminology to be used in these types of studies (Boulder Committee, 1970). Before this event, the first model was named the "Classic Radial View" (Fig. 2.5A). Basically, this model assumed the initial existence of a pseudo-stratified columnar neuroepithelium in which a germinative zone appeared at the *ventricular zone* (VZ), along with a clearly recognizable superficial layer that was designated as the *marginal zone* (MZ). At that time, it was thought that all cortical cells were generated in the VZ of this neuroepithelium, and that they ascended radially toward the pial surface, settling down in an inside-out gradient of different germinative waves (Angevine and Sidman 1961). In 1970, the Boulder Committee defined five different layers in the developing cortical neuroepithelium. The first of these were two deep germinative areas, the *ventricular* and *subventricular zones* (VZ, SVZ), followed by the *intermediate zone* (IZ), a mainly fibrous area from which some immature cell bodies migrated. Then there is the most important layer, the *cortical plate* (CP) that, although not well defined by the Boulder Committee, gave rise to cortical layers 2–6, and the *marginal zone* (MZ) against the pial membrane.

Some months later, when studying the early prenatal ontogenesis of the cat neocortex, Marín-Padilla (1971) showed that the arrival of the CP cells divides the MZ into two different strata, which he preferred to denominate as the *primordial plexiform layer* (PPL). Thus, the upper part of the CP remained as the MZ (future layer 1), with layer 6 below the CP. Soon after, another stratum was added to the Boulder descriptions, the *subplate zone* (SP), that corresponds to the lower area housing the neurons that the CP cells displaced when the PPL divided. Subsequently, the SP was no longer considered as layer 6 as Marín-Padilla had thought at the beginning. The interesting thing was that this author called his proposal the *dual origin of the mammalian neocortex* (Marín-Padilla 1978), because he thought that the most superficial layer (layer 1, or the MZ) and the deepest layer (layer 7, layer 6b, or SP) had a more primitive neuronal organization than layers 2–6 (CP-derived), and a distinct developmental origin. This is important because it is the first suggestion that some cortical cells can be generated outside the cortical mantle. Subsequently, this developmental model was named the "Dual Origin View," as completed by the description of Rakic (1972) of the role of radial glia as a scaffold used by the neuroblasts to ascend toward the pial surface (Fig. 2.5B).

These models remained stable until 1996, when our laboratory demonstrated for the first time that some cells generated in the ganglionic eminences of the basal telencephalon migrate tangentially, transgressing the cortico-striatal sulcus to incorporate into the developing cerebral cortex (De Carlos et al. 1996). A year later, further support for these findings was obtained and the cortical tangential migrating cells that originated in the basal telencephalon were identified as GABAergic interneurons (Anderson et al. 1997; Tamamaki et al. 1997). It is now accepted that the cortical projecting cells are generated in the germinative zone of the cortical neuroepithelium whereas the cortical interneurons are generated outside, in the subpallial ganglionic eminence. Consequently, we named this proposed model the "Tangential View" and showed that the tangentially migrating cells that enter the cortex via two separate pathways course through either the MZ or the lower IZ (Fig. 2.5C).

Finally, according to our most recent studies, we want to suggest a novel model to describe cortical development. This is our "Current View" model (Fig. 2.5D) in which two new discoveries have been added to the previous model: (1) the finding that Cajal–Retzius cells are mainly generated in the cortical hem (a structure outside the cortex), and that they reach and spread over the entire cortical surface through tangential migration (Takiguchi-Hayasi et al. 2004; García-Moreno et al. 2007a); and (2) the discovery that cells generated in many different germinative areas at the preplate stage spread out from the entire telencephalon, and they migrate tangentially and subpially following different stereotypic pathways to converge in the olfactory cortex (García-Moreno et al. 2007b). These two different systems (Cajal–Retzius cells and olfactory cell populations) migrate in the same time window using the same stratum but, whereas the first system runs through the upper part of the preplate and colonizes the entire cortical surface, the second system migrates through the lower part of the preplate. These latter cells do not remain at the cortical surface but rather they surpass this structure to colonize different olfactory cortical regions.

In summary, the complexity added to the initial model of cortical development comes from the abundant populations recently discovered that use tangential migration. In turn, this reflects the intricate pattern of tangential movements during early telencephalic development. Therefore, it is clear that although it was initially believed to be of little importance, this type of migration is fundamental during the earliest developmental stages. Moreover, it is also now clear that the origin of the different cephalic structures, in this case the cerebral and olfactory cortex, is not dual, as Marín-Padilla proposed (1971), but is multiple.

ACKNOWLEDGMENTS

We thank Laura López-Mascaraque and Maria Laura Ceci for helpful comments on the manuscript and Mark Sefton for editorial assistance. Our funding came from the Spanish Ministerio de Educación y Ciencia (BFU2007-60351/BFI) and the OLFACTOSENSE Consortium, Comunidad Autónoma de Madrid (P-SEM-0255-2006).

REFERENCES

Abu-Khalil, A., L. Fu, E. A. Grove, N. Zecevic, and D. H. Geschwind. 2004. Wnt genes define distinct boundaries in the developing human brain: implications for human forebrain patterning. *J Comp Neurol* 474:276–88.

Alcántara, S., M. Ruiz, G. D'Arcangelo, F. Ezan, L. de Lecea, T. Curran, C. Sotelo, and E. Soriano. 1998. Regional and cellular patterns of reelin mRNA expression in the forebrain of the developing and adult mouse. *J Neurosci* 18:7779–99.

Alvarez-Buylla, A., C.Y. Ling, W.S. Yu. 1994. Contribution of neurons born during embryonic, juvenile, and adult life to the brain of adult canaries: regional specificity and delayed birth of neurons in the song-control nuclei. *J Comp Neurol* 347:233–48.

Anderson, S.A., D.D. Eisenstat, L. Shi, and J.L.R. Rubenstein. 1997. Interneuron migration from basal forebrain to neocortex: Dependence on Dlx genes. *Science* 278:474–76.

Anderson, S.A., O. Marín, C. Horn, K. Jennings, and J.L.R. Rubenstein. 2001. Distinct cortical migrations from the medial and lateral ganglionic eminences. *Development* 128:353–63.

Angevine, J.B. and R.L. Sidman. 1961. Autoradiographic study of cell migration during histogenesis of cerebral cortex in the mouse. *Nature* 192:766–68.

Bayer, S.A., and J. Altman. 1991. *Neocortical development*. New York: Raven Press.

Borrell, V., and O. Marín. 2006. Meninges control tangential migration of hem-derived Cajal–Retzius cells via CXCL12/CXCR4 signaling. *Nat Neurosci* 9:1284–93.

Boulder Committee. 1970. Embryonic vertebrate central nervous system: Revised terminology. *Anat Record* 166:257–61.

Butt, S.J., M. Fuccillo, S. Nery, S. Noctor, A. Kriegstein, J.G. Corbin, and G. Fishell. 2005. The temporal and spatial origins of cortical interneurons predict their physiological subtype. *Neuron* 48:591–604.

Cajal, S.R. 1890. Sobre la existencia de células nerviosas especiales en la primera capa de las circunvoluciones cerebrales. *Gaceta Med Catalana* 13:737–39.

Cajal, S.R. 1892. La rétine des vertébrés. *La Cellule* 9:121–33.

Catalano, S.M., R.T. Robertson, and H.P. Killackey. 1991. Early ingrowth of thalamocortical afferents to the neocortex of the prenatal rat. *Proc Natl Acad Sci USA* 88:2999–3003.

Caviness, V.S., Jr. 1982. Neocortical histogenesis in normal and reeler mice: a developmental study based upon [3H]thymidine autoradiography. *Brain Res* 256:293–302.

Chisholm, A., and M. Tessier-Lavigne. 1999. Conservation and divergence of axon guidance mechanisms. *Current Opinion in Neurobiology* 9:603–15.

Corbin, J.G., N. Gaiano, R.P. Machold, A. Langston, and G. Fishell. 2000. The Gsh2 homeodomain gene controls multiple aspects of telencephalic development. *Development* 127:5007–20.

Corbin, J.G., S. Nery, and G. Fishell. 2001. Telencephalic cells take a tangent: non-radial migration in the mammalian forebrain. *Nature Neurosci* suppl 4:1177–82.

Corbin, J.G., M. Rutlin, N. Gaiano, and G. Fishell. 2003. Combinatorial function of the homeodomain proteins Nkx2.1 and Gsh2 in ventral telencephalic patterning. *Development* 130:4895–906.

De Carlos, J.A., L. López-Mascaraque, and F. Valverde. 1995b. The telencephalic vesicles are innervated by olfactory placode-derived cells: A possible mechanism to induce neocortical development. *Neuroscience* 68:1167–78.

De Carlos, J.A., L. López-Mascaraque, and F. Valverde. 1996a. Early olfactory fiber projections and cell migration into the rat telencephalon. *Int J Devl Neuroscience* 7/8:853–66.

De Carlos, J.A., L. López-Mascaraque, and F. Valverde. 1996b. Dynamics of cell migration from the lateral ganglionic eminence in the rat. *J Neurosci* 16:6146–56.

De Carlos, J.A., and D.D.M. O'Leary. 1992. Growth and targeting of subplate axons and establishment of major cortical pathways. *J Neurosci* 12:1194–1211.

De Carlos, J.A., B.L. Schlaggar, and D.D.M. O'Leary. 1995a. Development of acetylcholinesterase-positive thalamic and basal forebrain afferents to embryonic rat neocortex. *Exp Brain Res* 104:385–401.

Del Río, J.A., A. Martínez, M. Fonseca, C. Auladell, and E. Soriano. 1995. Glutamate-like immunoreactivity and fate of Cajal–Retzius cells in the murine cortex as identified with calretinin antibody. *Cereb Cortex* 5:13–21.

Fishell, G., C.A. Mason, and M.E. Hatten. 1993. Dispersion of neural progenitors within the germinal zones of the forebrain. *Nature* 362:636–38.

Flames, N., J.E. Long, A.N. Garratt, T.M. Fischer, M. Gassman, C. Birchmeier, C. Lai, J. L. Rubenstein, and O. Marín. 2004. Short- and long-range attraction of cortical GABAergic interneurons by neuregulin-1. *Neuron* 44:251–61.

Flames, N., R. Pla, D.M. Gelman, J.L. Rubenstein, L. Puelles, and O. Marín. 2007. Delineation of multiple subpallial progenitor domains by the combinatorial expression of transcriptional codes. *J Neurosci* 27:9682–95.

García-Moreno, F., L. López-Mascaraque, and J.A. De Carlos. 2007a. Origins and migratory routes of murine Cajal–Retzius cells. *J Comp Neurol* 500:419–32.

García-Moreno, F., L. López-Mascaraque, and J.A. De Carlos. 2007b. Early telencephalic migration topographically converging into the olfactory cortex. *Cerebral Cortex* (doi: 10.1093/cercor/bhm164).

Gorski, J.A., T. Talley, M. Qiu, L. Puelles, J.L.R. Rubenstein, and K.R. Jones. 2002. Cortical excitatory neurons and glia, but not GABAergic neurons, are produced in the Emx1-expressing lineage. *J Neurosci* 22:6309–14.

Grove, E.A., S. Tole, J. Limon, L. Yip, and C.W. Ragsdale. 1998. The hem of the embryonic cerebral cortex is defined by the expression of multiple Wnt genes and is compromised in Gli3-deficient mice. *Development* 125:2315–25.

Herms, J., B. Anliker, S. Heber, S. Ring, M. Fuhrmann, H. Kretzschmar, S. Sisodia, and U. Muller. 2004. Cortical dysplasia resembling human type 2 lissencephaly in mice lacking all three APP family members. *EMBO J* 23:4106–15.

Hevner, R.F., T. Neogi, C. Englund, R.A.M. Daza, and A. Fink. 2003. Cajal–Retzius cells in the mouse: transcription factors, neurotransmitters, and birthdays suggest a pallial origin. *Brain Res Dev Brain Res* 141:39–53.

Hiesberger, T., M. Trommsdorff, B.W. Howell, A. Goffinet, M.C. Mumby, J.A. Cooper, and J. Herz. 1999. Direct binding of Reelin to VLDL receptor and ApoE receptor 2 induces tyrosine phosphorylation of disabled-1 and modulates tau phosphorylation. *Neuron* 24:481–89.

Honig, M.G., and R.I. Hume. 1986. Fluorescent carbocyanine dyes allow living neurons of identified origin to be studied in long-term cultures. *J Cell Biol* 193:171–87.

Honig, M.G. and R.I. Hume. 1989. Carbocyanine dyes. Novel markers for labelling neurons. *Trends Neurosci* 12:336–38.

Howell, B.W., R. Hawkes, P. Soriano, and J.A. Cooper. 1997. Neuronal position in the developing brain is regulated by mouse disabled-1. *Nature* 389:733–37.

Hunter, K.E., and M.E. Hatten. 1995. Radial glial cell transformation to astrocytes in bidirectional: regulation by a diffusible factor in embryonic forebrain. *PROC NATL ACAD SCI* 92:2061–65.

Jiménez, D., L. López-Mascaraque, J.A. De Carlos, and F. Valverde. 2002b. Further studies on cortical tangential migration in wild type and Pax-6 mutant mice. *J Neurocytol* 31: 719–28.

Jiménez, D., L. López-Mascaraque, F. Valverde, and J.A. De Carlos. 2002a. Tangential migration in neocortical development. *Dev Biol* 244:155–69.

Jiménez, D., R. Rivera, L. López-Mascaraque, J.A. De Carlos. 2003. Origin of the cortical layer I in rodents. *Dev Neurosci* 25(2–4):105–15.

Kawasaki, T., K. Ito, and T. Hirata. 2006. Netrin 1 regulates ventral tangential migration of guidepost neurons in the lateral olfactory tract. *Development* 133:845–53.

König, N., J.P. Hornung, and H. Van der Loos. 1981. Identification of Cajal- Retzius cells in immature rodent cerebral cortex: a combined Golgi-EM study. *Neurosci Lett* 27:225–29.

Lavdas, A.A., M. Grigoriou, V. Pachnis, and J.G. Parnavelas. 1999. The medial ganglionic eminence gives rise to a population of early neurons in the developing cerebral cortex. *J Neurosci* 15:7881–88.

Lee, M.K., L.I. Rebhun, and A. Frankfurter. 1990. Posttranslational modification of class III beta-tubulin. *PROC NATL ACAD SCI* 87:7195–99.

Lois, C., and A. Alvarez-Buylla. 1994. Long-distance neuronal migration in the adult mammalian brain. *Science* 264:1145–48.

López-Bendito, G., K. Sturgess, F. Erdelyi, G. Szabo, Z. Molnar, and O. Paulsen. 2004. Preferential origin and layer destination of GAD65-GFP cortical interneurons. *Cereb Cortex* 14:1122–33.

López-Mascaraque, L., J.A. De Carlos, and F. Valverde. 1996. Early onset of the rat olfactory bulb projections. *Neuroscience* 70:255–66.

Magdaleno, S., L. Keshvara, and T. Curran. 2002. Rescue of ataxia and preplate splitting by ectopic expression of Reelin in reeler mice. *Neuron* 33:573–86.

Marín, O., and J.L.R. Rubenstein. 2001. A long, remarkable journey: tangential migration in the telencephalon. *Nature Rev Neurosci* 2:1–11.

Marín, O., and J.L.R. Rubenstein. 2002. Patterning, regionalization and cell differentiation in the forebrain. In Rossant and Tam 2002, 75–106.

Marín, O., A. Yaron, A. Bagri, M. Tessier-Lavigne, and J.L.R. Rubenstein. 2001. Sorting of striatal and cortical interneurons regulated by semaphorin/neuropilin interactions. *Science* 293:872–75.

Marín-Padilla, M. 1971. Early prenatal ontogenesis of the cerebral cortex (neocortex) of the cat (Felix domestica). A Golgi study. I. The primordial neocortical organization. *Z Anat Entwicklungsgesch* 134:117–45.

Marín-Padilla, M. 1978. Dual origin of the mammalian neocortex and evolution of the cortical plate. *Anat Embryol* 153:109–26.

Marín-Padilla, M. 1990. Three-dimensional structural organization of layer I of the human cerebral cortex: A Golgi study. *J Comp Neurol* 299:89–105.

Meyer, G., A. Cabrera Socorro, C.G. Perez Garcia, L. Martinez Millan, N. Walker, and D. Caput. 2004. Developmental roles of p73 in Cajal–Retzius cells and cortical patterning. *J Neurosci* 24:9878–87.

Meyer, G., C.G. Perez-Garcia, H. Abraham, and D. Caput. 2002. Expression of p73 and Reelin in the developing human cortex. *J Neurosci* 22:4973–86.

Nakajima, K. 2007. Control of tangential/non-radial migration of neurons in the developing cerebral cortex. *Neurochemistry International* 51:121–31.

Noctor, S.C., A.C. Flint, T.A. Weissman, R.S. Dammerman, and A.R. Kriegstein. 2001. Neuron derived from radial glial cells establishes radial units in neocortex. *Nature* 409:714–20.

Nomura, T., J. Holmberg, J. Frisen, and N. Osumi. 2006. Pax6-dependent boundary defines alignment of migrating olfactory cortex neurons via the repulsive activity of ephrin A5. *Development* 133:1335–45.

Nomura, T., and N. Osumi. 2004. Misrouting of mitral cell progenitors in the Pax6/small eye rat telencephalon. *Development* 131:787–96.

Ogawa, M., T. Miyata, K. Nakajima, K. Yagyu, M. Seike, K. Ikenaka, H. Yamamoto, and K. Mikoshiba. 1995. The reeler gene-associated antigen on Cajal–Retzius neurons is a crucial molecule for laminar organization of cortical neurons. *Neuron* 5: 899–912.

O'Rourke, N.A., M.E. Dailey, S.J. Smith, and S.K. McConnell. 1992. Diverse migratory pathways in the developing cerebral cortex. *Science* 258:299–30.

Paredes, M.F., G. Li, O. Berger, S.C. Baraban, and S.J. Pleasure. 2006. Stromal-derived factor-1 (CXCL12) regulates laminar position of Cajal–Retzius cells in normal and dysplastic brains. *J Neurosci* 26:9404–12.

Parnavelas, J.G., and S.M. Edmunds. 1983. Further evidence that Retzius-Cajal cells transform to nonpyramidal neurons in the developing rat visual cortex. *J Neurocytol* 12: 863–71.

Pencea, V., and M.B. Luskin. 2003. Prenatal development of the rodent rostral migratory stream. *J Comp Neurol* 463:402–18.

Pinto, L., and M. Götz. 2007. Radial glia cell heterogeneity-The source of diverse progeny in the CNS. *Progress Neurobiol* 83:2–23.

Pleasure, S.J., S. Anderson, R. Hevner, A. Bagri, O. Marín, D.H. Lowenstein, and J.L.R. Rubenstein. 2000. Cell migration from the ganglionic eminences is required for the development of hippocampal GABAergic interneurons. *Neuron* 28:727–40.

Polleux, F., K.L. Whitford, P.A. Dijkhuizen, T. Vitalis, and A. Ghosh. 2002. Control of cortical interneuron migration by neurotrophins and PI3-kinase signalling. *Development* 129:3147–60.

Powell, E.M., W.M. Mars, and P. Levitt. 2001. Hepatocyte growth factor/scatter factor is a motogen for interneurons migrating from the ventral to dorsal telencephalon. *Neuron* 30:79–89.

Pozas, E., and C.F. Ibáñez. 2005. GDNF and GFRalfa1 promote differentiation and tangential migration of cortical GABAergic neurons. *Neuron* 45:701–13.

Price, J., and L. Thurlow. 1988. Cell lineage in the rat cerebral cortex: a study using retroviral-mediated gene transfer. *Development* 104(3):473–82.

Puelles, L., E. Kuwana, E. Puelles, A. Bulfone, K. Shimamura, J. Keleher, S. Smiga, and J.L.R. Rubenstein. 2000. Pallial and subpallial derivatives in the embryonic chick and mouse telencephalon, traced by the expression of the genes Dlx-2, Emx-1, Nkx-2.1, Pax-6, and Tbr-1. *J Comp Neurol* 424:409–38.

Rakic, P. 1972. Mode of cell migration to the superficial layers of the fetal monkey neocortex. *J Comp Neurol* 145:61–84.

Retzius, G.M. 1893. Die Cajalschen Zellen der Grosshirnrinde beim Menschen und bei Säugetieren. *Biol Unters* 5:1–9.

Rossant, J., and P. Tam, eds. 2002. *Mouse development*. San Diego: Academic Press.

Rubenstein, J.L.R., S. Martínez, K. Shimamura, and L. Puelles. 1994. The embryonic vertebrate forebrain: the prosomeric model. *Science* 266:578–80.

Shigomori, T., V. Banuchi, H.Y. Ng, J.B. Strauss, and E. Grove. 2004. Embryonic signaling centers expressing BMP, WNT and FGF proteins interact to pattern the cerebral cortex. *Development* 131:5639–47.

Soriano, E., and J.A. Del Rio. 2005. The cells of Cajal–Retzius: still a mystery one century after. *Neuron* 46:389–94.

Stenman, J., H. Toresson, and K. Campbell. 2003. Identification of two distinct progenitor populations in the lateral ganglionic eminence: implications for striatal and olfactory bulb neurogenesis. *J Neurosci* 23:167–74.

Stumm, R.K., C. Zhou, T. Ara, F. Lazarini, M. Dubois-Dalcq, T. Nagasawa, V. Höllt, and S. Schulz. 2003. CXCR4 regulates interneuron migration in the developing neocortex. *J Neurosci* 23:5123–30.

Sussel, L., O. Marín, S. Kimura, and J.L.R. Rubenstein. 1999. Loss of Nkx2.1 homeobox gene function in a ventral to dorsal molecular respecification within the basal telencephalon: Evidence for a transformation of the pallidum into the striatum. *Development* 126:3359–70.

Takiguchi-Hayashi, K., M. Sekiguchi, S. Ashigaki, M. Takamatsu, H. Hasegawa, R. Suzuki-Migishima, M. Yokoyama, S. Nakanishi, and Y. Tanabe. 2004. Generation of reelin-positive marginal zone cells from the caudomedial wall of telencephalic vesicles. *J Neurosci* 24:2286–95.

Tamamaki, N., K.E. Fujimori, and R. Takauji. 1997. Origin and routes of tangentially migrating neurons in the developing neocortical intermediate zone. *J Neurosci* 17:8313–23.

Tamamaki, N., K. Nakamura, K. Okamoto, and T. Kaneko. 2001. Radial glia is a progenitor of neocortical neurons in the developing cerebral cortex. *Neurosci Res* 41:51–60.

Tissir, F., C.E. Wang, and A.M. Goffinet. 2004. Expression of the chemokine receptor Cxcr4 mRNA during mouse brain development. *Brain Res Dev Brain Res* 149:63–71.

Tomioka, N., N. Osumi, Y. Sato, T. Inoue, S. Nakamura, H. Fujisawa, and T. Hirata. 2000. Neocortical origin and tangential migration of guidepost neurons in the lateral olfactory tract. *J Neurosci* 20:5802–12.

Toresson, H., and K. Campbell. 2001. A role for Gsh1 in the developing striatum and olfactory bulb of Gsh2 mutant mice. *Development* 128:4769–80.

Trommsdorff, M., M. Gotthardt, T. Hiesberger, J. Shelton, W. Stockinger, J. Nimpf, R.E. Hammer, J.A. Richardson, and J. Herz. 1999. Reeler/Disabled-like disruption of neuronal migration in knockout mice lacking the VLDL receptor and ApoE receptor 2. *Cell* 97:689–701.

Tucker, E.S., F. Polleux, and A.S. LaMantia. 2006. Position and time specify the migration of a pioneering population of olfactory bulb interneurons. *Dev Biol* 297:387–401.

Valverde, F., and M. Santacana. 1994. Development and early postnatal maturation of the primary olfactory cortex. *Brain Res Dev Brain Res* 80:96–114.

Walsh, C., and C.L. Cepko. 1988. Clonally related cortical cells show several migration patterns. *Science* 241:1342–45.

Wichterle, H., D.H. Turbull, S. Nery, G. Fishell, and A. Alvarez-Buylla. 2001 In utero fate mapping reveals distinct migratory pathways and fates of neurons born in mammalian basal forebrain. *Development* 128:3759–71.

Xu, Q., C.P. Wonders, and S.A. Anderson. 2005. Sonic hedgehog maintains the identity of cortical interneuron progenitors in the ventral telencephalon. *Development* 132:4987–98.

Yoshida, M., S. Assimacopoulos, K.R. Jones, and E.A. Grove. 2006. Massive loss of Cajal–Retzius cells does not disrupt neocortical layer order. *Development* 133:537–45.

Yuan, S.S., L. Zhou, J.H. Chen, J.Y. Wu, Y. Rao, and D.M. Ornitz. 1999 The mouse SLIT family: secreted ligands for ROBO expressed in patterns that suggest a role in morphogenesis and axon guidance. *Dev Biol*, 15:290–306.

Yun, K., S. Garel, S. Fischman, J.L. Rubenstein. 2003. Patterning of the lateral ganglionic
    eminence by the Gsh1 and Gsh2 homeobox genes regulates striatal and olfactory bulb
    histogenesis and the growth of axons through the basal ganglia. *J Comp Neurol* 461:
    151–65.
Zhu, Y., H. Li, L. Zhou, J.Y. Wu, and Y. Rao. 1999. Cellular and molecular guidance of
    GABAergic neuronal migration from an extracortical origin to the neocortex. *Neuron*
    23:473–85.

Chapter Three

Genetic Control of Cajal–Retzius Cell Development

Amaya Miquelajáuregui and Alfredo Varela-Echavarría

INTRODUCTION

Cajal–Retzius cells are among the first neurons of the cerebral cortex to be generated and are responsible for its correct organization during embryonic development. They were discovered by Santiago Ramón y Cajal and Gustav Retzius in the mammalian cerebral cortex by means of Golgi's *reazione nera*, the black reaction staining of silver impregnation that revolutionized the study of the nervous system. Cajal–Retzius (C–R) cells are horizontally oriented neurons located unequivocally in the most superficial layer (I) of the developing cerebral cortex and possess long axonal plexuses and typical radial dendrites ascending toward the pial surface (Figure 3.1) (Marin-Padilla 1998; Meyer et al. 1999).

C–R cells exist transiently during corticogenesis and are characterized by the expression of reelin, a 400–450 kDa glycoprotein that is secreted into the extracellular matrix and is crucial for cortical development. Mutations of the reelin gene in humans account for a congenital form of lissencephaly associated with neuronal migration defects (Hong et al. 2000), and decreased levels of reelin have been found in patients with various developmental disorders, such as schizophrenia and autism (Fatemi 2001). Homozygous mutations of reelin, as in the spontaneous mouse mutant *reeler,* cause severe disorders in cortical lamination, as well as alterations in cerebellar and hippocampal development (Ogawa et al. 1995;

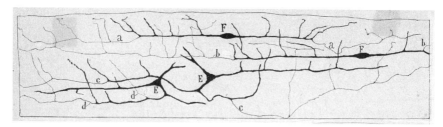

Figure 3.1. Cajal–Retzius cells in cortical layer I. Original drawing by Santiago Ramón y Cajal published originally in 1890 in "Textura de las circunvoluciones cerebrales de los mamíferos inferiores" (Gaceta Médica Catalana, pp. 22–31). Translation of the original figure legend: "Anteroposterior section of the molecular layer of the brain of a two-day old rabbit. F, fusiform cell; E, triangular cells; a, axons of a single fusiform cell; b, another pair of axons of a similar cell; d, axons emerging form the dendritic tree of a triangular cell; c, another pair of axons of a triangular cell." (See color Figure 3.1)

D'Arcangelo et al. 1997; Alcantara et al. 1998; Meyer et al. 1999; Soriano and Del Rio 2005).

At the beginning of corticogenesis, neurons born in the ventricular zone (VZ) of the neuroepithelium emigrate radially from this proliferative region to accumulate in the superficially located preplate. The preplate is subsequently split by a wave of cortical neurons. As a result, two layers of preplate derivatives embrace the newly formed cortical plate (CP): one layer above it, the C–R cell–containing marginal zone (MZ) and the subplate underneath (Marin-Padilla 1998; Bystron et al. 2008). In *reeler* mice, the neurons forming the CP do not respect the MZ boundary and migrate aberrantly to lie between the C–R cells. Hence, the *reeler* preplate fails to split, subplate cells intermingle with C–R cells, and CP neurons accumulate below in a disordered manner.

Corticogenesis normally proceeds after preplate splitting with the thickening of the CP. Newly generated neurons pass through cohorts of previously generated cells in the CP and settle below the MZ. This inside-first, outside-last gradient of formation assures that older neurons remain deep within the cortex (layers V and VI), while younger neurons settle above, forming upper layers II–IV (Hevner et al. 2003a). In the *reeler* mutant mouse, the inside-out cortical layering arrangement is inverted (Caviness and Sidman, 1973). Although neuronal phenotypes are generated on time and in the right proportions, late-born neurons seem to have difficulty passing their earlier siblings and accumulate in deeper locations in the *reeler* cortex (Caviness 1982; Pinto-Lord et al. 1982; Ogawa et al. 1995; Hevner et al. 2003a).

Putative cellular targets of reelin that possess the necessary molecular machinery for signal transduction in the cortex include CP neurons and radial glial cells. Mutations in different molecular components of the reelin signaling pathway induce *reeler*-like phenotypic traits, such as a failure to split the preplate and a rough inversion in cortical lamination, together with cellular hyperplasia of the

MZ and radial glia alterations (Forster et al. 2002; Frotscher et al. 2003; Hartfuss et al. 2003; Luque 2004; Kuo et al. 2005; Hack et al. 2007). Combined mutation of the reelin receptors VLDLR (very low density lipoprotein receptor) and ApoER2 (apolipoprotein E receptor 2), single mutation of the cytoplasmic adaptor Dab1 (Disabled-1), or double mutation of Src and Fyn kinases responsible for Dab1 phosphorylation and concomitant degradation, result in a phenocopy of the *reeler* phenotype, thereby confirming their participation in a common signaling pathway (Rice et al. 1998; D'Arcangelo et al. 1999; Hiesberger et al. 1999; Howell et al. 1999; Trommsdorff et al. 1999).

Radial glia serve as neuronal progenitors in all regions of the central nervous system (CNS) and give rise to the majority of pyramidal neurons in the cortex (Noctor et al. 2002; Fishell and Kriegstein 2003; Malatesta et al. 2003; Anthony et al. 2004). Radial glia serve not only as neuronal precursors but also as guides for migration. Each radial glial cell in the cortex extends a long radial process into the MZ that is used as migratory scaffold by newly generated neurons (Noctor et al. 2002; Malatesta et al. 2003; Kriegstein and Noctor 2004). Time-lapse studies revealed that late-generated neurons rely more on radial glia–directed locomotion than early-born cells, which preferentially use somal translocation to migrate toward the pial surface (Nadarajah et al. 2001; Nadarajah et al. 2003). During somal translocation, once the migrating neuron extends its leading process to the MZ, the cell body begins to move upward, independently of radial glia. Late-born neurons, in contrast, largely depend on radial glia to reach the lower CP and appear to proceed to the top by somal translocation. It seems that the glia-independent mode of radial migration may be necessary in the absence of a glial scaffold early in cortical development, whereas radial, glia-guided locomotion appears to be required later in order to sustain the increasingly long distances within a growing CP (Nadarajah and Parnavelas 2002; Kriegstein and Gotz 2003; Nadarajah et al. 2003; Tissir and Goffinet 2003). Based on these observations, it has been proposed that reelin acts on neurons whose leading processes reach the reelin-rich MZ, by stimulating two events in cortical development: detachment from radial glia and radial somal translocation (Cooper 2008).

In addition to radial migratory modes, C–R cells, interneurons, and locally derived cortical neurons have been shown to move tangentially within the cortex (de Carlos et al. 1996; Lavdas et al. 1999; Maricich et al. 2001; Nadarajah and Parnavelas 2002). As early as in the preplate stage, C–R cells born outside the cortex migrate tangentially along the subpial cortical space. Soon thereafter, the cortex starts receiving important contingents of tangentially migrating GABAergic interneurons (Bystron et al. 2008). Interneurons migrating into the cortical plate assume layer positions with isochronically generated, local cortical neurons, a process that seems to be reelin-independent. In *reeler* mutant mice, interneurons are generated at the same time and in the same proportions as in wild-type mice and they correctly position into the corresponding layer despite the cortical inversion.

Thus, the underlying relationship between the laminar fate of interneurons and projection neurons is preserved in *reeler* mutant mice (Hammond et al. 2001; Hevner et al. 2004; Metin et al. 2006; Pla et al. 2006).

Notably, both C–R and radial glial cells represent transient cell types in mammals in that they persist as long as corticogenesis takes place (Soriano and Del Rio 2005; Merkle and Alvarez-Buylla 2006). Perinatally, radial glia progenitors switch from a neurogenetic to gliogenetic program. Soon after birth, C–R cells gradually disappear from the cortex, as a population of GABA$^+$ and calbindin$^+$ interneurons co-expressing reelin start emerging within the cortical plate and MZ (Alcantara et al. 1998; Hevner et al. 2003b; Jimenez et al. 2003; Takiguchi-Hayashi et al. 2004).

Despite being represented by a relatively small neuronal population, C–R cells control important aspects of cortical development by secreting reelin into the extracellular matrix. In this chapter, we will discuss recent evidence on the genetic factors controlling C–R cell production, differentiation, and migration during corticogenesis.

GENETIC DETERMINANTS OF CAJAL–RETZIUS CELL DIFFERENTIATION

It used to be assumed that C–R cells in the cortex were generated locally throughout the ventricular zone, as are most of the cortical projection neurons (Marin-Padilla 1998). This view was recently modified by evidence showing that focal production sites in both pallial and subpallial areas generate C–R cells early in development and that they undergo extensive migration to quickly populate the entire dorsal telencephalon (Takiguchi-Hayashi et al. 2004; Bielle et al. 2005; Borrell and Marin 2006; Yoshida et al. 2006). The major sources of C–R cells so far identified in the mouse include the pallial cortical hem (Takiguchi-Hayashi et al. 2004; Yoshida et al. 2006), the subpallial septal/retrobulbar area (sep/RB) (Meyer and Goffinet 1998; Bielle et al. 2005), and the ventral pallium at the pallial–subpallial boundary (VP/PSB) (Bielle et al. 2005; Hanashima et al. 2007).

Important information on C–R cell differentiation and migration has been provided by manipulating gene expression in mice and by the use of cellular and genetic tracers. Following is a description of the genes, predominantly transcription factors, that have been associated with C–R cell development (see Table 3.1 for summary).

Tbr1

The T-box brain gene 1 (*Tbr1*) transcription factor has been directly implicated in the specification of C–R cells (Hevner et al. 2001). *Tbr1* is expressed in early glutamatergic cortical neurons including C–R and subplate (SP) cells. The earliest C–R cells found in the murine cortex (E10.5) are all *Tbr1*$^+$ (Hevner et al. 2003b).

TABLE 3.1 Genetic Factors Regulating Cajal–Retzius Cell Development

Gene (Mouse)	Early Expression (E10.5-E12.5)		Experimental Manipulations		Reeler-like Phenotype				Refs.
	Pallium	VP/PSB and Subpallium	Tracing	C-R cells (Reln+)	PP splitting defect	Laminar inversion	MZ cell invasion	Dab1 over-expression	
Coup-TFI	Non-C-R cells in preplate E12.5 (high caudolaterally).	E12.5 PSB, Ganglionic eminence	Subpallial CoupTFI+ neurons migrate to DP through MZ	Overexpression E12.5 in PP induces ↓ Cx++.	No	No	No	No	Adapted from Zhou et al. 1999; Tripodi et al. 2004; Studer et al. 2005
Coup-TFII	C-R cells in preplate E12.5	E12.5 PSB & Ganglionic eminences	No dorsal migration found in subpallial CoupTFII+ neurons	—	—	—	—	—	
Dbx1	—	Septum E10.5 C-R (reln+) PSB E11.5	Dbx1-derived cells invade cortex from Septum and PSB ›E12.5	Dbx1-DTA: ↓ Cx++ ↓ Septum+++ ↓ PSB+ ≈ hem	No	No	No	—	Adapted from Bielle et al. 2005
Emx2	VZ ›E11.5 (high caudo-medially). Reelin colocalizationE12	›E12.5 PSB & Ganglionic eminence	-	Emx2−/−:›E13.5 ↓ Cx++ (reminiscent cells restricted medially)	Yes (some areas)	Mild (Upper layer dispersion)	No	—	Adapted from Mallamaci et al. 2000; Hevner et al. 2003

(Continued)

TABLE 3.1 Genetic Factors Regulating Cajal–Retzius Cell Development (*Continued*)

Gene (Mouse)	Early Expression (E10.5-E12.5)		Experimental Manipulations		Reeler-like Phenotype				Refs.
	Pallium	VP/PSB and Subpallium	Tracing	C-R cells (Reln$^+$)	PP splitting defect	Laminar inversion	MZ cell invasion	Dab1 over-expression	
Emx1/2	Emx1: >E10.5 in the entire DP.	Emx1-lacz: E12.5 in some VP structures	—	In Emx1/2 double KO: C-R cells absent	Yes	—	—	—	Adapted from Gorski et al. 2002; Shinozaki et al. 2002
Foxg1	Proliferative neuroephitelium (high rostro-laterally)	Ganglionic eminence	—	In Foxg1$^{-/-}$: ↑ Cx^{+++} (Dorsalization f Cx)	—	—	—	—	Adapted from Hanashima et al. 2004; Muzio and Mallamaci 2005; Hanashima et al. 2007
Fzd10	Hem >E12.5 and caudo-medial cortex (Reelin coloc)	—	—	—	—	—	—	—	Adapted from Zhao et al. 2006
Lhx1	—	Septum >E10.5-PSB >E11.5	—	—	—	—	—	—	Adapted from Varela-Echavarria et al., unpublished data

Gene	Onset of expression	Septum & PSB expression	Migration	Knockout phenotype				References
Lhx5	Hem >E10.5	Septum & PSB >E11.5	—	In Lhx5−/−: ↓Cx++ ↓PSB+ ↓Septum+ ↓Hem+	—	—	—	Adapted from Zhou et al. 1999; Varela-Echavarria et al. unpublished data
p73	Hem >E10.5	Septum & PSB >E12	—	In p73−/−: ↓Cx++	No	No	No	Adapted from Meyer et al. 2002; Meyer et al. 2004
Pax6	Proliferative neuroepithelium (high rostro-laterally)	—	↑Migration across VP-DP (Ventralization of the cortex. PSB markers lost)	Pax6−/− Sey: ↑Cx+++	Yes (restricted to areas)	No	—	Adapted from Chapouton et al. 1999; Kim et al. 2001; Stoykova et al. 2003
Tbr1	>E10.5: In all post-mitotic neurons. Reelin colocalization	PSB >E11.5	—	In Tbr1−/−: ↓Cx++ ≈ hem	Yes (↓SP)	No	Yes	Adapted from Hevner et al. 2001; Hevner et al. 2003
Wnt3a	Hem >E10.5	—	—	Wnt3a -DTA: ↓Cx+++ ↓Hem+++ ↓PSB++ ≈ Septum	No	No	No	Adapted from Yoshida et al. 2006

In *Tbr1*-deficient mice, reelin expression is down-regulated in most of the dorsal telencephalon. Similarly affected is the expression of *Calretinin*, a marker for a subset of C–R cells. *Reelin* expression in the cortical hem, however, is detected in Tbr1$^{-/-}$ embryos, probably because *Tbr1* expression, which abuts this medial area, does not extend into it (Hevner et al. 2003b).

Although *Tbr1* has been commonly considered a pallial marker, some extra-cortical areas have been shown to express it early in development (Puelles et al. 2000; Hevner et al. 2003b). Indeed, double-labeled *Reelin*/Tbr1 cells were found to be more abundant in the subpallium than in the pallium at E11.5 (Hevner et al. 2003b). Moreover, the expression pattern of *Tbr1* largely resembles that of *Reelin* in both pallial and subpallial areas at E12.5 (compare Fig. 2 in Hevner et al. 2003b and Fig. 1d in Alcantara et al. 1998), overlapping the proposed VP/subpallial domains of C–R cell origin such as the sep/RB and VP/PSB (Bielle et al. 2005). Thus, alterations in the sites of origin of VP/subpallial C–R cells could account for the decreased numbers of C–R cells in the cortex and some *reeler*-like defects observed in *Tbr1* knock-out mice such as in preplate splitting and *Dab1* overexpression in cortical cells. In spite of the defective preplate splitting, layer formation occurs normally in *Tbr1*-deficient cortices, supporting the notion that preplate splitting and glia-dependent radial migration of cortical neurons are two independent developmental processes in which *Reelin* is involved (Soriano and Del Rio 2005).

p73

In addition to *Reelin*, an emerging bona fide marker for C–R cells is the transfor-mation-related protein 73, which belongs to the *p53* family of tumor suppressors (Yang et al. 2000; Meyer et al. 2002; Takiguchi-Hayashi et al. 2004; Hanashima et al. 2007). In the mouse cortex, *p73* expression is found in the medial roof plate from E10.5 and subsequently in the cortical hem and choroid plexus at E12.5 (Meyer et al. 2002; Takiguchi-Hayashi et al. 2004). At this stage, graded expression (high medially) along the pial cortical surface is evident. In the sub-pallium, *p73* is expressed in the septum forming a continuous domain that extends into the nearby retrobulbar area (together referred to as sep/RB), and the VP/PSB (Meyer et al. 2002; Meyer et al. 2004). Although co-localization of p73 and *Reelin* occurs in sep/RB and VP/PSB regions, it is more pronounced in the cortical hem and the adjacent hippocampal anlage (Meyer et al. 2002). In all locations, p73$^+$ cells seem to be outnumbered by *Reelin*$^+$ cells. Interestingly, pre-plate p73$^+$ cells usually do not express *Calretinin* at E12.5 (Meyer et al. 2002), whereas calretinin is usually detected *Reelin*$^+$ cells at this stage (Hevner et al. 2003b; Stoykova et al. 2003).

Gene inactivation of *p73* results in fewer *Reelin*$^+$ C–R cells in the preplate. In spite of the decreased number of C–R cells in the neocortical wall, cortical lamination is preserved in *p73* mutants (Meyer et al. 2002; Meyer et al. 2004), with no apparent disruption of sep/RB and VP/PSB C–R cell subpopulations. A dramatic increase in *Calretinin*⁺ cell abundance is observed in the entire mutant telencephalic wall at E12. It seems that the normal balance between cell populations in the outermost cortical layer is altered by compensatory mechanisms in *p73* knock-out mice.

Wnt3a

The role of dorso-medial signaling in C–R cell development was assessed with the help of genetically modified mice in which hem-derived cells were selectively depleted. The specific ablation of hem-derived C–R cells was achieved by directing the expression of diphtheria toxin–A (DTA) to the cortical hem cells using the *Wnt3a* promoter. *Wnt3a* is one of the various Wingless members of extracellular molecules expressed exclusively in the cortical hem from E10.5, and it has been shown to be required for normal hippocampal development (Lee et al. 2000). In *Wnt3a*-DTA mice, elimination of hem-derived cells results in an almost complete abolition of *Reelin* expression in the dorsal cortex (Yoshida et al. 2006). Strikingly, preplate splitting and layer formation proceeded normally in spite of the almost total absence of C–R cells. It might be that the small amount of *Reelin* produced in this hem-deficient cortex is sufficient to support the normal organizing function of C–R cells. Although the septal *Reelin*⁺ C–R cell subpopulation is present in *Wnt3a*-DTA mice, the VP/PSB area seems to be abnormal, as revealed by a decrease in *p73* expression by E12.5 (Fig. 4a–b Yoshida et al. 2006). This suggests that an interplay exists between hem-derived C–R cells and other C–R-rich areas.

Dbx1

Strong evidence supporting the VP and subpallial origin of C–R cells came from recent studies in which the developing brain homeobox 1 (*Dbx1*) gene was used to genetically trace C–R cells derived from this lineage (Bielle et al. 2005). In the septum, the earliest *Reelin*⁺ cells (E10.5–12.5) were shown to be *Calretinin*-negative and to derive almost entirely from *Dbx1* progenitors. The migration of C–R cells derived from *Dbx1* progenitors was assessed in embryonic brain slice culture assays that remain to be confirmed in whole brains. Septal *Dbx1*–derived cells appeared to migrate rostrodorsally up to the medial cortex and ventrally toward the piriform cortex (PC). From the VP/PSB, labeled *Dbx1*-derived cells were found to migrate to the dorsal pallium and to the PC, a major site of *Reelin* expression at embryonic stages. Notably, both *Dbx1*-derived septal and VP/PSB cells converge at the PC, a structure that has been shown to be composed of cells of mixed origin (Nomura et al. 2006; Garcia-Moreno et al. 2007). In contrast to septal *Dbx1*–derived C–R cells, those derived from the VP/PSB were shown to express *Calretinin* in addition to *Reelin* (Bielle et al. 2005). Thus, both septal/ *Calretinin*⁻ and VP/PSB/ *Calretinin*⁺ C–R neurons seem to populate cortical areas following stereotyped routes.

Genetic ablation experiments of *Dbx1*-derived cells using DTA induced a differential loss of *Reelin*⁺ cells in the specific regions of normal *Dbx1* expression. Whereas an almost complete loss of C–R cells occurred in the septal area, decreased *Reelin* expression in the PC was detected only in its most rostral and caudal ends. Overall C–R cell density on the cortical surface was largely diminished at E12.5, but it returned to normal levels by E14.5, most probably due to C–R cell compensation from the unaffected cortical hem (Bielle et al. 2005).

Lhx1/Lhx5

Early in corticogenesis, C–R cells up-regulate the LIM-homeodomain transcription factors *Lhx1* and *Lhx5* (Yamazaki et al. 2004). Both *Lhx1* and *-5* are expressed in postmitotic cells from the telencephalon and are expressed particularly in *Reelin*⁺ cells (Varela-Echavarria et al, unpublished data). Whereas *Lhx1* is only expressed in the sep/RB and VP/PSB populations of C–R cell origin, *Lhx5* is additionally expressed in the pallial cortical hem. Deletion of *Lhx5* impairs hippocampal development (Zhao et al. 1999) as well as the production and migration of C–R cells (Varela-Echavarria et al., unpublished data).

Notably, the number of C–R cells in the lateral cortex of E12.5 *Lhx5*⁻/⁻ embryos decreases by 60% when compared to control littermates. Caudomedial cortical areas are particularly affected in *Lhx5*⁻/⁻ embryos, because ectopic *Reelin*⁺ cell clusters appear consistently from early stages, suggesting that C–R migration is altered in these mutants. Presumably, the ectopic C–R cell clusters in *Lhx5*⁻/⁻ embryos have a ventral pallial origin, based on the expression of *Lhx1* and *Ebf2* (Varela-Echavarria et al., unpublished data). Whereas the VP/PSB region is altered in *Lhx5*⁻/⁻ mutant mice, the sep/RB C–R cell population seems less affected, as indicated by the expression of *Reelin, Lhx1,* and *p73*. Thus, C–R cell subpopulations seem to be differentially affected by *Lhx5* mutation. The combination of cell tracing and genetic markers in *Lhx5* mutants might shed some light on the mechanisms regulating C–R migration.

Foxg1

C–R cell fate has been shown to be inhibited by Fork head box G1 (*Foxg1*), which encodes a winged-helix transcriptional repressor. It is expressed in almost all mitotic and post-mitotic cells in the developing cortex, but it is excluded from the *Wnt3a*-expressing cortical hem and particularly from C–R cells (Hanashima et al. 2004; Hanashima et al. 2007). In *Foxg1* knock-out embryos, C–R cells are

supernumerary in the altered cortex (Hanashima et al. 2004; Muzio and Mallamaci 2005; Hanashima et al. 2007). Overexpression of *Reelin* in *Foxg1*⁻/⁻ mice is
accompanied by increased expression of *Calretinin* and *Cxcr4*. In these mice,
laminar specification is completely absent (Hanashima et al. 2004). Moreover,
overall area patterning is severely disturbed in *Foxg1*⁻/⁻ cortices, as the expression
of markers of the medial-hippocampal region extends into more dorsal regions
at the expense of lateral-neocortical areas (Muzio and Mallamaci 2005).
This patterning defect was shown by an expansion of the *Fzd10*⁺ cortical hem
region in *Foxg1*⁻/⁻ when crossed with a reporter *Fzd10*-lacz mouse (Zhao et al.
2006).

To better dissect the specific role of *Foxg1* in C–R cell differentiation and
overcome the problem of early cortical patterning, the gene was conditionally inactivated at E13.5, a stage when cortical patterning is mostly set and most C–R cells
have been already generated. Similar to the situation observed in *Foxg1* full
knock-out embryos, removal of *Foxg1* at E13.5 induced supernumerary and ectopic C–R cells within the CP. Notably, some of the ectopic *Reelin*⁺ cells found in
the conditional *Foxg1* mutant expressed the VP marker *Ebf2* and did not co-
express *p73*, suggesting a ventral pallial origin for some of the ectopic C–R
cells. This was confirmed by crossing *Foxg1* conditional mutants with two independent mutant mouse lines in which the dorsal midline signaling is known to be
affected (*Gli3* KO and *Bmpr1a/b* dKO). In spite of the absence of cortical hem
and dorsal midline signaling, *Foxg1* inactivation increased C–R cell numbers,
thereby suggesting that ectopic C–R cells originate in areas other than the cortical hem.

Thus, *Foxg1* negatively regulates C–R cell fate. The experimental inhibition of
Foxg1 expression in cortical progenitors after the normal birthdate of C–R cells
reactivates their capacity to generate C–R cells (Hanashima et al. 2004;
Hanashima et al. 2007). This has been further demonstrated in vitro by attenuat-
ing *Foxg1* signaling in isolated cortical progenitor cells (Shen et al. 2006). In culture conditions, cortical progenitors were shown to mimic the in vivo schedule
of neuronal subtype generation, giving rise to C–R cells only during the earliest
cell divisions. Upon *Foxg1* inhibition, cortical progenitors that would normally
generate cortical neurons of more advanced phenotype, instead resumed the production of C–R cells. Taken together, these results suggest that continued *Foxg1*
expression is required to suppress cortical progenitors from adopting a C–R neuronal fate later in development. It would be interesting to assess in the same culture
conditions the differences in the potential to generate C–R cells of progenitors isolated from various cortical areas and from the subcortical areas known to give
rise to C–R cells.

Recently, a precursor population accounting for approximately 3% of the total
progenitor pool was uncovered within the marginal zone during corticogenesis
(Costa et al. 2007). Fate-mapping experiments showed that these progenitors are

of mixed pallial (*Emx1*[+]) and subpallial (*Gsh*[+], *Nkx2.1*[+]) origin. The MZ progenitors express predominantly the transcription factor *Olig2*, suggesting that they are able to generate oligodendrocytes and astrocytes. In dissociated MZ cultures, this precursor population was shown to give rise to GABAergic interneurons but not to C–R *Reelin*[+] or *Calretinin*[+] neurons. In conclusion, the potential of cortical progenitors other than the cortical hem to generate C–R cells remains to be determined.

Coup-TFs

An interesting pair of *Coup-TF* orphan nuclear receptor transcription factors is expressed in a complementary manner in the preplate and seems to influence C–R cell fate. *CoupTFII* is expressed in C–R cells (Tripodi et al. 2004), showing a general expression pattern comparable to that of *Reelin* in both pallial and subpallial areas. In contrast, *CoupTFI* is expressed in the subplate but is excluded from C–R cells, and in the absence of *CoupTFI* subplate cells do not survive beyond E16.5 (Zhou et al. 1999). Conversely, sustained expression of *CoupTFI* in preplate cells induced by electroporation is able to repress C–R cell differentiation, as evidenced by *Reelin* and *Calretinin* down-regulation at E12.5 (Studer et al. 2005). Thus, whereas *CoupTFI* represses preplate cells to adopt a C–R cell fate, *CoupTFII* seems to regulate positively C–R cell development.

Later in cortical development the segregation of these factors is maintained, as *CoupTFII* expression remains confined to C–R cells, whereas *CoupTFI* is found in calbindin[+] and GABA[+] interneurons (Tripodi et al. 2004). Whether *CoupTFII* is involved in repressing *Foxg1* from C–R cell precursors and what the interplay is between the two *CoupTFs* are open issues that remain to be determined.

In addition to its role in specifying C–R cell identity, *CoupTFI* has been shown to be expressed preferentially in caudal areas and to be involved in repressing frontal/motor area fates (Zhou et al. 2001; Armentano et al. 2007). For this reason, *CoupTFI* has been classified within an emerging group of transcription factors involved in cortical arealization. Together with *Emx2*, *Pax6*, and *Sp8*, *CoupTFI* shows graded expression across the embryonic cortical axes and functions differentially to determine the size and location of the different functional cortical areas (for review see O'Leary et al. 2007).

Pax6 and Emx1/2

Given the opposed, graded expression of *Emx1/2* (high caudomedially) and *Pax6* (high rostrolaterally), together with the mutual repression of *Pax6* and *Emx2* (Muzio et al. 2002; Muzio and Mallamaci 2003), it has been suggested that the generation of *Reelin*[+] cells is regulated by opposing interactions between *Pax6* and *Emx1/2*. It has been reported that in the absence of *Pax6*, the number of

Reelin-positive cells is doubled in the mutant cortex (Stoykova et al. 2003; Costa et al. 2007). Conversely, from E16.5 a gradual decrease of C–R cells is observed upon deletion of *Emx2* (Mallamaci et al. 2000), whereas C–R cells are completely absent in the cortex of the *Emx1/2* double-mutant mice (Shinozaki et al. 2002).

Early in cortical development (E11.5 mouse) the onset of *Emx1* and *Emx2* expression overlaps in the cortical ventricular zone, coinciding with the generation of *Reelin*[+] cells (Mallamaci et al. 2000; Hevner et al. 2003b; Stoykova et al. 2003). *Emx2* expression is then confined to the VZ and the outer region of the preplate, where *Emx2* colocalizes with *Reelin* in many cells at E12.5 (Hevner et al. 2003b). In *Emx2* mutant mice *Reelin*[+] C–R cells are initially formed, but they are subsequently lost in the neocortical region, particularly in the lateral cortex (Mallamaci et al. 2000). In addition, the combined mutation of *Emx1/2* in mice results in abnormal specification of cortical areas and in non-cell-autonomous alterations in subpallial migration into the cortex, as shown by the impeded migration of wild-type cells within an *Emx1/2*[-/-] cortex (Mallamaci et al. 2000; Shinozaki et al. 2002).

In addition to the pallium, both *Emx1/2* genes have been found to be expressed in subpallial areas (Mallamaci et al. 2000; Tole et al. 2000; Gorski et al. 2002). *Emx1* has been specifically detected in some C–R cells derived from the *Dbx1* lineage in the septum early in development (Bielle et al. 2005) and might be used to label specific C–R cell subpopulations. *Emx2* is expressed in a subpopulation of C–R cells in the marginal zone and may be required for C–R cell maintenance and survival. In combination, *Emx1* and *Emx2* have important roles in cortical patterning that may influence C–R cell differentiation and migration either directly or indirectly.

Pax6 plays a significant regulatory role in the specification of rostrolateral cortical areas and in setting the boundary between dorsal and ventral telencephalon at the PSB (Stoykova et al. 2000; O'Leary et al. 2007). In *Pax6* mutants (*Sey* mice), ventral markers are extended dorsally, and focal markers normally expressed in the PSB are missing (Stoykova et al. 2000; Kim et al. 2001). Furthermore, the restricted migration of ventral cells to cortical territories is disrupted in the absence of *Pax6* function (Chapouton et al. 1999).

In *Pax6* mutants, the marginal zone was shown to contain significantly more Reelin[+] and Calretinin[+] cells compared to wild-type mice at E14.5 (Stoykova et al. 2003). Although the normal proportion of Reelin[+] cells expressing Calretinin was maintained in *Pax6* mutants, the numbers of double-labeled cells gradually increased throughout development. In addition, increased numbers of calbindin[+] cells were found in the mutant cortex (Chapouton et al. 1999), although this probably corresponds to an interneuronal population, as calbindin has never been found together with Reelin in either wild-type or mutant C–R cells (Hevner et al. 2003b; Stoykova et al. 2003).

BrdU chase experiments showed that although overall neuronal production at E11.5 was not altered in *Pax6* mutants, the proportion of BrdU-labeled cells ending up in the MZ greatly increased at the expense of subplate cells in the mutant as compared to wild-type mice. Interestingly, isolated cortical cells express the C–R cell markers Reelin and calretinin in similar amounts and proportions in *Pax6* mutant and control mice. However, when cells taken from the entire telencephalon (both pallial and subpallial regions) were grown in culture, the in vivo situation could be reproduced, as shown by the increased numbers of Reelin⁺ and calretinin⁺ cells (Stoykova et al. 2003). This finding suggests that the supernumerary C–R cells in the marginal zone of *Pax6* mutants have a subcortical origin.

Thus, *Pax6* is important in the establishment and maintenance of the PSB. Impaired PSB formation in *Pax6* mutants seemingly results in an increase of tangential migration of subpallial cells into the MZ. A non-cell-autonomous defect most likely underlies the abnormal migration found in *Pax6* mutant cortical neurons, as indicated by embryonic transplantation assays at early developmental stages (Nomura et al. 2006).

ROUTES OF CAJAL–RETZIUS CELL MIGRATION

Genetic manipulations designed to alter C–R cell production have provided two important lessons: First, C–R cells are generated at focal pallial and subpallial regions and then migrate to populate the cortex; and second, rapid compensatory mechanisms may increase the generation of C–R cells from different areas, allowing them to complete their main functions in the absence of particular C–R cell subsets (Figure 3.2). C–R migratory pathways have been recently studied by genetic tracing (in transgenic mice carrying a reporter gene or by vector electroporation), and/or assessed by dye labeling in either whole brains or slices.

Tangential migration is the main mode of migration used by C–R cells. It is now generally accepted that, unlike interneurons, C–R cells migrate exclusively within the MZ, regardless of their origin (Meyer et al. 2004; Takiguchi-Hayashi et al. 2004; Bielle et al. 2005; Garcia-Moreno et al. 2007). One of the mechanisms underlying the tangential migration of hem-derived cells is mediated by Cxcl12/Cxcr4 signaling from the meninges. This signaling was shown to be required for C–R cells to migrate from the cortical hem to the dorsal pallium within the MZ. Whereas the meninges secrete the chemokine Cxcl12, C–R cells bear its receptor, Cxcr4 (Stumm et al. 2003; Borrell and Marin 2006). Mechanical removal of the meninges as well as genetic and pharmacologic blockade of the receptor Cxcr4 impaired hem-derived C–R cell tangential migration; ectopic C–R cells were found within the cortical plate and intermediate zone of mice with disrupted Cxcr4 signaling (Borrell and Marin 2006). Interestingly, meninges from

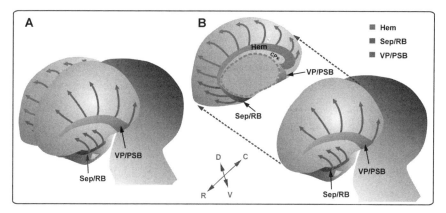

Figure 3.2. Routes of migration of Cajal–Retzius cells. Schematic representation of embryonic telencephalic vesicles (E10.5–12.5 mouse) viewed laterally in a diagram of the whole brain (**A**) and one in which the right telencephalic vesicle has been displaced laterally to view its medial side (**B**). C–R cells generated in the cortical hem in the medial wall (orange) migrate in a caudo-medial to rostro-lateral direction to cover most of the caudal regions of the cortex (only the early stages of migration out of the hem are shown). The septum/retrobulbar C–R cell progenitor domain (Sep/RB, blue) forms a continuous domain from the septum, through the retrobulbar region, and to the rostro-lateral side of the subpallium. C–R cells from this domain migrate dorsally and ventrally toward the rostro-lateral and piriform cortex, respectively. The ventral pallium and pallial–subpallial boundary domain (VP/PSB; green) extends from the caudo-ventral region of the medial telencephalic wall, turns around the ventral region of the telencephalic vesicle, and continues dorso-rostrally on the lateral side of the vesicle. C–R cells from the lateral aspect of this domain populate the piriform cortex and migrate dorsally to cover the lateral aspect of the cortex (CPx; choroid plexus). (See color Figure 3.2)

different cortical regions were shown to exert identical attraction on C–R cells from cortical hem explants, indicating that C–R cell dispersion does not depend on long-range meningeal cues, at least for hem-derived C–R cells. These results also suggest that C–R cell dispersion mediated by the Cxcl12/Cxcr4 pathway is nondirectional and that additional mechanisms are responsible for directing C–R cells to specific cortical regions. An additional mechanism of C–R cell dispersion could be mediated by cell repulsion, as C–R cells from cortical hem explants were shown to cease migrating as they approached cells from an adjacent explant (Borrell and Marin 2006).

In the pallium, a wave of cells migrating from the CMTW in a rostrolateral direction has been shown to include Reelin[+] and Calretinin[+] cells from early developmental stages (Takiguchi-Hayashi et al. 2004; Borrell and Marin 2006; Yoshida et al. 2006; C. Zhao et al. 2006; Garcia-Moreno et al. 2007). The Reelin[+] cells emanating from the CMTW, most likely originated in the cortical hem, follow the subpial surface and migrate tangentially in a rostrolateral direction. In this respect, it has been suggested that the migration from the CMTW occurs in streams of cells that do not seem to intermingle (Jimenez et al. 2003). Notably, a correlation has been observed between the initial position along the dorsoventral and rostrocaudal axes of the CMTW and the direction of migration toward the dorsal cortex (Takiguchi-Hayashi et al. 2004; Garcia-Moreno et al. 2007). These studies indicate that the migration of hem-derived C–R cells in the CMTW follows predominantly a caudomedial to rostrolateral direction covering most of the caudal telencephalic region.

Migratory pathways followed by cells from additional regions have been uncovered recently. It was shown that C–R cells from the sep/RB and the VP/PSB areas populate the dorsal pallium. Sep/RB C–R cells migrate dorsally toward the dorsal cortex and ventrally to the piriform cortex, a subpallial area close to the VP/PSB that is rich in *Reelin*+ cells (Alcantara et al. 1998). In turn, VP/PSB C–R cells migrate dorsomedially to cover the lateral aspect of the dorsal telencephalon, and ventrally to populate the PC (Bielle et al. 2005).

Hence, C–R cells generated from the various progenitor cell domains follow different routes into the cortex and each one eventually reaches a different distribution. Caudally, C–R cells from the cortical hem migrate in a caudomedial to rostrolateral direction populating predominantly the caudal cortex. Rostrally, C–R cells from the sep/RB region populate the rostral aspect of the cortex. In turn, C–R cells from the VP/PSB preferentially migrate dorsally and populate lateral regions of the cortex. The complementary and, to some extent, overlapping patterns of C–R cell migration result in the total coverage of the cortical surface during early stages of corticogenesis. It is not yet known, however, whether the migratory pathways taken by C–R cells are a consequence of intrinsic mechanisms, such as C–R dispersion by cellular repulsion, or an effect of extrinsic, long-range guidance cues that act differentially upon C–R cell subtypes.

DISTINCT PROGENITOR DOMAINS GENERATE SUBTYPES OF CAJAL–RETZIUS CELLS

Based on differential gene expression, onset of generation, and migratory routes, it has been suggested that C–R cells generated at different sites represent distinct neuronal subpopulations (Meyer et al. 2004; Yamazaki et al. 2004; Bielle et al. 2005; Hanashima et al. 2007). However, these subpopulations are able to carry out similar functions, because compensatory mechanisms rescue general C–R function in the absence of a particular C–R cell subset. Behind this apparent redundancy, it remains to be investigated whether C–R cell subpopulations confer distinct regional identities to cortical regions or C–R cells from a particular subpopulation influence the identity or migration of C–R cells that originate from distinct sites.

Birth-dating studies have shown that the generation of the entire C–R cell population in the developing mouse cortex occurs in a relatively short time window (E10.5–E12.5 in the mouse), based on Reelin and Calretinin expression. Importantly, Reelin$^+$ cells often co-localize with Calretinin (80%), although single-labeled cells have also been identified (Hevner et al. 2003b; Stoykova et al. 2003; Takiguchi-Hayashi et al. 2004; Garcia-Moreno et al. 2007). Thus, the use of Calretinin alone as a marker of C–R cells might be misleading because many Reelin$^+$ cells do not express Calretinin, and vice versa. Indeed, subpopulations of Reelin$^-$ cells expressing either Calretinin or calbindin have been found interspersed with C–R cells in the subpial cortical space, and they likely correspond to interneurons and subplate cells (Hevner et al. 2003b; Stoykova et al. 2003; Garcia-Moreno et al. 2007).

Currently, C–R cells are best identified by the expression of Reelin and, as described above, the vast majority can be also detected by the co-expression of Calretinin. Other genetic markers have been shown to be expressed in particular subsets of C–R cells, depending on their site of generation (see Table 3.1). Markers that identify a particular subpopulation, however, are rather uncommon because they usually label more than one subpopulation. Although little information exists regarding the molecular identity of each of the C–R cell subtypes, we can attempt to unify data from several laboratories in order to better define the gene repertoire of specific C–R cell subtypes.

Cortical Hem

C–R cells from the cortical hem express *Calretinin, p73, Lhx5,* and *Fzd10,* although only the latter is exclusively expressed in this region of the telencephalon. Genetic disruption of *p73* and *Lhx5* causes an overall decrease in *Reelin$^+$* cells in the cortex, particularly in caudal regions. Upon cortical hem deletion in *Wnt3a*-DTA mice, *Reelin$^+$* cells are almost absent by E12.5, but nevertheless an important number of *p73* cells seem to accumulate in the medial aspect of the cortex (Yoshida et al. 2006). It is possible that *p73* expression reflects an immature state of C–R cell development, as its expression precedes that of *Reelin* in the cortical hem (Takigushi-Hayashi 2004). Importantly, p73 rarely co-expresses with Calretinin, suggesting that they might label different C–R cell subsets within the cortical hem. This idea is further supported by the differential effect of the absence of *p73*: Whereas Reelin$^+$ cells decrease in *p73$^{-/-}$* cortices, Calretinin is strongly overexpressed as early as E12.5 (Meyer et al. 2002). In addition, the cortical hem is negative for *Tbr1* and *Foxg1* expression. The exclusion from this cortical region of *Foxg1*, a repressor of C–R cell fate, might allow the differentiation of C–R neurons from the cortical hem (Hanashima et al. 2004).

Septal/Retrobulbar Area

C–R cells originating in the septal/retrobulbar area express *Dbx1*, *p73*, *Tbr1*, *Lhx1*, and *Lhx5*. Notably, most C–R cells in the septum (98%) have been shown to derive from *Dbx1*⁺ precursors and to lack Calretinin expression. This Reelin⁺/Calretinin⁻ subpopulation appears early in development (E10.5). Moreover, upon ablation of the *Dbx1*⁺ progenitor domains, C–R cells in the septal region and in the rostral cortex are primarily affected (Bielle et al. 2005). Also, because septal C–R cells migrate to the VP/PSB area, it is likely that most Reelin⁺/Calretinin⁻ cells in the ventral pallium have a septal origin (Bielle et al. 2005). Thus, the C–R subset originating in the sep/RB arises almost entirely from *Dbx1* progenitors and lacks Calretinin expression.

Ventral Pallium/PSB

Another C–R cell subset emerging from the VP/PSB, and migrating toward the piriform cortex and dorsal cortex, express *Dbx1*, *p73*, *Tbr1*, *Foxg1*, *Lhx1*, *Lhx5*. A vast majority (around 80%) of C–R cells in the PC have been shown to derive from the *Dbx1*⁺ lineage and express Calretinin. C–R cells that do not express Calretinin in the PC may partially originate in the sep/RB area, as cells migrating from this area have been shown to settle in the PC (Bielle et al. 2005; Garcia-Moreno et al. 2007). Unlike the cortical hem, both VP/PSB and sep/RB areas express Tbr1, and in the embryonic cortex Tbr1 has been shown to be expressed in most of the Reelin⁺ C–R cells since early stages of corticogenesis (Hevner et al. 2001; Hevner et al. 2003b). Thus, C–R cells from subpallial *Tbr1*⁺ origin might largely contribute to the C–R cells populating all cortical regions.

CONCLUDING REMARKS

Although Cajal–Retzius-like cells are found in all amniotes and *Reelin* is present in the nervous system of all vertebrates, it is believed that the unique mammalian inside-out pattern of cortical lamination required an expansion of *Reelin* signaling during evolution (Tissir and Goffinet 2003). In mammals, C–R cells and Reelin secretion are critical during corticogenesis, as their absence severely disrupts cortical lamination (Caviness 1982; Soriano and Del Rio 2005).

In an attempt to find a molecular fingerprint of C–R cells and the factors that regulate *Reelin* expression in these neurons, an increasing number of genes preferentially expressed in C–R cells have been analyzed (Yamazaki et al. 2004). A picture is now emerging of C–R cells being a heterogeneous population formed by distinct subtypes generated in different focal sites at pallial and subpallial locations that migrate toward the dorsal pallium following stereotyped routes

(Jimenez et al. 2003; Takiguchi-Hayashi et al. 2004; Bielle et al. 2005; Soriano and Del Rio 2005; Borrell and Marin 2006).

C–R cell subtypes differ not only in their place of origin and migratory routes but also in their gene expression profile. Some of the genetic factors that regulate directly C–R development by promoting C–R cell fate include *Tbr1*, *p73*, *Dbx1*, *Lhx5*, and *CoupTFII*. In contrast, *Foxg1* and *CoupTFI* repress C–R cell fate. In addition, genes involved in general cortical patterning such as *Pax6*, *Emx1/2*, *Foxg1*, and *CoupTFI* might also influence indirectly C–R cell differentiation and migration. It is still unknown whether epistatic relationships exist between all these factors and whether the differences in the expression profile of C–R cell subgroups are translated into relevant functional properties, thereby conferring different regional identities to the cortex.

In the near future, the combined spatio-temporal analysis of expression of these transcription factors, the study of their regulatory interactions, and lineage tracing analysis, will shed light into the mechanisms controlling C–R differentiation and migration. This will, in turn, bring us closer to understanding how the mammalian cortex developed its characteristic inside-out mechanism of cortical lamination during evolution.

ACKNOWLEDGMENTS

A.V.-E. receives support from the Wellcome Trust (GR071174AIA) and CONACYT (40286M, 46754Q). A.M. is a recipient of a postdoctoral fellowship from UNAM. We thank the Instituto Cajal for the authorization to use one of S. Ramón y Cajal's original drawings and Juan A. de Carlos for the information regarding the figure.

REFERENCES

Alcantara, S., M. Ruiz, G. D'Arcangelo, F. Ezan, L. de Lecea, T. Curran, C. Sotelo and E. Soriano (1998). Regional and cellular patterns of reelin mRNA expression in the forebrain of the developing and adult mouse. *J Neurosci* 18(19):7779–99.

Anthony, T. E., C. Klein, G. Fishell and N. Heintz (2004). Radial glia serve as neuronal progenitors in all regions of the central nervous system. *Neuron* 41(6):881–90.

Armentano, M., S. J. Chou, G. S. Tomassy, A. Leingartner, D. D. O'Leary and M. Studer (2007). COUP-TFI regulates the balance of cortical patterning between frontal/motor and sensory areas. *Nat Neurosci* 10(10):1277–86.

Bielle, F., A. Griveau, N. Narboux-Neme, S. Vigneau, M. Sigrist, S. Arber, M. Wassef and A. Pierani (2005). Multiple origins of Cajal–Retzius cells at the borders of the developing pallium. *Nat Neurosci* 8(8):1002–12.

Borrell, V. and O. Marin (2006). Meninges control tangential migration of hem-derived Cajal–Retzius cells via CXCL12/CXCR4 signaling. *Nat Neurosci* 9(10):1284–93.

Bystron, I., C. Blakemore and P. Rakic (2008). Development of the human cerebral cortex: Boulder Committee revisited. *Nat Rev Neurosci* 9(2):110–22.

Caviness, V. S., Jr. (1982). Neocortical histogenesis in normal and reeler mice: a developmental study based upon [3H]thymidine autoradiography. *Brain Res* 256(3):293–302.

Chapouton, P., A. Gartner and M. Gotz (1999). The role of Pax6 in restricting cell migration between developing cortex and basal ganglia. *Development* 126(24):5569–79.

Cooper, J. A. (2008). A mechanism for inside-out lamination in the neocortex. *Trends Neurosci* 31(3):113–9.

Costa, M. R., N. Kessaris, W. D. Richardson, M. Gotz and C. Hedin-Pereira (2007). The marginal zone/layer I as a novel niche for neurogenesis and gliogenesis in developing cerebral cortex. *J Neurosci* 27(42):11376–88.

D'Arcangelo, G., R. Homayouni, L. Keshvara, D. S. Rice, M. Sheldon and T. Curran (1999). Reelin is a ligand for lipoprotein receptors. *Neuron* 24(2):471–9.

D'Arcangelo, G., K. Nakajima, T. Miyata, M. Ogawa, K. Mikoshiba and T. Curran (1997). Reelin is a secreted glycoprotein recognized by the CR-50 monoclonal antibody. *J Neurosci* 17(1):23–31.

de Carlos, J. A., L. Lopez-Mascaraque and F. Valverde (1996). Dynamics of cell migration from the lateral ganglionic eminence in the rat. *J Neurosci* 16(19):6146–56.

Fatemi, S. H. (2001). Reelin mutations in mouse and man: from reeler mouse to schizophrenia, mood disorders, autism and lissencephaly. *Mol Psychiatry* 6(2):129–33.

Fishell, G. and A. R. Kriegstein (2003). Neurons from radial glia: the consequences of asymmetric inheritance. *Curr Opin Neurobiol* 13(1):34–41.

Forster, E., A. Tielsch, B. Saum, K. H. Weiss, C. Johanssen, D. Graus-Porta, U. Muller and M. Frotscher (2002). Reelin, Disabled 1, and beta 1 integrins are required for the formation of the radial glial scaffold in the hippocampus. *Proc Natl Acad Sci USA* 99(20):13178–83.

Frotscher, M., C. A. Haas and E. Forster (2003). Reelin controls granule cell migration in the dentate gyrus by acting on the radial glial scaffold. *Cereb Cortex* 13(6):634–40.

Garcia-Moreno, F., L. Lopez-Mascaraque and J. A. de Carlos (2007). Early Telencephalic Migration Topographically Converging in the Olfactory Cortex. *Cereb Cortex*

Garcia-Moreno, F., L. Lopez-Mascaraque and J. A. de Carlos (2007). Origins and migratory routes of murine Cajal-Retzius cells. *J Comp Neur* 500:419–32.

Gorski, J. A., T. Talley, M. Qiu, L. Puelles, J. L. Rubenstein and K. R. Jones (2002). Cortical excitatory neurons and glia, but not GABAergic neurons, are produced in the Emx1-expressing lineage. *J Neurosci* 22(15):6309–14.

Hack, I., S. Hellwig, D. Junghans, B. Brunne, H. H. Bock, S. Zhao and M. Frotscher (2007). Divergent roles of ApoER2 and Vldlr in the migration of cortical neurons. *Development* 134(21):3883–91.

Hammond, V., B. Howell, L. Godinho and S. S. Tan (2001). disabled-1 functions cell autonomously during radial migration and cortical layering of pyramidal neurons. *J Neurosci* 21(22):8798–808.

Hanashima, C., M. Fernandes, J. M. Hebert and G. Fishell (2007). The role of Foxg1 and dorsal midline signaling in the generation of Cajal–Retzius subtypes. *J Neurosci* 27(41):11103–11.

Hanashima, C., S. C. Li, L. Shen, E. Lai and G. Fishell (2004). Foxg1 suppresses early cortical cell fate. *Science* 303(5654):56–9.

Hartfuss, E., E. Forster, H. H. Bock, M. A. Hack, P. Leprince, J. M. Luque, J. Herz, M. Frotscher and M. Gotz (2003). Reelin signaling directly affects radial glia morphology and biochemical maturation. *Development* 130(19):4597–609.

Hevner, R. F., R. A. Daza, C. Englund, J. Kohtz and A. Fink (2004). Postnatal shifts of interneuron position in the neocortex of normal and reeler mice: evidence for inward radial migration. *Neuroscience* 124(3):605–18.

Hevner, R. F., R. A. Daza, J. L. Rubenstein, H. Stunnenberg, J. F. Olavarria and C. Englund (2003a). Beyond laminar fate: toward a molecular classification of cortical projection/pyramidal neurons. *Dev Neurosci* 25(2–4):139–51.

Hevner, R. F., T. Neogi, C. Englund, R. A. Daza and A. Fink (2003b). Cajal–Retzius cells in the mouse: transcription factors, neurotransmitters, and birthdays suggest a pallial origin. *Brain Res Dev Brain Res* 141(1–2):39–53.

Hevner, R. F., L. Shi, N. Justice, Y. Hsueh, M. Sheng, S. Smiga, A. Bulfone, A. M. Goffinet, A. T. Campagnoni and J. L. Rubenstein (2001). Tbr1 regulates differentiation of the preplate and layer 6. *Neuron* 29(2):353–66.

Hiesberger, T., M. Trommsdorff, B. W. Howell, A. Goffinet, M. C. Mumby, J. A. Cooper and J. Herz (1999). Direct binding of Reelin to VLDL receptor and ApoE receptor 2 induces tyrosine phosphorylation of disabled-1 and modulates tau phosphorylation. *Neuron* 24(2):481–9.

Hong, S. E., Y. Y. Shugart, D. T. Huang, S. A. Shahwan, P. E. Grant, J. O. Hourihane, N. D. Martin and C. A. Walsh (2000). Autosomal recessive lissencephaly with cerebellar hypoplasia is associated with human RELN mutations. *Nat Genet* 26(1):93–6.

Howell, B. W., T. M. Herrick and J. A. Cooper (1999). Reelin-induced tyrosine [corrected] phosphorylation of disabled 1 during neuronal positioning. *Genes Dev* 13(6): 643–8.

Jimenez, D., R. Rivera, L. Lopez-Mascaraque and J. A. De Carlos (2003). Origin of the cortical layer I in rodents. *Dev Neurosci* 25(2–4):105–15.

Kim, A. S., S. A. Anderson, J. L. Rubenstein, D. H. Lowenstein and S. J. Pleasure (2001). Pax-6 regulates expression of SFRP-2 and Wnt-7b in the developing CNS. *J Neurosci* 21(5):RC132.

Kriegstein, A. R. and M. Gotz (2003). Radial glia diversity: a matter of cell fate. *Glia* 43(1):37–43.

Kriegstein, A. R. and S. C. Noctor (2004). Patterns of neuronal migration in the embryonic cortex. *Trends Neurosci* 27(7):392–9.

Kuo, G., L. Arnaud, P. Kronstad-O'Brien and J. A. Cooper (2005). Absence of Fyn and Src causes a reeler-like phenotype. *J Neurosci* 25(37):8578–86.

Lavdas, A. A., M. Grigoriou, V. Pachnis and J. G. Parnavelas (1999). The medial ganglionic eminence gives rise to a population of early neurons in the developing cerebral cortex. *J Neurosci* 19(18):7881–8.

Lee, S. M., S. Tole, E. Grove and A. P. McMahon (2000). A local Wnt-3a signal is required for development of the mammalian hippocampus. *Development* 127(3):457–67.

Luque, J. M. (2004). Integrin and the Reelin-Dab1 pathway: a sticky affair? *Brain Res Dev Brain Res* 152(2):269–71.

Malatesta, P., M. A. Hack, E. Hartfuss, H. Kettenmann, W. Klinkert, F. Kirchhoff and M. Gotz (2003). Neuronal or glial progeny: regional differences in radial glia fate. *Neuron* 37(5):751–64.

Mallamaci, A., S. Mercurio, L. Muzio, C. Cecchi, C. L. Pardini, P. Gruss and E. Boncinelli (2000). The lack of Emx2 causes impairment of Reelin signaling and defects of neuronal migration in the developing cerebral cortex. *J Neurosci* 20(3):1109–18.

Maricich, S. M., E. C. Gilmore and K. Herrup (2001). The role of tangential migration in the establishment of mammalian cortex. *Neuron* 31(2):175–8.

Marin-Padilla, M. (1998). Cajal–Retzius cells and the development of the neocortex. *Trends Neurosci* 21(2):64–71.

Merkle, F. T. and A. Alvarez-Buylla (2006). Neural stem cells in mammalian development. *Curr Opin Cell Biol* 18(6):704–9.

Metin, C., J. P. Baudoin, S. Rakic and J. G. Parnavelas (2006). Cell and molecular mechanisms involved in the migration of cortical interneurons. *Eur J Neurosci* 23(4):894–900.

Meyer, G., A. Cabrera Socorro, C. G. Perez Garcia, L. Martinez Millan, N. Walker and D. Caput (2004). Developmental roles of p73 in Cajal–Retzius cells and cortical patterning. *J Neurosci* 24(44):9878–87.

Meyer, G. and A. M. Goffinet (1998). Prenatal development of reelin-immunoreactive neurons in the human neocortex. *J Comp Neurol* 397(1):29–40.

Meyer, G., A. M. Goffinet and A. Fairen (1999). What is a Cajal–Retzius cell? A reassessment of a classical cell type based on recent observations in the developing neocortex. *Cereb Cortex* 9(8):765–75.

Meyer, G., C. G. Perez-Garcia, H. Abraham and D. Caput (2002). Expression of p73 and Reelin in the developing human cortex. *J Neurosci* 22(12):4973–86.

Morante-Oria, J., A. Carleton, B. Ortino, E. J. Kremer, A. Fairen and P. M. Lledo (2003). Subpallial origin of a population of projecting pioneer neurons during corticogenesis. *Proc Natl Acad Sci USA* 100(21):12468–73.

Muzio, L., B. DiBenedetto, A. Stoykova, E. Boncinelli, P. Gruss and A. Mallamaci (2002). Conversion of cerebral cortex into basal ganglia in Emx2(-/-) Pax6(Sey/Sey) double-mutant mice. *Nat Neurosci* 5(8):737–45.

Muzio, L. and A. Mallamaci (2003). Emx1, emx2 and pax6 in specification, regionalization and arealization of the cerebral cortex. *Cereb Cortex* 13(6):641–7.

Muzio, L. and A. Mallamaci (2005). Foxg1 confines Cajal–Retzius neuronogenesis and hippocampal morphogenesis to the dorsomedial pallium. *J Neurosci* 25(17): 4435–41.

Nadarajah, B., P. Alifragis, R. O. Wong and J. G. Parnavelas (2003). Neuronal migration in the developing cerebral cortex: observations based on real-time imaging. *Cereb Cortex* 13(6):607–11.

Nadarajah, B., J. E. Brunstrom, J. Grutzendler, R. O. Wong and A. L. Pearlman (2001). Two modes of radial migration in early development of the cerebral cortex. *Nat Neurosci* 4(2):143–50.

Nadarajah, B. and J. G. Parnavelas (2002). Modes of neuronal migration in the developing cerebral cortex. *Nat Rev Neurosci* 3(6):423–32.

Noctor, S. C., A. C. Flint, T. A. Weissman, W. S. Wong, B. K. Clinton and A. R. Kriegstein (2002). Dividing precursor cells of the embryonic cortical ventricular zone have morphological and molecular characteristics of radial glia. *J Neurosci* 22(8):3161–73.

Nomura, T., J. Holmberg, J. Frisen and N. Osumi (2006). Pax6-dependent boundary defines alignment of migrating olfactory cortex neurons via the repulsive activity of ephrin A5. *Development* 133(7):1335–45.

Ogawa, M., T. Miyata, K. Nakajima, K. Yagyu, M. Seike, K. Ikenaka, H. Yamamoto and K. Mikoshiba (1995). The reeler gene-associated antigen on Cajal–Retzius neurons is a crucial molecule for laminar organization of cortical neurons. *Neuron* 14(5): 899–912.

O'Leary, D. D., S. J. Chou and S. Sahara (2007). Area patterning of the mammalian cortex. *Neuron* 56(2):252–69.

Pinto-Lord, M. C., P. Evrard and V. S. Caviness, Jr. (1982). Obstructed neuronal migration along radial glial fibers in the neocortex of the reeler mouse: a Golgi-EM analysis. *Brain Res* 256(4):379–93.

Pla, R., V. Borrell, N. Flames and O. Marin (2006). Layer acquisition by cortical GABAergic interneurons is independent of Reelin signaling. *J Neurosci* 26(26):6924–34.

Puelles, L., E. Kuwana, E. Puelles, A. Bulfone, K. Shimamura, J. Keleher, S. Smiga and J. L. Rubenstein (2000). Pallial and subpallial derivatives in the embryonic chick and mouse telencephalon, traced by the expression of the genes Dlx-2, Emx-1, Nkx-2.1, Pax-6, and Tbr-1. *J Comp Neurol* 424(3):409–38.

Rice, D. S., M. Sheldon, G. D'Arcangelo, K. Nakajima, D. Goldowitz and T. Curran (1998). Disabled-1 acts downstream of Reelin in a signaling pathway that controls laminar organization in the mammalian brain. *Development* 125(18):3719–29.

Shen, Q., Y. Wang, J. T. Dimos, C. A. Fasano, T. N. Phoenix, I. R. Lemischka, N. B. Ivanova, S. Stifani, E. E. Morrisey and S. Temple (2006). The timing of cortical neurogenesis is encoded within lineages of individual progenitor cells. *Nat Neurosci* 9(6):743–51.

Shinozaki, K., T. Miyagi, M. Yoshida, T. Miyata, M. Ogawa, S. Aizawa and Y. Suda (2002). Absence of Cajal–Retzius cells and subplate neurons associated with defects of tangential cell migration from ganglionic eminence in Emx1/2 double mutant cerebral cortex. *Development* 129(14):3479–92.

Soriano, E. and J. A. Del Rio (2005). The cells of Cajal–Retzius : still a mystery one century after. *Neuron* 46(3):389–94.

Stoykova, A., O. Hatano, P. Gruss and M. Gotz (2003). Increase in reelin-positive cells in the marginal zone of Pax6 mutant mouse cortex. *Cereb Cortex* 13(6):560–71.

Stoykova, A., D. Treichel, M. Hallonet and P. Gruss (2000). Pax6 modulates the dorso-ventral patterning of the mammalian telencephalon. *J Neurosci* 20(21):8042–50.

Studer, M., A. Filosa and J. L. Rubenstein (2005). The nuclear receptor COUP-TFI represses differentiation of Cajal–Retzius cells. *Brain Res Bull* 66(4–6):394–401.

Stumm, R. K., C. Zhou, T. Ara, F. Lazarini, M. Dubois-Dalcq, T. Nagasawa, V. Hollt and S. Schulz (2003). CXCR4 regulates interneuron migration in the developing neocortex. *J Neurosci* 23(12):5123–30.

Takiguchi-Hayashi, K., M. Sekiguchi, S. Ashigaki, M. Takamatsu, H. Hasegawa, R. Suzuki-Migishima, M. Yokoyama, S. Nakanishi and Y. Tanabe (2004). Generation of reelin-positive marginal zone cells from the caudomedial wall of telencephalic vesicles. *J Neurosci* 24(9):2286–95.

Tissir, F. and A. M. Goffinet (2003). Reelin and brain development. *Nat Rev Neurosci* 4(6):496–505.

Tole, S., C. W. Ragsdale and E. A. Grove (2000). Dorsoventral patterning of the telencephalon is disrupted in the mouse mutant extra-toes(J). *Dev Biol* 217(2):254–65.

Tripodi, M., A. Filosa, M. Armentano and M. Studer (2004). The COUP-TF nuclear receptors regulate cell migration in the mammalian basal forebrain. *Development* 131(24): 6119–29.

Trommsdorff, M., M. Gotthardt, T. Hiesberger, J. Shelton, W. Stockinger, J. Nimpf, R. E. Hammer, J. A. Richardson and J. Herz (1999). Reeler/Disabled-like disruption of neuronal migration in knockout mice lacking the VLDL receptor and ApoE receptor 2. *Cell* 97(6):689–701.

Yamazaki, H., M. Sekiguchi, M. Takamatsu, Y. Tanabe and S. Nakanishi (2004). Distinct ontogenic and regional expressions of newly identified Cajal–Retzius cell-specific genes during neocorticogenesis. *Proc Natl Acad Sci USA* 101(40):14509–14.

Yang, A., N. Walker, R. Bronson, M. Kaghad, M. Oosterwegel, J. Bonnin, C. Vagner, H. Bonnet, P. Dikkes, A. Sharpe, F. McKeon and D. Caput (2000). p73-deficient mice have neurological, pheromonal and inflammatory defects but lack spontaneous tumours. *Nature* 404(6773):99–103.

Yoshida, M., S. Assimacopoulos, K. R. Jones and E. A. Grove (2006). Massive loss of Cajal–Retzius cells does not disrupt neocortical layer order. *Development* 133(3): 537–45.

Zhao, C., W. Guan and S. J. Pleasure (2006). A transgenic marker mouse line labels Cajal–Retzius cells from the cortical hem and thalamocortical axons. *Brain Res* 1077(1):48–53.

Zhao, Y., H. Z. Sheng, R. Amini, A. Grinberg, E. Lee, S. Huang, M. Taira and H. Westphal (1999). Control of hippocampal morphogenesis and neuronal differentiation by the LIM homeobox gene Lhx5. *Science* 284(5417):1155–8.

Zhou, C., Y. Qiu, F. A. Pereira, M. C. Crair, S. Y. Tsai and M. J. Tsai (1999). The nuclear orphan receptor COUP-TFI is required for differentiation of subplate neurons and guidance of thalamocortical axons. *Neuron* 24(4):847–59.

Zhou, C., S. Y. Tsai and M. J. Tsai (2001). COUP-TFI: an intrinsic factor for early regionalization of the neocortex. *Genes Dev* 15(16):2054–9.

Chapter Four

_____

Development of the Paraventricular Nucleus of the Hypothalamus

Larry W. Swanson

INTRODUCTION

The mammalian paraventricular nucleus of the hypothalamus (PVH) is ripe for systematic analysis with the molecular genetics tools of modern developmental neuroscience. The stage has been set by over 30 years of extensive research demonstrating that the PVH is a microcosm of hypothalamic structure-function relationships in the adult. On the functional side it coordinates behavioral, autonomic, and neuroendocrine responses critical for the homeostatic control of metabolism and body water—which are the very cornerstones of an individual's survival—and on the structural side it contains three distinct classes of neurons that are responsible for magnocellular neuroendocrine, parvicellular neuroendocrine, and autonomic-behavioral responses (Swanson and Sawchenko 1983; Armstrong 2004; Bota and Swanson 2007). The purpose of this chapter is to outline briefly the structure-function organization of the adult PVH, and then to review some highlights of what has already been learned about its pre- and postnatal development, with an eye toward providing a conceptual framework for broader experimental examination of molecular mechanisms underlying the progression from differentiated neuroepithelium to adult three-dimensional structure, axonal connections, and function.

WHAT IS THE PARAVENTRICULAR NUCLEUS?

As its name implies, the PVH lies adjacent to the third ventricle in all mammals. It is particularly obvious and well differentiated in the adult rat (Figure 4.1), where it is a roughly wing-shaped, bilateral region of highly differentiated, compact gray matter along rostral and dorsal aspects of the hypothalamic part of the third ventricle, commencing dorsally just ventral to the hypothalamic sulcus and containing on the order of 10,000 neurons in somewhat less than 0.5 mm³ on each side of the brain (Swanson and Sawchenko 1983; Swanson and Simmons 1989). A combination of data based on experimental pathway tracing, histochemical (immuno- and hybridization), and normal neuroanatomical staining (for example, Nissl and Golgi/single-cell filling) analyses has led to the detailed parceling of the rat PVH into on the order of 10 divisions and parts (see Figures 4.2 and 4.3), with different authors providing significantly different interpretations (recently reviewed in Simmons and Swanson 2008).

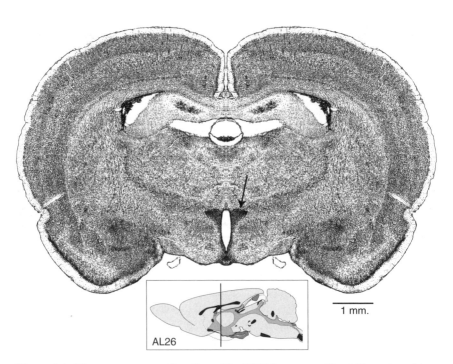

Figure 4.1. The appearance and location of the PVH (arrow; see Fig. 4.6) as viewed in a Nissl-stained transverse section of the adult rat forebrain (location in sagittal inset at bottom). Note in this photomicrograph that the PVH is one of the most obvious cell aggregates at this level of the brain. Photo of right side flipped to create pseudo-bilateral view of Atlas Level 26 (AL26) in Swanson (2004). Adapted from Swanson (2004).

The data as a whole indicate that the rat PVH has three separate though partly overlapping structure-function divisions (Swanson 1991, 1992). One is magnocellular neuroendocrine, with normally separate populations of oxytocin- and vasopressin-synthesizing neurons projecting to the posterior pituitary; another is parvicellular neuroendocrine, with neuron populations influencing anterior pituitary hormone secretion via the hypophysial portal system; and yet another has descending projections to midbrain behavior-related regions and most midbrain-hindbrain-spinal components of the central autonomic system. Each of these divisions is further parceled, and of particular relevance here, there is in the rat a partial spatial segregation of different magnocellular and parvicellular neuroendocrine neuron types that forms a regular, distinct, reproducible pattern (Figs. 4.2 and 4.3).

In any analysis of the PVH it is useful to take account of the supraoptic nucleus, because it can be viewed as a simplified version of the PVH with only a magnocellular neuroendocrine component containing partly segregated populations of oxytocin and vasopressin neurons; and like the PVH it apparently does not even harbor local interneurons. Finally, it is important to note that in the adult hypothalamus there are scattered individual, and small groups of, magnocellular

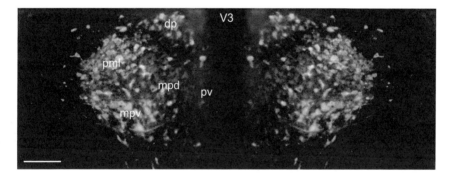

Figure 4.2. Cellular differentiation of the rat PVH at approximately the level illustrated in Fig. 4.1. In this photomicrograph, green neurons were labeled with an antiserum to vasopressin and mark part of the magnocellular neuroendocrine division. At this level, antisera to oxytocin label a thin ring of neurons partly surrounding the vasopressin population (see Fig. 4.3). Red neurons were labeled with an antiserum to corticotrophin-releasing hormone (CRH) and thus mark part of the parvicellular neuroendocrine division. Thyrotropin-releasing hormone (TRH) parvicellular neuroendocrine neurons (not labeled here) form a population centered just medial to (and partly intermixed with) the CRH neurons, and somatostatin (SS) parvicellular neuroendocrine neurons are centered even more medially, in the periventricular part (pv) of the PVH. The two regions of blue neurons were labeled with the retrograde tracer, True Blue, injected into upper thoracic levels of the spinal cord. Other abbreviations: dp, dorsal parvicellular part; mpd, medial parvicellular part, dorsal zone; mpv, medial parvicellular part, ventral zone; pml, posterior magnocellular part, lateral zone; V3, third ventricle (hypothalamic part). Photo of right side flipped to create pseudobilateral view. Scale bar = 200 μm. Adapted from Swanson et al. (1986). (See color Figure 4.2)

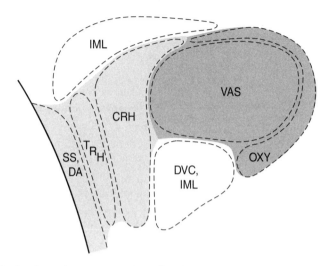

Figure 4.3. A schematic transverse view of rat PVH structure-function parcellation, emphasizing predominantly neuroendocrine regions (gray). In this drawing, which is at about the level illustrated in Fig. 4.2, three PVH divisions are indicated. The light gray region corresponds to the parvicellular neuroendocrine division at this level, which consists of neuron populations expressing either CRH, TRH, somatostatin (SS), or dopamine (DA, which inhibits prolactin release). The darker gray region corresponds to the magnocellular neuroendocrine division at this level, which consists of vasopressin (VAS) and oxytocin (OXY) neuron populations. The two unshaded regions are parts of the descending division that innervate the spinal intermediolateral column (IML) and the IML plus the dorsal vagal complex (DVC). For clarity, the various neuron populations have been depicted as entirely segregated, which is not the case; there is some intermixing between them. Adapted from Swanson (1986).

neurosecretory neurons commonly known as the accessory supraoptic nucleus, essentially between the PVH and supraoptic nucleus (see Swanson 1886; Markakis and Swanson 1997; Armstrong 2004).

WHAT NEUROEPITHELIAL REGION
GENERATES THE PVH?

Based on location, histological appearance, and CRH mRNA expression patterns, the PVH can be identified unequivocally on embryonic day 17 (E17; time of insemination considered beginning on E0) in the rat (Grino et al. 1989; Alvarez-Bolado et al. 1995; Alvarez-Bolado and Swanson 1996). A detailed analysis of spatiotemporal expression patterns of POU-III homeobox genes throughout forebrain development first suggested the location of a neuroepithelial patch giving rise to the paraventricular nucleus (Alvarez-Bolado et al. 1995). Overall, the evidence suggests that three of these genes—Brain-1 (Brn-1), Brain-2 (Brn-2), and Brain-4 (Brn-4)—are expressed at the anterior hypothalamic level of the rat only in the PVH and companion supraoptic nucleus (and the accessory supraoptic nucleus) of the adult (He et al. 1989; Mathis et al. 1992) and embryo (Alvarez-Bolado et al. 1995), whereas a fourth member of this gene family, Testes-1 (Tst-1), is never expressed in the PVH and supraoptic nucleus (He et al. 1989; Alvarez-Bolado et al. 1995).

Starting with the ventricular layer, the gene expression pattern develops as follows for the hypothalamic anterior level (Alvarez-Bolado et al. 1995). On E10 and E11 (the earliest times examined), dense Brn-1 and Brn-2 hybridization is dorsally restricted in the presumptive anterior level, whereas Brn-4 hybridization also extends more ventrally. On E12 and E13 moderate Brn-2 expression extends throughout the dorsal half of the anterior level, whereas moderate Brn-1 (Figures 4.4a and 4.5) and Brn-4 hybridization has become narrowed to a strip of the ventricular zone just ventral to the dorsocaudal end of the optic sulcus and rostral end of the hypothalamic sulcus. Between E14 and E17 all three genes are expressed just in the definitive region of the PVH (Fig. 4.4b).

Turning to the mantle layer, which is formed by young neurons born in, and migrating out of, the ventricular layer, the Brn-1 gene expression pattern is most clear. On E12 a tiny patch of mantle layer between the optic and hypothalamic sulci is weakly hybridized, and this localization pattern is maintained into adulthood (Figs. 4.4a and 4.5). Moderate Brn-2 hybridization is found in the dorsal half of the hypothalamic anterior level mantle layer on E12 and E13, and becomes confined to the region of the PVH (and supraoptic nucleus, see below) from E14 through adulthood. The Brn-4 expression pattern is similar though not

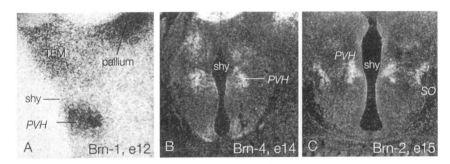

Figure 4.4. Expression patterns of POU-III homeobox genes in early developmental stages of the rat PVH. (**A**) Three patches of Brn-1 expression (black regions in this bright-field photomicrograph) are found near the rostral end of the third ventricle on embryonic day 12: in the thalamic eminence (TEM), presumptive PVH (separated by the hypothalamic sulcus, shy), and pallium. (**B**) On embryonic day 14, Brn-4 clearly labels a patch in lateral regions of the presumptive PVH mantle layer (white labeling below the hypothalamic sulcus in this dark-field photomicrograph). (**C**) On embryonic day 15, Brn-2 labels a distinctive band in the presumptive PVH, the supraoptic nucleus (SO), and a "stream" of neurons between them. This stream probably indicates young neurons migrating radially from the region of the PVH to the SO, and remnants of the stream probably form the adult accessory supraoptic nucleus. Transverse histological sections treated for in situ hybridization. Adapted from Alvarez-Bolado et al. (1995).

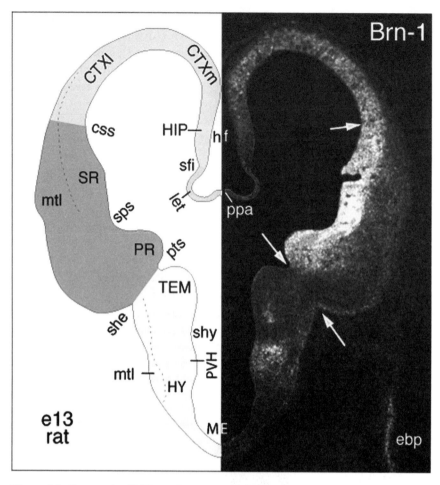

Figure 4.5. Presumptive PVH ventricular layer and mantle layer (mtl) marked by Brn-1 expression (white label in this dark-field photomicrograph, on the right) on embryonic day 13. Note that expression of this homeobox gene also clearly distinguishes the telencephalic vesicle (pink in schematic anatomical drawing on the left) from the diencephalic vesicle (yellow) at this transverse level of the forebrain treated for in situ hybridization. Other abbreviations: css, corticostriatal sulcus; CTXl,m, cortex, median and lateral regions; ebp, epibranchial placodes; hf, hippocampal fissure; HIP, hippocampus; HY, hypothalamus; let, epithelial lamina; ME, median eminence; ppa, parahypophysial arch; PR, pallidal (medial ventricular) ridge; pts, pallidothalamic sulcus; sfi, fimbrial sulcus; she, hemispheric sulcus; SR, striatal (lateral ventricular) ridge; TEM, thalamic eminence. Adapted from Swanson (2000). (See color Figure 4.5)

identical to that for Brn-2, with hybridization on E12 not quite restricted to the presumptive PVH region of the mantle layer. From E14 on, it is clear that whereas Brn-1, Brn-2, and Brn-3 are all expressed in the PVH, their precise spatial patterns are different, and their precise patterns of co-expression may play a role in the maturation of specific neuronal types within the nucleus (Alvarez-Bolado et al. 1995; Schonemann et al. 1995).

In the adult, Brn-1 and Brn-2 are expressed most abundantly in magnocellular neuroendocrine oxytocin and vasopressin neurons, and in parvicellular neuroendocrine corticotropin-releasing hormone (CRH) neurons (Swanson 1992; Schonemann et al. 1995). A series of experiments in mice homozygous null for Brn-2 demonstrated that CRH neurons in the PVH, and oxytocin and vasopressin neurons in the PVH and supraoptic nucleus, failed to mature properly and did not survive into postnatal life—and that these effects appeared to be specific in the sense that non-neuroendocrine neurons expressing CRH, oxytocin, and vasopressin were intact, other hypothalamic neuroendocrine cell types were normal, and other parts of the brain expressing Brn-2 also appeared normal (Nakai et al. 1995; Schonemann et al. 1995). Later it was shown that expression of two other genes, Sim1 and Arnt2, is necessary for maintaining Brn-2 expression, so that mice lacking these factors eventually lose Brn-2 expression along with oxytocin, vasopressin, and CRH neurons in the PVH (Michaud et al. 1998, 2000; Keith et al. 2001). Finally, it has been shown that null mutant mice for the paired-type homeobox gene Opt also lack the same three neuroendocrine cell types as found in Brn-2 null mutants, as well as the adjacent thyrotropin-releasing hormone (TRH) and somatostatin parvicellular neuroendocrine populations (Acampora et al. 1999).

In summary, POU-III homeobox genes provide expression markers for the earliest developmental stages of the PVH, in rodents at least, and at least one of them, Brn-2, appears to be necessary for the maturation and survival of three neuroendocrine cell populations—CRH, oxytocin, and vasopressin in mice. Certain other genes expressed in the developing PVH are reviewed by Markakis (2002), Asbreuk et al. (2006), and Zhu et al. (2007).

WHEN ARE PVH NEURONS BORN?

Initial studies using ^{3}H-thymidine to determine the embryonic generation time for PVH neurons—that is, the final mitosis time or birthdate of its young neurons from the ventricular zone—did not take into account modern parceling of the nucleus, but did suggest a peak period between E13 and E15 in the rat (Ifft 1972; Altman and Bayer 1978a, 1986). Later, a systematic, comprehensive birthdating analysis of all PVH parvicellular neuroendocrine neuron types was carried out using a triple fluorescence labeling method consisting of bromodeoxyuridine (BrdU) birthdating, peptide immunolabeling for phenotyping, and retrograde labeling from the blood to confirm neuroendocrine identity (Markakis and Swanson 1997). This paper also contains an analysis of parvicellular neuroendocrine neuron birthdates throughout the rest of the hypothalamus, and a thorough review of the earlier literature.

The work of Markakis and Swanson (1997) indicates that all four parvicellular neuroendocrine populations in the PVH are generated essentially simultaneously, presumably from the adjacent proliferative neuroepithelium of the third ventricle

(Figs. 4.4 and 4.5). Cell counts showed that a vast majority of these neurons undergo their final division between E12 and E14, with a peak on E13. Interestingly, this is also the same peak day for magnocellular neuroendocrine birthdays in the PVH (Ifft 1972). Thus, to a first order of approximation, all neuroendocrine neurons in the PVH appear to be generated at about the same time, although a weak dorsolateral to ventromedial gradient of neurogenesis between E12 and E14 is displayed by CRH neurons and TRH neurons (Figure 4.6), as has been reported for the PVH as a whole (Altman and Bayer 1986).

This early generation of neuroendocrine motoneurons in the PVH is an exception to the general "outside-in" pattern of hypothalamic neurogenesis whereby peak lateral zone birthdays occur on E12–E13, peak medial nuclei birthdays occur on E14–E15, and peak periventricular region birthdays occur on E16–E17 (Ifft 1972; Altman and Bayer 1986). This suggests that neuroendocrine neurons in the PVH, and in the rest of the hypothalamic periventricular region (Markakis

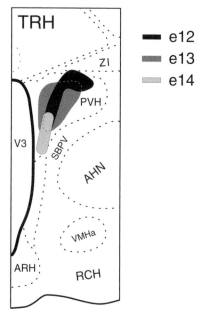

Figure 4.6. A dorsolateral to ventromedial gradient of parvicellular neuroendocrine TRH neuron generation in the rat PVH. This pattern of neurogenesis is displayed in the adult population of TRH neurons, based on injections of BrdU in the mother on either embryonic day 12, 13, or 14. The data are presented on a transverse projection or compression map, summarized on Atlas Level 26 (see Fig. 4.1). Abbreviations: AHN, anterior hypothalamic nucleus; ARH, arcuate nucleus; RCH, retrochiasmatic area; SBPV, subparaventricular zone; V3, third ventricle; VMHa, ventromedial nucleus, anterior part; ZI, zona incerta. Adapted from Markakis and Swanson (1997).

and Swanson 1997), display a form of arrested migration and may constitute "pioneer neurons" for the various anatomically distinct parts of the mature periventricular region, many of which arc generated later, on E16–E17 (above).

There is thus little evidence for sequential generation of the various neuroendocrine cell types that display partial spatial segregation—essentially from medial to lateral, with respect to the third ventricle—in the adult rat PVH (Fig. 4.3). In addition, while the parvicellular neuroendocrine populations are being generated, intermixed neuron populations expressing the same neurotransmitters but apparently not projecting to the median eminence are being born at the same time in the PVH (Markakis and Swanson 1997). Thus, intermixed populations of parvicellular neuroendocrine neurons and non-neuroendocrine neurons (within the parvicellular neuroendocrine division) are not generated at different times early in the development of the PVH. This evidence suggests that the differentiation of various PVH neuron populations is not determined by simple morphogen gradients, which may be necessary but not sufficient. An alternate mechanism could involve some degree of preprogramming in the neuroepithelium or ventricular layer itself, possibly involving the homeobox genes mentioned above (Alvarez-Bolado et al. 1995; Schonemann et al. 1995).

Nothing is currently known with certainty about the important question of when neurons of the PVH descending division are generated relative to those of the neuroendocrine divisions.

HOW ARE PVH AND SUPRAOPTIC NUCLEUS DEVELOPMENT RELATED?

The starting point here is evidence suggesting that magnocellular neuroendocrine neurons of the supraoptic nucleus (there is no good evidence for significant numbers of other neuron types in the nucleus) are generated in the same neuroepithelial patch generating magnocellular neuroendocrine and other neuron types of the PVH, and that they simply migrate along radial glial processes to the lateral edge of the mantle layer (Altman and Bayer 1978a, 1978b, 1986). Our results indicate that there is a major peak of rat supraoptic neurogenesis restricted to E12–E13, with a peak on E13 (Markakis and Swanson 1997), a conclusion that is corroborated by earlier ^{3}H-thymidine analysis (Ifft 1972). Thus, it would appear that the great majority of magnocellular neuroendocrine neurons in the PVH and supraoptic nucleus are generated from the same neuroepithelial patch at the same developmental time. We did, however, observe low but significant and increasing amounts of BrdU labeling in the rat supraoptic nucleus between E15 and E17 the last day examined (Markakis and Swanson 1997). Whether this labeling continues postnatally is not known, and exactly what cell types are involved remains to be determined. Intriguingly, though, evidence for postpubertal generation of supraoptic neurons has been reported in the female pig (van Eerdenburg and Swaab 1994), and neurogenesis and DNA synthesis have been reported in the supraoptic nucleus of adult primates (van Eerdenburg and Rakic 1994).

More direct evidence for this model of supraoptic nucleus development emerged from studies of POU-III gene expression reviewed above (Alvarez-Bolado et al. 1995). Specifically, Brn-2 and Brn-4 hybridization was observed clearly in the supraoptic nucleus, and in the accessory supraoptic nucleus between it and the PVH, from embryonic day 13 on into adulthood (Fig. 4.4c), and in mice homozygous null for Brn-2, supraoptic neurons failed to differentiate and survive after birth (Schonemann et al. 1995). In contrast to the PVH, Brn-1 expression was not detected in the supraoptic and accessory supraoptic nuclei during embryogenesis, suggesting perhaps that it is not involved critically in the development of magnocellular neurosecretory neurons (Alvarez-Bolado 1995). Conversely, Brn-1 is expressed in adult supraoptic neurons, suggesting a function in mature magnocellular neurosecretory neurons (He et al. 1989).

These insights into supraoptic nucleus development offer further support for the hypothesis mentioned above that neuroendocrine neurons remaining in the periventricular region are subject to a mechanism of arrested migration after their birth in the adjacent ventricular layer (Markakis and Swanson 1997). The basic observation is that magnocellular neuroendocrine neurons of the PVH and supraoptic nucleus appear to be born simultaneously in the same patch of rostro-dorsal hypothalamic ventricular layer, and yet roughly half of them migrate radially to the lateral edge of the diencephalic vesicle to form the supraoptic nucleus while the other half remain adjacent to the ventricular layer to form the PVH magnocellular division—and a small fraction of the migrating young neurons never make it to the supraoptic nucleus, forming instead the intervening accessory supraoptic nucleus of the adult.

WHEN DO PVH EXTRINSIC AXONAL CONNECTIONS MATURE?

The PVH establishes extensive axonal connections with the pituitary and other parts of the hypothalamus, with the lower brain stem and spinal cord, and with the cerebral hemispheres (see reviews in Sawchenko and Swanson 1981; Swanson 1987, 1991, 2005; Sawchenko 1998; Dong and Swanson 2006). Insights into the maturation of three especially functionally significant pathways have begun to emerge: PVH projections to the median eminence and posterior pituitary, descending PVH projections to autonomic centers in the medulla, and a projection from the arcuate nucleus of the hypothalamus to the PVH.

The critically important parvicellular neuroendocrine PVH projections to the median eminence—involving primarily CRH, TRH, and somatostatin neuron populations—have not been examined carefully with respect to axon growth, guidance, and targeting to the internal layer of the median eminence. However, it is clearly established that in rats hypothalamic axons begin reaching the median eminence on E14 (Makarenko et al. 2001), and that gene expression for the phenotype-specific peptides in PVH neurons generally can be detected 2–3 days after birth of the neurons (reviewed in Swanson 1991; Markakis and Swanson 1997). It is not known when axons from these PVH neurons functionally release hypophysiotropic hormones, although CRH immunoreactivity has been detected there on E16, the same day peptides can be detected with this method in the cell bodies themselves (Daikoku et al. 1984). In contrast, TRH immunoreactivity has been detected in PVH neurons on E17, but not in the median eminence until birth (Nishiyama et al. 1984); and somatostatin has been detected in PVH neurons also on E17 (Daikoku et al. 1983), and in the median eminence a day later on E18 (Adachi et al. 1984).

Turning to the other, magnocellular, neuroendocrine projection, DiI retrograde tracer analysis indicates that in the rat, axons from the supraoptic nucleus may reach the region of the presumptive posterior pituitary as early as E15, those from accessory supraoptic neurons as early as E16, and those from the PVH as early as E17 (Makarenko et al. 2000), and the functional maturation of this system has been reviewed (Ugrumov 2002). In mice homozygous null for Brn-2, there is a postnatal atrophy and loss of the posterior lobe altogether, suggesting that axons from magnocellular neuroendocrine neurons secrete trophic factor(s) critical for posterior lobe differentiation and/or maintenance, in particular the survival of pituicytes (Schonemann et al. 1995).

The third major PVH division consists of a neuron population that, instead of projecting to the median eminence and posterior pituitary, sends axons to the thalamus, midbrain, hindbrain, and spinal cord. One major function of this PVH projection system is to coordinate neuroendocrine responses (effected by the other two PVH divisions) with autonomic responses from the hindbrain and spinal cord (for example, see Saper et al. 1976; Swanson and Hartman 1980; Sawchenko and Swanson, 1981). Imaginative experiments using viruses that are transported retrogradely across multiple synapses as a function of survival time indicate clearly that a major component of PVH axonal projections to the dorsal vagal complex are established during the first 10 days postnatally (Rinaman et al. 2000; Rinaman 2004). This conclusion is based on virus tracer injections in the ventral stomach wall on various postnatal days of life, and observing the accumulation of label first in the dorsal vagal complex, and then in the PVH and other forebrain regions.

Finally, the third set of connections that has been examined carefully is also of considerable functional significance. It involves a direct axonal projection from the arcuate nucleus of the hypothalamus to the PVH. This particular projection is of special interest because it binds circulating leptin, and uses neuropeptide Y (and several other molecules) as a neurotransmitter. Leptin, of course, is a hormone secreted from fat cells that acts (in part) on the arcuate nucleus to reduce food intake, and neuropeptide Y is a neuropeptide that stimulates eating when injected into the PVH (see Sawchenko 1998). Using DiI as an anterograde axonal tracer, Simerly and colleagues have shown, surprisingly, that under normal circumstances in the rat this arcuate nucleus "humerosensory" projection containing NYP only reaches the PVH on about postnatal day 8 and achieves a mature pattern of innervation by day 16 (Bouret et al. 2004). Furthermore, this projection is underdeveloped in leptin-deficient mice, although it can be rescued by leptin treatment during a neonatal critical period but not in adulthood (Bouret et al. 2004; Simerly 2008).

WHAT IS THE RELATIONSHIP BETWEEN DEVELOPING PVH AND PITUITARY?

Developmental and adult relationships between parvicellular neuroendocrine neurons with axon terminals in the median eminence, and the cell types they control in the anterior pituitary via the hypophysial portal system, is a problem of fundamental importance for almost all aspects of physiology. The basic morphological features of rat pituitary development have been known for some time, and indicate that the infundibular recess, the first indication of the presumptive posterior pituitary, appears on E12, along with an identifiable Rathke's pouch, which will form the anterior and intermediate lobes of the pituitary (Schwind 1928).

A systematic in situ hybridization study (Simmons et al. 1990) indicated that within the developing rat anterior lobe, transcripts for ßTSH are detected on E14 in the anterior tip of the incipient anterior lobe, whereas POMC transcripts are localized just caudal to them. This implies that thyrotropes and corticotropes are the first hormone-specific cell types to differentiate in the anterior lobe, and that this differentiation is spatially restricted and segregated. Recall from the discussion above that TRH and CRH parvicellular neuroendocrine neuron populations in the PVH both have peak birthdays on E13, and that CRH and TRH peptide can be detected immunohistochemically in median eminence axon terminals on E16, and around the time of birth, respectively. Returning to the anterior lobe, it is not until 2 or 3 days later, on E16 and E17, that transcripts for the ß-subunits of luteinizing hormone and follicle-stimulating hormone are detected, in ventral regions of the developing anterior lobe, indicating the molecular differentiation of gonadotropes; and then on E17/E18 cells expressing growth hormone or prolactin begin to be detected in dorsocaudal regions of the anterior lobe, reflecting the appearance of somatotropes and lactotropes, respectively.

These results indicate that spatiotemporal patterns of hormone-specific gene expression in the developing mammalian anterior lobe are relatively clear and differentiated, in contrast to the extensive intermingling of the five classic cell types found in the adult. Recent concepts about the molecular physiology of pituitary cell type development, including influences of hypothalamic factors on early pituitary differentiation, have been reviewed by Zhu et al. (2007).

CONCLUSIONS

The PVH provides a rich, deep test bed for clarifying mechanisms underlying the differentiation and maturation of complex central nervous system circuitry that is essential for survival of the individual. On one hand, certain basic information about this problem has emerged, especially in the rodent. Molecular markers have been identified for the patch of neuroepithelium that appears to generate the presumptive PVH early in the embryo, the time of final mitosis (birthdates) for all major magnocellular and parvicellular neuroendocrine neuron populations in the PVH has been established, certain key regulatory genes involved in the differentiation and maturation of neuroendocrine neuron populations in the PVH have been identified, and the general developmental features of a few key axonal outputs and inputs of the PVH have been characterized. On the other hand, every bit of data so painstakingly obtained thus far raises far more questions that it answers. To what extent are PVH neuronal cell types preprogrammed in the neuroepithelium? What controls the migration of PVH (and supraoptic) young neurons after their final mitosis? Do neurons of the PVH neuroendocrine and descending divisions have fundamentally different origins in the neuroepithelium, and fundamentally different maturation processes in the PVH mantle layer? What parenchymal factors guide the axon of some PVH neurons to the posterior pituitary, the axon of other neurons to the median eminence, and the axon of yet other neurons to the spinal cord? The tools are now available to approach these and other questions experimentally, and the answers will undoubtedly hold many surprises.

ACKNOWLEDGMENTS

Experimental work from the author's laboratory reviewed here was supported in part by NINDS grant NS-16686.

REFERENCES

Acampora, D., M.P. Postiglione, V. Avantaggiato, M. Di Bonito, F.M. Vaccarino, J. Michaud, A. Simeone, Progressive impairment of developing neuroendocrine cell lineages in the hypothalamus of mice lacking the Orthopedia gene. *Genes Dev* 13 (1999) 2787–2800.

Adachi, T., M. Ohtsuka, S. Hisano, Y. Tsuruo, S. Daikoku, Ontogenetic appearance of somatostatin-containing nerve terminals in the median eminence of rats, *Cell Tissue Res* 236 (1984) 47–51.

Altman, J., S.A. Bayer, Development of the diencephalon in the rat. I. Autoradiographic study of the time of origin and settling patterns of neurons of the hypothalamus, *J Comp Neurol* (1978a) 945–72.

Altman, J., S.A. Bayer, Development of the diencephalon in the rat. II. Correlation of the embryonic development of the hypothalamus with the time of origin of its neurons, *J Comp Neurol* (1978b) 973–94.

Altman, J., S.A. Bayer, *The Development of the Rat Hypothalamus*, New York, Springer-Verlag, 1986, 178 pp.

Alvarez-Bolado, G., M.G. Rosenfeld, L.W. Swanson, Model of forebrain regionalization based on spatiotemporal patterns of POU-III homeobox gene expression, birthdates, and morphological features, *J Comp Neurol* 355 (1995) 237–95.

Alvarez-Bolado, G., L.W. Swanson, *Developmental Brain Maps: Structure of the Embryonic Rat Brain*, Elsevier, Amsterdam, 1996, 154 pp.

Armstrong, W.E., Hypothalamic supraoptic and paraventricular nuclei. In: G. Paxinos (Ed.), *The Rat Nervous System*, 3rd Edn., Elsevier, Amsterdam, 2004, pp. 369–88.

Asbreuk, C.H.J., J.H. van Doorninck, A. Mansouri, M.P. Smidt, J.P.H. Burbach, Neurohypophysial dysmorphogenesis in mice lacking the homeobox gene Uncx4.1, *J Mol Endocrinol* 36 (2006) 65–71.

Bota, M., L.W. Swanson, The neuron classification problem, *Brain Res Rev* 56 (2007) 79–88.

Bouret, S.G., S.J. Draper, R.B. Simerly, Trophic action of leptin on hypothalamic neurons that regulate feeding, *Science* 304 (2004) 108–10.

Daikoku, S., S. Hisano, H. Kawano, Y. Okamura, Y. Tsuro, Ontogenetic studies on the topographical heterogeneity of somatostatin-containing neurons in rat hypothalamus, *Cell Tissue Res* 233 (1983) 347–54.

Daikoku, S., Y. Okamura, H. Kawano, Y. Tsuruo, M. Maegaws, T. Shibasaki, Immunohistochemical study on the development of CRF-containing neurons in the hypothalamus of the rat, *Cell Tissue Res* 238 (1984) 539–44.

Dong, H.-W., L.W. Swanson, Projections from bed nuclei of the stria terminalis, anteromedial area: cerebral hemisphere integration of neuroendocrine, autonomic, and behavioral aspects of energy balance, *J Comp Neurol* 494 (2006) 142–78.

Grino, M., W.S. Young, Jr., J.-M. Burgunder, Ontogeny of expression of the corticotropin-releasing factor gene in the hypothalamic paraventricular nucleus and of the proopiomelanocortin gene in rat pituitary. *Endocrinol* 124 (1989) 60–8.

He, X., M.N. Treacy, D.M. Simmons, H.A. Ingraham, L.W. Swanson, M.G. Rosenfeld, Expression of a large family of POU-domain regulatory genes in mammalian brain development, *Nature* 340 (1989) 35–42.

Ifft, J.D., An autoradiographic study of the time of final division of neurons in the rat hypothalamic nuclei, *J Comp Neurol* 144 (1972) 193–204.

Keith, B., D.M. Adelman, M.C. Simon, Targeted mutation of the murine arylhydrocarbon receptor nuclear translocator 2 Arnt2 gene reveals partial redundancy with Arnt. *Proc Natl Acad Sci* 98 (2001) 6692–97.

Makarenko, I.G., M.V. Ugrumov, A. Calas, Axonal projections from the hypothalamus to the median eminence in rats during ontogenesis: DiI tracing study, *Anat Embryol* 204 (2001) 239–52.

Makarenko, I.G., M.V. Ugrumov, P. Derer, A. Calas, Projections from the hypothalamus to the posterior lobe in rats during ontogenesis: 1, 1'-dioctadecyl-3, 3, 3', 3'-tetramethylindocarbocyanine perchlorate tracing study, *J Comp Neurol* 422 (2000) 327–37.

Markakis, E., Development of the neuroendocrine hypothalamus, *Front Neuroendocrinol* 23 (202) 257–91.

Mathis, J.M., D.M. Simmons, X. He, L.W. Swanson, M.G. Rosenfeld, Brain-4: a novel mammalian POU domain transcription factor exhibiting restricted brain-specific expression, *EMBO J* (1992) 2551–61.

Michaud, J.L., C. DeRossi, N.R. May, B.C. Holdener, C. Fan, ARNT2 acts as the dimerization partner of SIM1 for the development of the hypothalamus. *Mech Dev* 90 (2000) 253–61.

Michaud, J.L., T. Rosenquist, N.R. May, C.M. Fan, Development of neuroendocrine lineages requires the bHLH-PAS transcription factor SIM1. *Genes Dev* 12 (1998) 3264–75.

Nakai, S., H. Kawano, T. Yudate, M. Nishi, J. Kuno, A. Nagata, K. Jishage, H. Hamada, H. Fujii, K. Kawamura, The POU domain transcription factor Brn-2 is required for the determination of specific neuronal lineages in the hypothalamus of the mouse. *Genes Dev* 9 (1995) 3109–21.

Nishiyama, T., Y. Heike, T. Matsuzaki, H. Kawano, S. Daikoku, M. Suzuki, Immunoreactive TRH-containing neurons in the rat hypothalamus, *Biomed Res* Suppl. 4 (1984) 65–74.

Rinaman, L., Postnatal development of central feeding circuits. In: E.M. Stricker, S.C. Woods (Eds.), *Handbook of Behavioral Neurobiology*, vol. 14, *Neurobiology of Food and Fluid Intake*, 2nd Edn., Kluwer Academic/Plenum Publishers, New York, 2004, pp. 159–94.

Rinaman, L., P. Levitt, J.P. Card, Progressive postnatal assembly of limbic-autonomic circuits revealed by central transneuronal transport of pseudorabies virus, *J Neurosci* 20 (2000) 2731–41.

Saper, C.B., A.D. Loewy, L.W. Swanson, W.M. Cowan, Direct hypothalamo-autonomic connections, *Brain Res* 117 (1976) 305–12.

Sawchenko, P.E., Toward a new neurobiology of energy balance, appetite, and obesity: the anatomists weigh in, *J Comp Neurol* 402 (1998) 435–41.

Sawchenko, P.E., L.W. Swanson, Central noradrenergic pathways for the integration of hypothalamic neuroendocrine and autonomic responses, *Science* 214 (1981) 685–7.

Schonemann, M.D., A.K. Ryan, R.J. McEvilly, S.M. O'Connell, C.A. Arias, K.A. Kalla, P.E. Sawchenko, M.G. Rosenfeld, Development and survival of the endocrine hypothalamus and posterior pituitary gland requires the neuronal POU domain factor Brn-2, *Genes Dev* 9 (1995) 3122–35.

Schwind, J., The development of the hypophysis cerebri of the albino rat, *Am J Anat* 41 (1928) 295–319.

Simerly, R.B., Hypothalamic substrates of metabolic imprinting, *Physiol Behav* (in press).

Simmons, D.M., L.W. Swanson, High resolution paraventricular nucleus serial section model constructed within a traditional rat brain atlas. *Neurosci Lett* (in press).

Simmons, D.M., J.W. Voss, H.A. Ingraham, J.M. Holloway, R.S. Broide, M.G. Rosenfeld, L.W. Swanson, Pituitary cell phenotypes involve cell-specific Pit-1 mRNA translation and synergistic interactions with other classes of transcription factors, *Genes Dev* 4 (1990) 695–711.

Swanson, L.W., Organization of mammalian neuroendocrine system. In: F.E. Bloom (Ed.), *Handbook of Physiology—The Nervous System IV*, Waverly Press, Baltimore, 1986, pp. 317–63.

Swanson, L.W., The hypothalamus. In: T. Hökfelt, A. Björklund, L.W. Swanson (Eds.), *Handbook of Chemical Neuroanatomy*, Vol. 5, *Integrated Systems of the CNS, Part I*, Elsevier, Amsterdam, 1987, pp. 1–124.

Swanson, L.W., Biochemical switching in hypothalamic circuits mediating responses to stress, *Prog Brain Res* 87 (1991) 181–200.

Swanson, L.W., Spatiotemporal patterns of transcription factor gene expression accompanying the development and plasticity of cell phenotypes in the neuroendocrine system, *Prog Brain Res* 92 (1992) 97–113.

Swanson, L.W., Cerebral hemisphere regulation of motivated behavior, *Brain Res* 886 (2000) 113–64.

Swanson, L.W., *Brain Maps: Structure of the Rat Brain. A Laboratory Guide with Printed and Electronic Templates for Data, Models and Schematic*, 3rd. Edn. with CD-ROM, Elsevier, Amsterdam, 2004, 215 pp.

Swanson, L.W., Anatomy of the soul as reflected in the cerebral hemispheres: neural circuits underlying voluntary control of basic motivated behaviors, *J Comp Neurol* 493 (2005) 122–31.

Swanson, L.W., B.K. Hartman, Biochemical specificity in central pathways related to peripheral and intracerebral homeostatic functions, *Neurosci Lett* 16 (1980) 55–60.

Swanson, L.W., P.E. Sawchenko, Hypothalamic integration: organization of the paraventricular and supraoptic nuclei, *Annu Rev Neurosci* 6 (1983) 269–324.

Swanson, L.W., P.E. Sawchenko, R.W. Lind, Regulation of multiple peptides in CRF parvocellular neurosecretory neurons: implications for the stress response, *Prog Brain Res* 68 (1986) 169–90.

Swanson, L.W., D.M. Simmons, Differential steroid hormone and neural influences on peptide mRNA levels in CRH cells of the paraventricular nucleus: a hybridization histochemical study in the rat, *J Comp Neurol* 285 (1989) 413–35.

Ugrumov, M.V., Magnocellular vasopressin system in ontogenesis: development and regulation, *Microsc Res Tech* 56 (2002) 164–71.

van Eerdenburg, F.J., P. Rakic, Neurogenesis and postnatal DNA synthesis in the anterior hypothalamus of the monkey. *Abstr Am Soc Neuroscience* (1994).

van Eerdenburg, F.J., D.F. Swaab, Postnatal development and sexual differentiation of pig hypothalamic nuclei, *Psychoneuroendocrinol* 19 (1994) 471–84.

Zhu, X., A.S. Gleiberman, M.G. Rosenfeld, Molecular physiology of pituitary development: signaling and transcriptional networks, *Physiol Rev* 87 (2007) 933–63.

Chapter Five

Neural Tube Defects: New Insights on Risk Factors

Enrique Pedernera, Rodrigo Núñez Vidales, and Carmen Méndez

INTRODUCTION

Neural-tube defects (NTDs) include a group of congenital malformations that mainly affect the structure of the central nervous system (CNS). Etiology of these pathologies is complex because in most cases malformations are not limited to neural-tube derivatives (from which most of the CNS is originated), but it also affects other embryonic structures such as the meninges, the spine, and the skull. Each of the pathologies included in the NTDs shows a wide spectrum of involvement that mainly depends on the damaged CNS element. Consequently this leads to pathologies that range from asymptomatic and described only as radiographic abnormalities, to other severe sensory and motor deficiencies that mainly involve lower extremities, all the way through pathologies that affect intra- and extra-uterine mortality. This chapter will describe the main entities that comprise NTDs, provide population-based statistics, present advances in the elucidation of their etiology, and discuss associated risk factors.

CLINICAL AND PATHOLOGICAL FEATURES

Based on their frequency, the main NTDs are anencephaly, spina bifida, and encephalocele.

Anencephaly is a malformation that affects brain, skull, meninges, scalp and its derivatives presenting a failure of closure in the rostral portion of the head. If not stillborn, this condition will commonly cause the infant's death shortly after birth. Ten to 20% of cases have additional abnormalities in the ear, the palate, and theheart. Polyhydramnios is associated in 50% of anencephaly cases (Johnston and Kinsman 2004).

Spina bifida is found in two varieties, closed and open. Closed spina bifida is an entity that basically modified the spine but usually the spinal cord is not affected. It commonly involves the vertebral arches and laminae between L5 and S1. Other CNS pathologies associated with it are syringomyelia, lipoma, and dermoid sinus, which is a fistula that communicates the exterior to the medullary cavity, allowing recurrent CNS infections (Johnston and Kinsman 2004). Diverse visible skin stigmas have been associated with spina bifida such as hypertrichosis, caudal appendage or human tail, angioma, and Wilms tumor (Garcia-Álix et al. 2005).

Open spina bifida is grouped into entities that involve the spinal cord, the spine, the meninges, and occasionally the skin. Meningocele is a hernia of meninges and cerebrospinal fluid that protrude through a defect in the vertebrae. It is observed as a tumor usually in the lumbrosacral region of the spine that contains fluid and no neural tissue. Most meningoceles are covered with skin and may be accompanied by other anomalies such as urinary dysfunction, rectovaginal fistula diastematomyelia, and tethered spinal cord. There have been reports in which patients who did not have the lesion removed developed other lesions such as dermoid and epidermoid tumor, meningioma, neurofibroma, chordoma, chondroma, lipoma, and teratoma (Johnston and Kinsman 2004; Rivero et al. 2006).

Myelomeningocele is similar to meningocele but it includes the protrusion of a fragment of the spinal cord. Approximately 70–75% of cases have the defect in the lumbosacral region, and the neurological lesion may cause motor and sensory deficits of the lower limbs and bowel and bladder incontinence due to the loss of control over external sphincters.

Approximately 80% of myelomeningocele cases are associated with the Arnold-Chiari type II malformation, a condition with hydrocephaly due to a disruption of the medullary canal, leading to hindbrain dysfunction (Medina et al. 2001; Johnston and Kinsman 2004).

Encephalocele is a malformation that affects bone tissue, the meninges, and the brain. It presents as a protrusion of a meningeal sac that contains brain tissue; it may be covered by skin and usually projects through a bone defect of the skull in the midline. It affects mainly the occipital region, even though the fronto-ethmoidal lesion is more common in Asian countries. This pathology may be worsened by hydrocephaly due to aqueduct stenosis, by developing an Arnold-Chiari type II malformation when there is a hernia of the cerebellum and the medulla, or by microcephaly increasing the risk for seizures and failure to thrive (Johnston and Kinsman 2004; Kanev 2007).

In order to reach a diagnosis of these defects, maternal serum concentrations of alpha fetoprotein (AFP) are taken between the 15th and 20th week. An NTD is suspected when the levels of this protein are above 2.5 MOM (multiples of the median) or evidence is found via ultrasound and magnetic resonance imaging (Kanev 2007). In 2006, Dashe and colleagues described that AFP has a sensibility between 79% and 86%, which can improve with the proper use of ultrasound detecting approximately 88% of NTDs (anencephaly and open spina bifida). It is important to note that AFP failed to detect 25% of NTD cases (Norem et al. 2005) and that the estimate of AFP is modified by gestational age, maternal weight, race, maternal diabetes, multiple pregnancy, and the use of phenothiazines (Salas et al. 2003). The use of ultrasound for the early detection of anencephaly (between the 11th and 14th week of gestation) requires adequate training of the person that performs the ultrasonography in order to observe the characteristic "Mickey Mouse" sign that corresponds to the brain hemispheres in a coronal section (Chatzipapas et al. 1999).

EPIDEMIOLOGY

Many population-based studies have been published describing the incidence and prevalence of NTDs, in particular statistics on the effects of vitamin supplementation. However, five points must be considered when evaluating epidemiological data of NTDs in order to understand the relevance of the problem.

1. NTDs include a group of entities of which most studies only report three: anencephaly, open spina bifida, and encephalocele. Because these three are considered the lesions with the highest prevalence, other NTDs are left out.
2. Some lesions such as anencephaly are not compatible with life and the fetus may die before birth. This is important because some studies have reported a mortality rate that only accounts for newborns and stillbirths, leaving out spontaneous or elective abortions (Velie and Shaw 1996; Gucciardi et al. 2002; Alfaro et al. 2004). In 1996 Velie and Shaw reported that using NTD prevalence in births, NTDs in newborns only comprise 48.8% of total anencephaly cases, 70.2% of spina bifida, and 57.7% of other NTDs when all newborns, stillbirths, and abortions were taken into account. It must be noted that these statistics might be influenced by the abortion policy that exists in the United States. In Ontario, Canada, Gucciardi and colleagues reported for 1999 that the total prevalence of NTDs was 8.6 × 10,000 pregnancies. Newborn NTD prevalence was 5.3 × 10,000 births, for stillbirths 159 × 10,000, and for abortions 28.7 × 10,000. Of the total of NTDs, 75% in the newborn cases were spina bifida, whereas in the case of stillbirths 57% corresponded to anencephaly.

3. The incidence of NTDs seems to vary in time and location, hence, low rates may be obtained if only these populations are studied (Stevenson et al. 2000; Busby et al. 2005). Based on a database from 17 European countries known as EUROCAT, it was reported that between 2000 and 2002 the prevalence of NTDs was 8.31 × 10,000 births. This database takes into account all newborns, stillbirths, and abortions after prenatal diagnosis (Busby et al. 2005). The cases of NTDs seem to be distributed irregularly in the European continent, even within countries like Spain, Germany, France, Belgium, Switzerland, and Denmark that registered total prevalence between 11.44 (Basque country, Spain) and 27.01 × 10,000 births (Mainz, Germany).

4. Approximately 20% of NTDs cases are associated with other congenital malformations, anencephaly 16%, spina bifida 12%, and encephalocele 38% (Stevenson et al. 2000), suggesting a different etiology of the NTD. By taking this into account NTD statistics might be modified.

5. Finally, an important aspect to note is the difference in NTD frequency by gender that might suggest a biological influence on the etiology of these malformations. Anencephaly and spina bifida are more frequent among women (Martínez et al. 2002; Lisi et al. 2005; Li et al. 2006; Tan et al. 2007).

PATHOGENESIS

Just like most congenital malformations, it is widely accepted that the etiology of NTDs is multifactorial. In other words, numerous environmental, maternal, and genetic variables are involved to various degrees in their development. The neural tube is the precursor of the entire central nervous system. The development of this structure involves complex interactions among tissues and a large list of signaling molecules that go beyond the scope of this chapter and are reviewed elsewhere (Botto et al. 1999; Detrait et al. 2005). However, crucial steps in neural tube development, like folding, may be implicated in the genesis of NTDs. As the neural tube is closing, it is known that the cranial and caudal ends remain open and are known as cranial and caudal neuropores, respectively. They usually close between the 24th and 27th day of gestation, respectively. The closure of the neural tube is a fundamental process that might be the most studied mechanism of pathogenesis of NTDs. It is postulated that the failure to close one of the neuropores is the direct cause of NTDs, either due to lack of fusion or due to cellular death in the edge of the borders, or earlier due to the lack of elevation of the folds of the neural streak. Perhaps the clearest relations would be: the one between the lack of closure of the cranial neuropore and the presentation of anencephaly, as well as the lack of closure of the caudal neuropore and open spina bifida. However, a great deal of controversy lies in the location of these closure points. In 1993 Van Allen and colleagues postulated the existence of five closure points in different regions of the neural tube, relating them to the different clinical presentations observed. Nonetheless, in 1998 Sulik and colleagues demonstrated experimentally in humans the existence of two fusion points and a closure mechanism similar to a zipper along the tube. This view was revised in the studies by Nakatsu and colleagues (2000) and O'Rahilly and colleagues (2002), who confirmed some of the previous findings and suggested modifications to the closure points.

Of the possible mechanisms implicated in the pathogenesis of NTDs, three important observations are underscored:

1. Shum and Copp (1996) proposed different forms of neural tube closure conditioned by the mechanism implicated in the folding, and relating each of them with a spectrum of pathologies specific to each zone. For example, the failure that occurs at a higher spine level is related to craneo-rachischisis (Shum and Copp 1996; Detrait et al. 2005).
2. The work of Matsumoto and colleagues related a particular type of exencephaly with the final presentation of anencephaly, suggesting that the disruption of the neural tube morphology and adjacent tissues was due to the excessive growth of the mesencephalon.
3. Lastly, another element studied in the pathogenesis of the NTDs is the cytoskeleton. Various studies have manifested the importance of microfilaments in different processes of normal neural tube development, emphasizing the role of actin filaments during the closure of the anterior neural tube, participating in the fusion of the neural folds, though not their elevation (Ybot-González and Copp 1999; Lu et al. 2004).

GENETIC FACTORS

NTD animal models have been developed and, among those, the murine models are outstanding because they number close to 200. In these models, many genes that have been studied relate mainly to the development of exencephaly and open spina bifida. The great majority of modified genes are known to code for proteins involved in diverse signaling pathways such as Wnt, Shh, BMP, apoptosis, cellular polarity, and cellular adhesion, among others (Harris and Juriloff 2007; Lu et al. 2004; Chi et al. 2005; Greene et al. 2005; Wlodarczyk et al. 2006).

The prevention of the defect development in some of these models after the administration of vitamins and micronutrients supports the role that these (mainly folates) play in the prevention of neural damage as it has been proposed in the human population (Wlodarczyk et al. 2006; Harris and Juriloff 2007). Furthermore, the following data are of importance: exencephaly is much more frequent in females (2/3) than in males in 11 animal models, and open spina bifida has approximately the same distribution between genders and mimicks what is observed in human populations (Lisi et al. 2005; Harris and Juriloff 2007).

The study of these genes could possibly expose the underlying mechanism behind the percentage of NTDs that does not respond to peri-conceptional administration of folates, which in humans is between 20% and 80% (Czeizel and Dudas 1992; Bekkers and Eskes 1999; Tissir and Goffinet 2006; Pitkin 2007).

A gene that has been studied in human populations due to its impact in studies about the use of folic acid and its metabolism and that possess a high prevalence in populations with a great number of NTDs is the one that codifies the protein 5,10-methylenetetrahydrofolate reductase (MTHFR). This enzyme converts methylenetetrahydrofolate to methyltetraydrofolate, which is a donor of methyl groups used during the re-methylation of homocysteine and methionine. The mutation most studied in this gene is C677T, which encodes a thermolabile protein with a 50% activity reduction. The prevalence of this variant is very high in countries like Mexico and is significantly associated with NTDs (Botto et al. 1999; Mutchinik et al. 1999; Martínez et al. 2001). In the familial presentation of NTDs it is necessary to emphasize that some NTDs present within the spectrum of well-defined syndromes like Meckel-Gruber, Waardenburg, Kippel-Feil syndromes, and trisomies such as those of chromosomes 13 and 18.

The risk of recurrence is between 3% and 4% after a birth with an NTD and about 10% after two births with a type of NTD. Additionally, between 60% to 70% of the recurrent malformations affect almost the same area as in the first case (Johnston and Kinsman 2004; Detrait et al. 2005; Mitchell 2005).

MATERNAL FACTORS

In 2003 Watkins and colleagues proved in their study the relationship between obesity and congenital defects, using the data from the Birth Defects Risk Factors Surveillance Study in Atlanta, Georgia (USA). They reported that an obese mother would have a 2.7-fold increased risk of having a child with an NTD, particularly spina bifida with a 3.5-fold risk (CI 1.2–10.3). In the case of anencephaly the risk was 2.9-fold; however, the confidence interval limited the conclusions (CI 0.7–2.3). Other defects were found to be associated with cardiac malformations and omphalocele (RM: 3.3 CI 1.0–10.3). Previous studies demonstrated a similar relationship between NTDs and a body mass index of 29. This could be explained in terms of the metabolic changes due to insulin resistance, hyperglycemia, or nutritional deficiency (Shaw et al. 1996; Watkins et al. 2003).

Another factor associated with NTDs is maternal diabetes. Based on epidemiological studies, it is known that the risk of a diabetic mother having a child with an NTD is between 2.5 and 4.5 times greater, depending on the stage at which glycemic levels were controlled and the amount of therapy. The studies based on animal models have opened a new perspective on the etiology of NTDs. Recently, it was proven in animal models that the oxidative damage produced by the metabolic changes secondary to maternal hyperglycemia (and subsequently in the child) leads to cellular death mediated by p53. Under normal oxidative conditions, p53 could be controlled by the transcription factor Pax-3. Hyperglycemia was associated with a reduction in the expression of Pax-3 and a rise in cellular death mediated by p53. These changes could be prevented in different proportions by: the administration of antioxidants, the reduction in the tubular reabsorption of glucose, and also in genetically modified mouse strains without Pax-3 or p53 genes. These studies, when added to the population studies described previously, bring us closer to understanding NTD physiopathology, particularly in situations such as an obese or diabetic mother (Phelan et al. 1997; Loeken 2005).

USE OF FOLIC ACID AND OTHER VITAMINS

The first suggestions about a relationship between folic acid and congenital malformations began during the 1960s with a study conducted by Hibbard in 1964. Subsequent studies followed by others, such as Laurence and colleagues (1981), Smithells and colleagues (1983), from the Medical Research Counsel (MRC 1991), and Czeizel and Dudas (1992). They showed a protective effect of folic acid in the incidence of NTDs. These studies differed in the reduction of the incidence of NTD attributable to the use of folic acid during peri-conception period, being between 35% and 75% in observational studies and around 80% in clinical studies (Pitkin 2007).

Following the publication of the results of the MRC in 1991 and Czeizel and Dudas in 1992, some countries implemented a widespread supplementation of folic acid in the diet so that pregnant women with no history of births with NTDs would ingest 0.4 mg of folic acid per day during the peri-conceptional period (3 months before and after conception) and 4 mg/day in women with a history of affected children. These recommendations were released in the United States, Britain, and Ireland toward the end of 1992, Holland in 1993 (with doses of 0.5 mg/day), Hungary in 1995, and other countries after 1996 (with doses of 0.4 mg/day), among them Mexico. Some of these countries decided to fortify flour with folic acid in various amounts (approximately 140 mcg/100g of flour), such as in the United States (1998) and Latin America (Mexico, 1999, with 2 mg of folic acid/1000g of flour), but not others, including Britain and Ireland. In addition to the supplementation and fortification some of these countries added a campaign to promote a better diet (Bekkers and Eskes 1999; Rosano et al. 1999; Martínez 2002; Busby et al. 2005; Pitkin 2007).

In the United States toward the end of 2001 was reported a 19% reduction in the incidence of NTDs over a 10-year period (1990–1999) out of the cases reported in birth certificates. Whereas spina bifida cases showed a 23% reduction, anencephaly only showed an 11% reduction (Honein et al. 2001). In 2002 this reduction in the incidence of NTDs was kept between 20% and 30%.

The reduction in NTD incidence has been corroborated by other international studies, in particular in populations like Ontario, Canada; Nuevo Leon, Mexico; and European countries considered in the EUROCAT. Later multicentric reports, like the one from Botto and colleagues in 2005 and Busby and colleagues in 2005, published the results of the statistics on NTDs in selected populations, showing a reduction in the incidence of NTDs. Each of these regions has some peculiarities to be noted:

1. The group of Gucciardi, based in Ontario, Canada, showed a reduction in the incidence of NTDs in newborns and stillbirths and products of abortion from 1986 to 1999. The reduction was around 42–53%, being most notorious in the stillbirths group (Gucciardi et al. 2002).
2. The group of Martínez Villareal based in Nuevo León, Mexico, in 2002 demonstrated a reduction in the incidence of NTDs of 43% being greater in females as a result of a campaign started in 1999 in which low-income women from the region were given 5 mg of folic acid per week or 5 mg per day in those with a history of an affected child (Martínez et al. 2002).
3. In the case of the group of Busby and the EUROCAT registry, the authors observed a reduction in the prevalence of NTDs, comparing the period of 1981–1991 and 2000–2002, of 30% for the United Kingdom and Ireland, 43% for Holland, and between 16% and 32% for some other European countries. It is interesting to note that the reduction of NTDs in the United Kingdom had been progressively descending in the past 20 years, long before the introduction of folic acid supplementation. Meanwhile this reduction became evident in Holland almost simultaneously with the introduction of the supplementation (Busby et al. 2004).

It is noteworthy that the reduction of NTD incidence through the use of folates in the diet could be due to their role as antioxidants, in that they lower the serum concentration of homocysteine, an oxidant. This information opens a line of research to etiology and prevention of NTDs (Nakano et al. 2001).

ASSOCIATED RISK FACTORS AND OUR EXPERIENCE

Even though a better understanding of the etiology and pathogenesis of NTDs has been obtained, there still is not enough information to explain the actual cause of NTDs. An extensive list of associated risk factors includes several conditions, from those affecting the maternal condition, such as age (Vieira et al. 2005), race (Canfield 1996), dietary intake and nutritional state (Shaw et al. 2001; Carmichael et al. 2003; Missmer et al. 2006), obstetrics history (Whiteman 2000), and use of drugs (Blatter et al. 1994). Many of these associations arise from observational studies and lack a well-defined biological explanation. However, many chemicals, mainly neuromodulator drugs and some chemotherapeutic agents, have been documented to have a teratogenic effect. One of the most studied anticonvulsants, valproic acid, showed a complex array of disruptive effects through the interference with the Wnt signaling pathway (Wiltse 2005) and the impairment of the neural crest cells' normal morphology and motility (Fuller et al. 2002). In contrast, others, such as phenytoin and the fungicide vinclozilin, affect the expression and regulation (Gehlhaus et al. 2007) as well as the signaling transactivation capacity of the androgen receptor (AR) (Kavlock and Cummings 2005).

A clue for neurogenesis may reside in the presence and metabolism of steroid hormones within neural tissue. The steroid hormones, such as androgen, estrogen, and progesterone, have been documented to play a role in the development of sexual behavior, gonadal control axis, and reproductive organ development (Rahman 2005; Weiser 2007). These substances can easily enter the neuroepithelium. However, the neural tissue can also produce its own steroid, known as neurosteroids (Mensah et al. 1999; Compagnone and Mellon 2000). The importance of these substances in neural tissue has been carefully studied in animal models at late developmental stages and were found to have a series of actions that influence the development of neural tissue, such as cellular proliferation (Wang et al. 2005), differentiation, and response to toxic insults (Núñez and McCarthy 2008).

Our work has focused on the influences of androgens. These substances are thought to have some effect on nervous system patterning shortly after neural tube closure. However, recent studies have described the presence of steroid receptors in neural stem cells (Brännvall et al. 2005), particularly the AR, but its expression, presence, and role(s) during early embryogenesis remain uncertain.

The AR is a member of the nuclear receptors family and acts as a ligand-dependent transcriptional factor mediating the actions of endogenous androgens such as testosterone (Gao et al. 2005) and neurosteroids such as DHEA (Mo et al. 2004). Androgens acting through the AR promote the transcription of several genes including those involved in cellular growth (Estrada 2005; Chang 2005), differentiation (Zhang 2000; Narayanan 2006), morphogenesis (Gomez and Newman 1991), and neuroprotection against cytotoxic insults (Hammond 2001; Mantoni 2006; Pike 2007). The AR has been found throughout the nervous system of prenatal/postnatal and adult animals (Murphy et al. 1999; Núñez et al. 2003; Milner et al. 2007). However, the role of the AR in early periods of development has not been described.

Assuming that the AR mediates the action of endogenous androgens and can also participate in alternative signaling pathways through its co-activators, its possible role in early neurogenesis needed to be examined. To accomplish this goal, we based our experiments in chicken and mouse embryos whose neural tissue was processed to qualitatively assess the presence of the AR (Figure 5.1). Using cDNA of the three cerebral vesicles of the embryos through RT-PCR, we described a similar pattern of expression of a fragment of the AR's mRNA. There was no apparent difference among cerebral vesicles of both chicken and mouse embryos, and also no difference in the sex of the embryo. We sequenced this fragment for each of the species and found a 100% match with the reported sequence. This information was completed by searching for the AR's protein through peroxidase- and fluorescence-based immunohistochemistry. The AR's protein, considered as a positive nuclear staining, was found to be localized in the three cerebral vesicles and throughout the neuroepithelium, along with other surrounding structures including the notochord, somites, and mesonephros (Figure 5.2). The presence of the protein was assessed using western blot technique, and the data confirmed the positive results from immunohistochemistry.

These results suggest a possible role for the AR in neurogenesis. Its role could include several possibilities, ranging from those of the maternal steroids to the recent and better documented co-activating, ligand-independent capacity of the AR. Interactions between the AR and the Wnt signaling pathway have been studied, not only because of the relative proximity of expression (Machon et al. 2007), but also because of the interactions between the AR and β-catenin in a co-activation manner (Verras 2004; Yardi and Brewster 2005). Another important action of the AR is its protection against cytotoxic insults, favoring the survival of the cell (Figure 5.3) (Hammond et al. 2001; Comstock and Knudsen 2007).

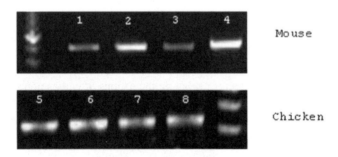

Figure 5.1. Representative RT-PCR analysis of a fragment of the AR mRNA in cerebral vesicles of chicken and mouse embryos. Photograph of agarose gel electrophoresis showing prosencephalon and mesencephalon of mouse embryos E9.5, male (lanes 1,2) and female (lanes 3,4). Prosencephalon of chicken embryos HH 13 (lane 5), HH 18 (lane 6), mesencephalon of chicken embryos HH 18 (lane 7), and rombencephalon of chicken embryos HH18 (lane 8).

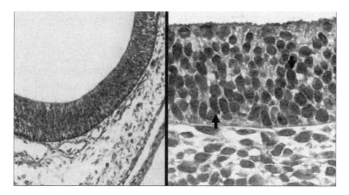

Figure 5.2. Immunohistochemistry for androgen receptor revealing positive nuclear staining. The presence of the protein in the neuroepithelium is observed in paraffin embedded samples of the forebrain of chicken (HH13) and mouse (E9.5) embryos. (See color Figure 5.2)

The AR, as stated above, is linked to the expression of several genes whose actions, along with those of its co-factors, are important in the mechanisms that are thought to fail and cause NTDs: cellular proliferation, cellular death, regulation of the cytoskeleton, and cellular adhesion (Chi et al. 2005). Our main focus has been centered on the role of the AR in the early stages of neural development. Although the AR does not play a primary role in neurulation, it may be involved in the modulation of the normal development of the neural tube.

CONCLUSIONS AND PERSPECTIVES

Congenital malformations command attention due to the importance they have taken, not only as a cause of death among children under 4 years of age, but also

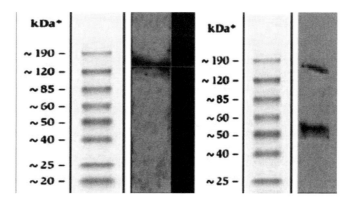

Figure 5.3. Representative western blot of the AR protein from homogenates of cerebral vesicles of the mouse embryo E9.5 observing the presence of a band of ≈110 kDa expected for the AR protein (left); mouse prostate was used as positive control (right). (See color Figure 5.3)

for the impact that they have on the surviving newborns and their families. Prevention before conception, the supplementation of folic acid, and the fortification of flour requires an informed population that takes the necessary action to lower the probabilities of giving birth to a child with an NTD. It is hard to calculate the social, emotional, and economic impact on the family of a child with an NTD.

There are several research groups that have studied in utero repair of spina bifida, particularly the open variant, and have made suggestions about the possibility that the neurological damage could be due to the traumatic action of the uterine environment and the toxicity of amniotic fluid over the neural tissue. The group of Meuli et al. (1996) observed an improvement in the motor and sensory functions after sheep fetuses with an induced NTD were repaired in utero. This finding was corroborated by Yoshizawa et al. (2004), who observed the maintenance of the structure of the anal sphincter using a different surgery technique for the in utero repair of the NTD. In 1998 a repair in utero of a human fetus was performed successfully and preserved some neurological function (Adzick et al. 1998). These surgical approaches open a new field of therapeutic possibilities for patients with NTDs that could not have been prevented with the therapies described in this chapter.

ACKNOWLEDGMENTS

We thank QFB. Carmen Mondragón and Od. María José Gómora for their technical help. The present work was supported by SDI-PTID.05.01 "Nuevas Estrategias Epidemiológicas Genómicas y Proteómicas en Salud Pública" from the Universidad Nacional Autónoma de México.

REFERENCES

Adzick NS, Sutton LN, Crombleholme TM, Flake AW. Successful fetal surgery for spina bifida. *Lancet* 1998; 352:1675–6.

Alfaro N, Pérez JJ, Valadéz I, González T Y. Malformaciones congénitas externas en la zona metropolitana de Guadalajara. Diez años de estudio. *Investigación en Salud* 2004; 6:180–7.

Bekkers RL, Eskes TK. Periconceptional folic acid intake in Nijmegen, Netherlands. *Lancet* 1999; 353:292.

Blatter B, van der Star M, Roeleveld N. Review of neural tube defects: risk factors in parental occupation and the environment. *Environ Health Perspect* 1994; 102(2):140–5.

Botto LD, Lisi A, Robert-Gnansia E, Erickson JD, Vollset SE, Mastroiacovo P, Botting B, Cocchi G, de Vigan C, de Walle H, Feijoo M, Irgens LM, McDonnell B, Merlob P, Ritvanen A, Scarano G, Siffel C, Metneki J, Stoll C, Smithells R, Goujard J. International retrospective cohort study of neural tube defects in relation to folic acid recommendations: are the recommendations working? *BMJ* 2005; 330:571.

Botto LD, Moore CA, Khoury MJ, Erickson JD. Neural-tube defects. *N Engl J Med* 1999; 341:1509–19.

Brännvall K, Bogdanovic N, Korhonen L, Lindholm D.19-Nortestosterone influences neural stem cell proliferation and neurogenesis in the rat brain. *Eur J Neurosci* 2005 Feb; 21(4):871–8.

Busby A, Abramsky L, Dolk H, Armstrong B. Preventing neural tube defects in Europe: a missed opportunity. *Reprod Toxicol* 2005; 20:393–402.

Busby A, Abramsky L, Dolk H, Armstrong B. Eurocat Folic Acid Working Group. Preventing neural tube defects in Europe. population based study. *BMJ* 2005; 330:574–5

Canfield M, Annegers J, Brender J, Cooper S, Greenberg F. Hispanic origin and neural tube defects in Houston/Harris County, Texas. II. Risk factors. *Am J Epidemiol* 1996; 143(1):12–24.

Carmichael S, Shaw G, Schaffer D, Laurent C, Selvin S. Dieting behaviors and risk of neural tube defects. *Am J Epidemiol* 2003; 158(12):1127–31.

Chang C, Hsuuw Y, Huang F, Shyr C, Chang S, Huang C, Kang H, Huang K. Androgenic and antiandrogenic effects and expression of androgen receptor in mouse embryonic stem cells. *Fertil Steril* 2006; 85 Suppl 1:1195–1203.

Chatzipapas IK, Whitlow BJ, Economides DL. The "Mickey Mouse" sign and the diagnosis of anencephaly in early pregnancy. *Ultrasound Obstets Gynecol* 1999; 13:196–9.

Chi H, Sarkisian M, Rakic P, Flavell R. Loss of mitogen-activated protein kinase kinase kinase 4 (MEKK4) results in enhanced apoptosis and defective neural tube development. *Proc Natl Acad Sci U S A* 2005; 102(10):3846–51.

Compagnone NA, Mellon SH. Neurosteroids: biosynthesis and function of these novel neuromodulators. *Front Neuroendocrinol* 2000; 21(1):1–56.

Comstock C, Knudsen K. The complex role of AR signaling after cytotoxic insult: implications for cell-cycle-based chemotherapeutics. *Cell Cycle* 2007; 6(11):1307–13.

Czeizel AE, Dudas I. Prevention of the first occurrence of neural-tube defects by periconceptional vitamin supplementation. *N Engl J Med* 1992; 327:1832–5.

Dashe J, Twickler D, Santos-Ramos R, McIntire D, Ramus R. Alpha-fetoprotein detection of neural tube defects and the impact of standard ultrasound. *Am J Obstets Gynecol* 2006; 195:1623–8.

Detrait ER, George TM, Etchevers HC, Gilbert JR, Vekemans M, Speer MC. Human neural tube defects: developmental biology, epidemiology, and genetics. *Neurotoxicol Teratol* 2005; 27:515–24.

Dubrovsky B. Steroids, neuroactive steroids and neurosteroids in psychopathology. *Prog Neuropsychopharmacol Biol Psychiatry* 2005 Feb; 29(2):169–92.

Fuller L, Cornelius S, Murphy C, Wiens D. Neural crest cell motility in valproic acid. *Reprod Toxicol* 2002; 16(6):825–39.

García A, Lucas R, Quero J. La piel como expresión de alteraciones neurológicas en el recién nacido. *Anales de Pediatría* 2005; 62:548–63.

Gehlhaus M, Schmitt N, Volk B, Meyer R. Antiepileptic drugs affect neuronal androgen signaling via a cytochrome P450-dependent pathway. *J Pharmacol Exp Ther* 2007; 322(2):550–9.

Gomez DM, Newman SW. Medial nucleus of the amygdala in the adult Syrian hamster: a quantitative Golgi analysis of gonadal hormonal regulation of neuronal morphology. *Anat Rec* 1991; 231(4):498–509.

Greene ND, Copp AJ. Mouse models of neural tube defects: investigating preventive mechanisms. *Am J Med Genet C Semin Med Genet* 2005; 135:31–41.

Gucciardi E, Pietrusiak MA, Reynolds DL, Rouleau J. Incidence of neural tube defects in Ontario, 1986–1999. *CMAJ* 2002; 167:237–40.

Hammond J, Le Q, Goodyer C, Gelfand M, Trifiro M, LeBlanc A.Testosterone-mediated neuroprotection through the androgen receptor in human primary neurons. *J Neurochem* 2001; 77(5):1319–26.

Harris MJ, Juriloff DM. Mouse mutants with neural tube closure defects and their role in understanding human neural tube defects. *Birth Defects Res A Clin Mol Teratol* 2007; 79:187–210.

Hernández S, Werler M, Walker A, Mitchell A. Neural tube defects in relation to use of folic acid antagonists during pregnancy. *Am J Epidemiol* 2001; 153(10):961–8.

Hibbard BM. The role of folic acid in pregnancy. *J Obstet Gynaecol Br Commonw* 1964; 71:529–42.

Honein MA, Paulozzi LJ, Mathews TJ, Erickson JD, Wong LY. Impact of folic acid fortification of the US food supply on the occurrence of neural tube defects. *JAMA* 2001; 285:2981–6.

Johnston M, Kinsman S. Congenital Anomalies of the Central Nervous System. En Behrman, Nelson Textbook of Pediatrics, 17th ed. Elsevier, USA, 2004, Cap. 585.

Kanev PM. Congenital Malformations of the Skull and Meninges. *Otolaryngol Clin North Am* 2007; 40:9–26.

Kavlock R, Cummings A. Mode of action: inhibition of androgen receptor function: vinclozolin-induced malformations in reproductive development. *Crit Rev Toxicol* 2005; 35(8–9):721–6.

Li Z, Ren A, Zhang L, Ye R, Li S, Zheng J, Hong S, Wang T, Li Z. Extremely high prevalence of neural tube defects in a 4-county area in Shanxi Province, China. *Birth Defects Res A Clin Mol Teratol* 2006; 76:237–40.

Lisi A, Botto LD, Rittler M, Castilla E, Bianchi F, Botting B, de Walle H, Erickson JD, Gatt M, de Vigan C, Irgens L, Johnson W, Lancaster P, Merlob P, Mutchinick OM, Ritvanen A, Robert E, Scarano G, Stoll C, Mastroiacovo P. Sex and congenital malformations: an international perspective. *Am J Med Genet A* 2005; 134:49–57.

Loeken MR. Current perspectives on the causes of neural tube defects resulting from diabetic pregnancy. *Am J Med Genet C Semin Med Genet* 2005; 135:77–87.

Lu X, Borchers AG, Jolicoeur C, Rayburn H, Baker JC, Tessier-Lavigne M. PTK7/CCK-4 is a novel regulator of planar cell polarity in vertebrates. *Nature* 2004; 430:93–8.

Mantoni T, Reid G, Garrett M. Androgen receptor activity is inhibited in response to genotoxic agents in a p53-independent manner. *Oncogene* 2006; 25(22):3139–49.

Martínez L, Delgado I, Valdez R. Folate levels and N(5),N(10)-methylenetetrahydrofolate reductase genotype (MTHFR) in mothers of offspring with neural tube defects: a case-control study. *Arch Med Res* 2001; 32:277–82.

Martínez L, Perez JZ, Vazquez PA. Decline of neural tube defects cases after a folic acid campaign in Nuevo Leon, Mexico. *Teratology* 2002; 66:249–56.

Matsumoto A, Hatta T, Moriyama K, Otani H. Sequential observations of exencephaly and subsequent morphological changes by mouse exo utero development system: analysis of the mechanism of transformation from exencephaly to anencephaly. *Anat Embryol (Berl)* 2002; 205:7–18.

Medina A, Coutiño B, Alvarado G, Ramírez J. Epidemiología del mielomeningocele en niños menores de un año de edad en el Instituto Nacional de Pediatría. *Revista Mexicana de Medicina Física y Rehabilitación* 2001; 13:50–4.

Mensah-Nyagan AG, Do-Rego JL, Beaujean D, Luu-The V, Pelletier G, Vaudry H. Neurosteroids: expression of steroidogenic enzymes and regulation of steroid biosynthesis in the central nervous system. *Pharmacol Rev* 1999; 51(1):63–81.

Meuli M, Meuli-Simmen C, Yingling C, Hutchins GM, Timmel GB, Harrison MR, Adzick NS. In utero repair of experimental myelomeningocele saves neurological function at birth. *J Pediatr Surg* 1996; 31:397–402.

Milner TA, Hernandez FJ, Herrick SP, Pierce JP, Iadecola C, Drake CT. Cellular and subcellular localization of androgen receptor immunoreactivity relative to C1 adrenergic neurons in the rostral ventrolateral medulla of male and female rats. *Synapse* 2007; 61(5):268–78.

Mitchell LE. Epidemiology of neural tube defects. *Am J Med Genet C Semin Med Genet* 2005; 135:88–94.

Mo Q, Lu S, Hu S, Simon N. DHEA and DHEA sulfate differentially regulate neural androgen receptor and its transcriptional activity. *Brain Res Mol Brain Res* 2004; 126(2):165–72.

MRC Vitamin Research Group. Prevention of neural tube defects: results of the Medical Research Council Vitamin Study. *Lancet* 1991; 338:131–7.

Murphy A, Shupnik M, Hoffman G. Androgen and estrogen (alpha) receptor distribution in the periaqueductal gray of the male rat. *Horm Behav* 1999; 36(2):98–108.

Mutchinick OM, Lopez MA, Luna L, Waxman J, Babinsky VE. High prevalence of the thermolabile methylenetetrahydrofolate reductase variant in Mexico: a country with a very high prevalence of neural tube defects. *Mol Genet Metab* 1999; 68:461–7.

Nakano E, Higgins JA, Powers HJ. Folate protects against oxidative modification of human LDL. *Br J Nutr* 2001; 86:637–9.

Narayanan B, Narayanan NK, Davis L, Nargi D. RNA interference-mediated cyclooxygenase-2 inhibition prevents prostate cancer cell growth and induces differentiation: modulation of neuronal protein synaptophysin, cyclin D1, and androgen receptor. *Mol Cancer Ther* 2006; 5(5):1117–25.

Norem CT, Schoen EJ, Walton DL, Krieger RC, O'Keefe J, To TT, Ray GT. Routine ultrasonography compared with maternal serum alpha-fetoprotein for neural tube defect screening. *Obstet Gynecol* 2005; 106:747–52.

Nuñez J, Huppenbauer C, McAbee M, Juraska J, DonCarlos L. Androgen receptor expression in the developing male and female rat visual and prefrontal cortex. *J Neurobiol* 2003; 56(3):293–302.

Nuñez, J., McCarthy M., Androgens predisposemales to GABAA-mediated excitotoxicity in the developing hippocampus. *Experimental Neurology* 2008, doi: 10.1016/j.expneurol.2008.01.001

O'Rahilly R, Muller F. The two sites of fusion of the neural folds and the two neuropores in the human embryo. *Teratology* 2002; 65:162–70.

Phelan SA, Ito M, Loeken MR. Neural tube defects in embryos of diabetic mice: role of the Pax-3 gene and apoptosis. *Diabetes* 1997; 46:1189–97.

Pike C, Nguyen T, Ramsden M, Yao M, Murphy M, Rosario E. Androgen cell signaling pathways involved in neuroprotective actions. *Hormones and Behavior* 2007, doi:10.1016/j.yhbeh.2007.11.006

Pitkin R. Folate and neural tube defects. *Am J Clin Nutr* 2007; 85:528–88.

Rahman Q. The neurodevelopment of human sexual orientation. *Neurosci Biobehav Rev* 2005; 29(7):1057–66.

Rivero D, Carcavilla L, Marin M. Tumoral degeneration occurring over a non-healing meningocele: report of two cases. *Neurocirugia (Astur)* 2006; 17:532–7.

Rosano A, Smithells D, Cacciani L, Botting B, Castilla E, Cornel M, Erickson D, Goujard J, Irgens L, Merlob P, Robert E, Siffel C, Stoll C, Sumiyoshi Y. Time trends in neural tube defects prevalence in relation to preventive strategies: an international study. *J Epidemiol Community Health* 1999; 53:630–5.

Salas P, Rodriguez S, Cunningham L, Castro I. Utilidad de la alfa-fetoporteína en el diagnóstico prenatal de defectos del tubo neural y anomalías cromosómicas. *Revista Biomédica* 2003; 14:5–10.

Shaw G, Selvin S, Carmichael S, Schaffer D, Nelson V, Neri E. Assessing combined chemical exposures as risk factors for neural tube defects. *Reprod Toxicol* 2001; 15(6):631–5.

Shaw G, Todoroff K, Carmichael S, Schaffer D, Selvin S. Lowered weight gain during pregnancy and risk of neural tube defects among offspring. *Int J Epidemiol* 2001; 30(1):60–5.

Shaw G, Velie E, Schaffer D. Risk of neural tube defect-affected pregnancies among obese women. *JAMA* 1996; 275:1093–6.

Shum A, Copp A. Regional differences in morphogenesis of the neuroepithelium suggest multiple mechanisms of spinal neurulation in the mouse. *Anat Embryol (Berl)* 1996; 194:65–73.

Smithells R, Nevin N, Seller M, Sheppard S, Harris R, Read A, Fielding D, Walker S, Schorah C, Wild J. Further experience of vitamin supplementation for prevention of neural tube defect recurrences. *Lancet* 1983; 1:1027–31.

Stevenson R, Allen W, Pai G, Best R, Seaver L, Dean J, Thompson S. Decline in prevalence of neural tube defects in a high-risk region of the United States. *Pediatrics* 2000; 106:677–83.

Tan K, Tan S, Tan K, Yeo G. Anencephaly in Singapore: a ten-year series 1993–2002. *Singapore Med J* 2007; 48:12–15.

Tissir F, Goffinet A. Expression of planar cell polarity genes during development of the mouse CNS. *Eur J Neurosci* 2006; 23:597–607.

Van Allen M, Kalousek D, Chernoff G, Juriloff D, Harris M, McGillivray B, Yong S, Langlois S, MacLeod P, Chitayat D, et al. Evidence for multi-site closure of the neural tube in humans. *Am J Med Genet* 1993; 47:723–43.

Velie E, Shaw G. Impact of prenatal diagnosis and elective termination on prevalence and risk estimates of neural tube defects in California, 1989–1991. *Am J Epidemiol* 1996; 144:473–9.

Verras M, Brown J, Li X, Nusse R, Sun Z. Wnt3a growth factor induces androgen receptor-mediated transcription and enhances cell growth in human prostate cancer cells. *Cancer Res* 2004; 64(24):8860–6.

Vieira A, Castillo S. Edad materna y defectos del tubo neural: evidencia para un efecto mayor en espina bífida que anencefalia. *Rev Méd Chile* 2005; 133:62–70.

Wang J, Johnston P, Ball B, Brinton R. The neurosteroid allopregnanolone promotes proliferation of rodent and human neural progenitor cells and regulates cell-cycle gene and protein expression. *J Neurosci* 2005; 25(19):4706–18.

Watkins M, Rasmussen S, Honein M, Botto L, Moore CA. Maternal obesity and risk for birth defects. *Pediatrics* 2003; 111:1152–8.

Weiser M, Foradori C, Handa R. Estrogen receptor beta in the brain: From form to function. *Brain Res Rev* 2008; 57(2):309–20.

Whiteman D, Murphy M, Hey K, O'Donnell M, Goldacre M. Reproductive factors, subfertility, and risk of neural tube defects: a case-control study based on the Oxford Record Linkage Study Register. *Am J Epidemiol* 2000; 152(9):823–8.

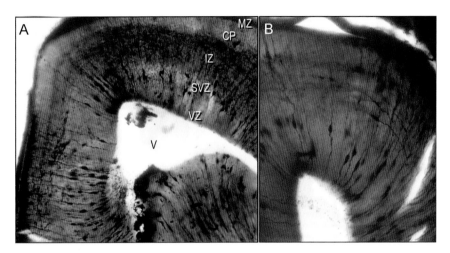

Figure 2.1. Coronal sections through the telencephalon of a rodent embryo impregnated using the Golgi method and showing the two types of cell displacement, radial and tangential. Microphotographs taken from some original histological preparations made by Cajal more than 100 years ago and conserved at the Cajal Institute. In picture (**A**) we have labelled the different layers of the developing neuroepithelium as we know them today: marginal zone (MZ), cortical plate (CP), intermediate zone (IZ) with many impregnated fibers and the germinative areas, the subventricular and ventricular zones (SVZ, VZ). The ventricle (V) is also labeled above the ganglionic eminence. Medial is left, and dorsal is up. Picture (**B**) shows several labeled cells undergoing radial migration and two cells migrating tangentially through the lower intermediate zone, at higher magnification.

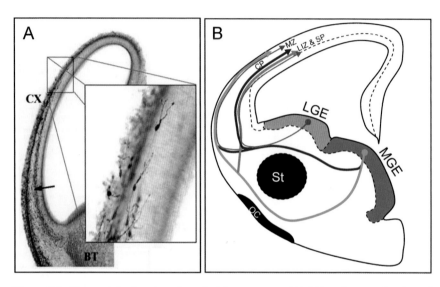

Figure 2.2. Tangential migration of cortical interneurons. **(A)** Microphotograph taken of a coronal section from the telencephalon of an E15 rat embryo immunostained with an antibody against the neurotransmitter GABA. The migratory GABAergic cells coming from the basal telencephalon (BT) enter the cortex (CX) through the marginal and intermediate zone (arrow). The box in the dorsal telencephalon shows a higher magnification of the leading tangential migrating cells as they progress toward the hippocampal anlage, bearing a fine trailing process and a robust and sometimes bifurcated leading process. **(B)** Cartoon representation of a coronal section from the left hemisphere of a mouse embryo at E14–E15 of development. Green arrows trace the migratory routes taken by the cortical cells generated in the medial ganglionic eminence (MGE; blue) and bordering the developing dorsal and ventral striatum (St). Both dorsal and ventral routes bifurcate at the level of the pallial–subpallial boundary to reach the cortex through the marginal zone (MZ) or the lower intermediate zone (LIZ). Red arrows trace the migratory routes following by the cortical interneurons generated in the lateral ganglionic eminence (LGE; orange), which also bifurcate as they enter the cortex. The striatum (St) and the olfactory cortex (OC) are chemorepellent areas for cortical interneurons generated in the basal telencephalon (see Marín and Rubenstein, 2001). CP, cortical plate; SP, subplate.

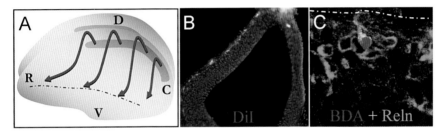

Figure 2.3. Origin of Cajal–Retzius cells and their tangential migration. (**A**) Cartoon representing a view of the telencephalon of an E11 mouse embryo from the left side. Cajal–Retzius cells originate in the cortical hem (purple band). The blue arrows indicate the migratory routes taken by Cajal–Retzius cells to cover the entire telencephalic surface. The migration is in an oblique caudal to rostral direction. (**B**) Coronal section from the telencephalon of an E10 mouse embryo injected with DiI in the cortical hem and cultured in toto for 24 hours. Cells generated in the cortical hem (injection site) migrate toward the basal telencephalon through the upper part of the preplate (red). The section was counterstained with DAPI (blue nuclei). (**C**) Migrating cell labelled with BDA injected in the cortical hem (red). The section was immunostained for *Reelin*, which labels the Cajal–Retzius cells (green) in the cortical preplate. Migrating cells express *Reelin*.

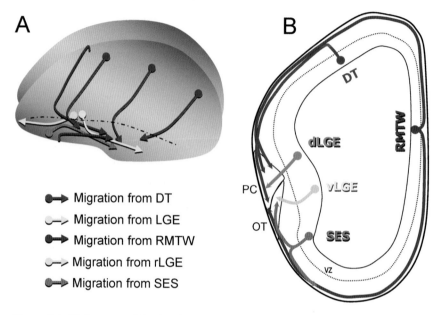

Figure 2.4. Early tangential migrations in the telencephalon converging in the olfactory cortex. **(A)** Cartoon of the telencephalon of an E11 mouse embryo, a lateral view of the left hemisphere. The different migratory routes identified in our studies are represented with a color code. Each cell population generated at E11 that was studied converges in the area of the developing olfactory cortex. Migration from the dorsal telencephalon (DT) and the rostromedial telencephalic wall (RMTW; red and blue arrows, respectively) crosses the cortical preplate initially following a rostral course. When the cells reach the pallial–subpallial boundary (dashed line), they change their migratory direction toward the caudal pole, together with some cell populations that originated in the lateral ganglionic eminence (LGE; yellow arrow) and in the septo-eminential sulcus (SES; orange arrow). In turn, a cell population emerges from the rostral area of the lateral ganglionic eminence (LGE; light blue arrow) that migrates rostrally, below the pallial–subpallial boundary, to the area of the prospective olfactory bulb (pOB). **(B)** Drawing representing a coronal section through the telencephalon of an E11 embryo. Diverse cell populations emerge from all proliferative telencephalic regions that use tangential displacement through the superficial preplate to reach the two main areas of the olfactory cortex, the piriform cortex (PC), and/or the olfactory tubercle (OT). VZ, ventricular zone.

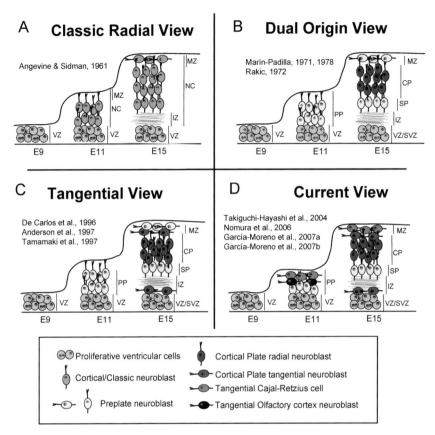

A Classic Radial View

Angevine & Sidman, 1961

MZ
NC
MZ
NC
IZ
VZ VZ VZ

E9   E11   E15

B Dual Origin View

Marín-Padilla, 1971, 1978
Rakic, 1972

MZ
CP
SP
PP
IZ
VZ   VZ   VZ/SVZ

E9   E11   E15

C Tangential View

De Carlos et al., 1996
Anderson et al., 1997
Tamamaki et al., 1997

MZ
CP
SP
PP
IZ
VZ   VZ   VZ/SVZ

E9   E11   E15

D Current View

Takiguchi-Hayashi et al., 2004
Nomura et al., 2006
García-Moreno et al., 2007a
García-Moreno et al., 2007b

MZ
CP
SP
PP
IZ
VZ   VZ   VZ/SVZ

E9   E11   E15

Proliferative ventricular cells

Cortical/Classic neuroblast

Preplate neuroblast

Cortical Plate radial neuroblast

Cortical Plate tangential neuroblast

Tangential Cajal-Retzius cell

Tangential Olfactory cortex neuroblast

Figure 2.5. Evolution of our understanding of cerebral cortex development through different models. (**A**) Model validated up to 1970. All the cortical cells are generated in the germinative area of the neocortical (NC) epithelium, the ventricular zone (VZ). The first layer to develop, the marginal zone (MZ), and the inside-out gradient (radial migration) of the different waves of cell generations, are indicated. (**B**) Model validated from 1970 to 1996. Following the revised nomenclature of the Boulder Committee, this model establish the *dual origin theory*, whereby the cortical plate (CP; source of cortical layers 2–6) originated in the ventricular and subventricular zones (VZ, SVZ), and ascended using the radial glia to colonize the preplate (PP), which is considered of different origin. The PP is divided into an upper marginal zone (MZ; future layer 1) and a lower subplate zone (SP). (**C**) Model validated from 1996 to 2007. Introducing the arrival of different GABAergic cell populations that come from the basal telencephalon and reach the neuroepithelium by tangential migration. (**D**) The current view incorporates the latest discoveries on the early tangential migrations at preplate stages into the previous model; these cells converge at the olfactory cortex. The intermediate zone (IZ) is a fibrous layer present in all the models that will be the white matter in the adult. The lower bar in each model represents different embryonic ages (E9, E11, E15).

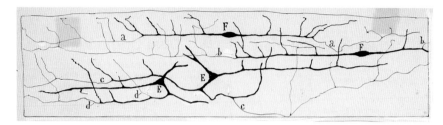

Figure 3.1. Cajal–Retzius cells in cortical layer I. Original drawing by Santiago Ramón y Cajal published originally in 1890 in "Textura de las circunvoluciones cerebrales de los mamíferos inferiores" (Gaceta Médica Catalana, pp. 22–31). Translation of the original figure legend: "Anteroposterior section of the molecular layer of the brain of a two-day old rabbit. F, fusiform cell; E, triangular cells; a, axons of a single fusiform cell; b, another pair of axons of a similar cell; d, axons emerging form the dendritic tree of a triangular cell; c, another pair of axons of a triangular cell."

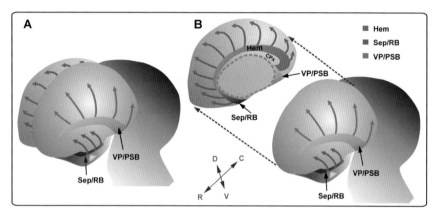

Figure 3.2. Routes of migration of Cajal–Retzius cells. Schematic representation of embryonic telencephalic vesicles (E10.5–12.5 mouse) viewed laterally in a diagram of the whole brain (**A**) and one in which the right telencephalic vesicle has been displaced laterally to view its medial side (**B**). C–R cells generated in the cortical hem in the medial wall (orange) migrate in a caudo-medial to rostro-lateral direction to cover most of the caudal regions of the cortex (only the early stages of migration out of the hem are shown). The septum/retrobulbar C–R cell progenitor domain (Sep/RB, blue) forms a continuous domain from the septum, through the retrobulbar region, and to the rostro-lateral side of the subpallium. C–R cells from this domain migrate dorsally and ventrally toward the rostro-lateral and piriform cortex, respectively. The ventral pallium and pallial–subpallial boundary domain (VP/PSB; green) extends from the caudo-ventral region of the medial telencephalic wall, turns around the ventral region of the telencephalic vesicle, and continues dorso-rostrally on the lateral side of the vesicle. C–R cells from the lateral aspect of this domain populate the piriform cortex and migrate dorsally to cover the lateral aspect of the cortex (CPx; choroid plexus).

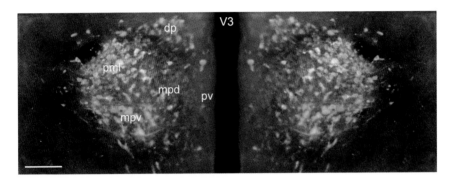

Figure 4.2. Cellular differentiation of the rat PVH at approximately the level illustrated in Fig. 4.1. In this photomicrograph, green neurons were labeled with an antiserum to vasopressin and mark part of the magnocellular neuroendocrine division. At this level, antisera to oxytocin label a thin ring of neurons partly surrounding the vasopressin population (see Fig. 4.3). Red neurons were labeled with an antiserum to corticotrophin-releasing hormone (CRH) and thus mark part of the parvicellular neuroendocrine division. Thyrotropin-releasing hormone (TRH) parvicellular neuroendocrine neurons (not labeled here) form a population centered just medial to (and partly intermixed with) the CRH neurons, and somatostatin (SS) parvicellular neuroendocrine neurons are centered even more medially, in the periventricular part (pv) of the PVH. The two regions of blue neurons were labeled with the retrograde tracer, True Blue, injected into upper thoracic levels of the spinal cord. Other abbreviations: dp, dorsal parvicellular part; mpd, medial parvicellular part, dorsal zone; mpv, medial parvicellular part, ventral zone; pml, posterior magnocellular part, lateral zone; V3, third ventricle (hypothalamic part). Photo of right side flipped to create pseudobilateral view. Scale bar = 200 μm. Adapted from Swanson et al. (1986).

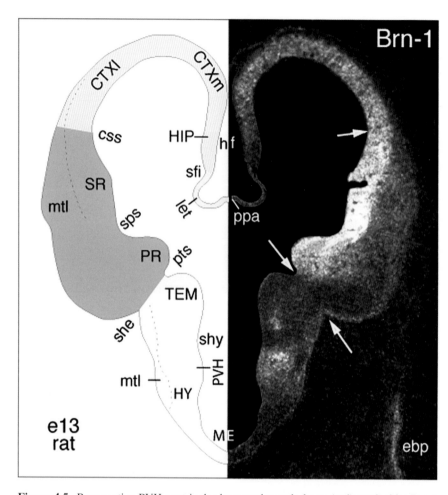

Figure 4.5. Presumptive PVH ventricular layer and mantle layer (mtl) marked by Brn-1 expression (white label in this dark-field photomicrograph, on the right) on embryonic day 13. Note that expression of this homeobox gene also clearly distinguishes the telencephalic vesicle (pink in schematic anatomical drawing on the left) from the diencephalic vesicle (yellow) at this transverse level of the forebrain treated for in situ hybridization. Other abbreviations: css, corticostriatal sulcus; CTXl,m, cortex, median and lateral regions; ebp, epibranchial placodes; hf, hippocampal fissure; HIP, hippocampus; HY, hypothalamus; let, epithelial lamina; ME, median eminence; ppa, parahypophysial arch; PR, pallidal (medial ventricular) ridge; pts, pallidothalamic sulcus; sfi, fimbrial sulcus; she, hemispheric sulcus; SR, striatal (lateral ventricular) ridge; TEM, thalamic eminence. Adapted from Swanson (2000).

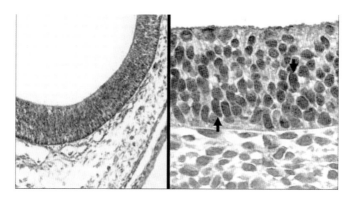

Figure 5.2. Immunohistochemistry for androgen receptor revealing positive nuclear staining. The presence of the protein in the neuroepithelium is observed in paraffin embedded samples of the forebrain of chicken (HH13) and mouse (E9.5) embryos.

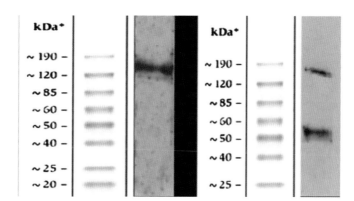

Figure 5.3. Representative western blot of the AR protein from homogenates of cerebral vesicles of the mouse embryo E9.5 observing the presence of a band of ≈110 kDa expected for the AR protein (left); mouse prostate was used as positive control (right).

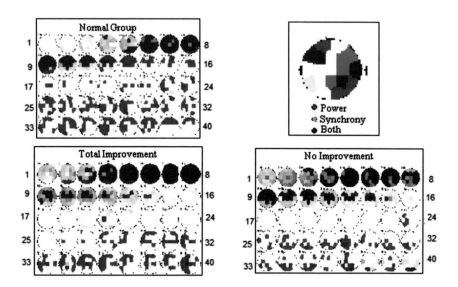

Figure 6.1. Display of significant (p < 0.01) increases in power and synchrony from 3 months to 12 months old in the different groups. Each circle corresponds to a head (front in the upper portion) at different frequencies from 1 Hz to 40 Hz. Magenta color indicates a significant (p < 0.01) increase in power. Cyan color corresponds to a significant (p < 0.01) increase in synchrony. Blue stands for common increases in power and synchrony.

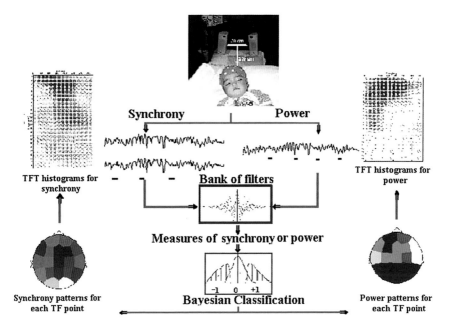

Figure 6.2. Analysis pathway. Selected EEG recordings (one channel for computation of power, two channels for the calculation of phase synchrony) are passed through a bank of band-pass filters (SQFs) centered at 1 Hz intervals (from 1 Hz to 40 Hz). Power analysis is performed by taking the log-power of each filtered signal and subtracting the pre-stimulus average. Phase-synchrony is obtained by estimating the mean phase difference, baseline-corrected by subtracting its pre-stimulus average. Baseline log-power and synchrony values are classified using a Bayesian estimation procedure, indicating significantly (p<0.01) higher (+1), equal (0), or lower (-1) values than pre-stimulus values. In this way, maps for increasing or decreasing values are constructed (not shown in the diagram). For each frequency and time it is possible to display a simple head diagram. In this illustration significant (p<0.01) increasing values for both power and synchrony were selected. However, differential colors indicate the stimulus condition, magenta for syllables, cyan for tones, and blue when in both conditions values increased in relation to baseline. A time-frequency topography (TFT) or multitoscopic display is obtained by dividing the time-frequency plane into cells for each Hz and every 50 ms. Thus, a representative head diagram at each cell (the mode of all class values within the cell) is produced.

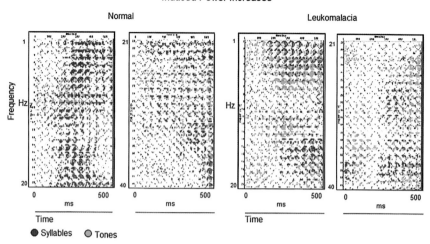

Figure 6.3. Multitoposcopic display of significant (p<0.01) increases in power. Time is plotted in the x-axis and frequency in the y-axis. Magenta color indicates an increase in power only in the syllables condition. Cyan color corresponds to an increase in power only in the tones condition. Blue indicates common increases in power.

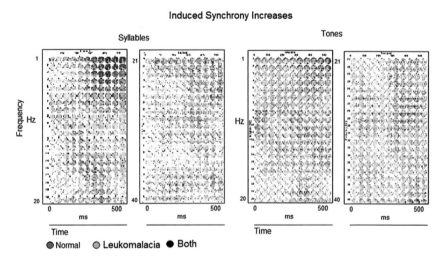

Figure 6.4. Multitoposcopic display of significant (p<0.01) increases in synchrony. Time is plotted in the x-axis and frequency in the y-axis. Magenta color indicates an increase in synchrony only in the syllables condition. Cyan color corresponds to an increase in synchrony only in the tones condition. Blue indicates common increases in synchrony.

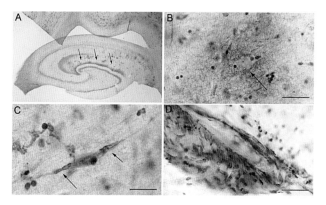

Figure 9.2. Aβ pathology in the aged canine brain. (**A**) Aβ accumulates as diffuse plaques and within the outer molecular layer in the hippocampus (arrows). (**B**) At higher magnification, Aβ within a diffuse plaque appears fibrillar but intact neurons (arrow) can be found within these deposits. (**C**) A subset of neurons in the entorhinal cortex show Aβ accumulation on dendrites (arrow). (**D**) Cerebrovascular Aβ can be observed in the walls of leptomeningeal blood vessels. All sections were immunolabeled with anti-Aβ1-42 after 90% formic acid pretreatment and counterstained with cresyl violet. Bars in B, C, D = 20μm.

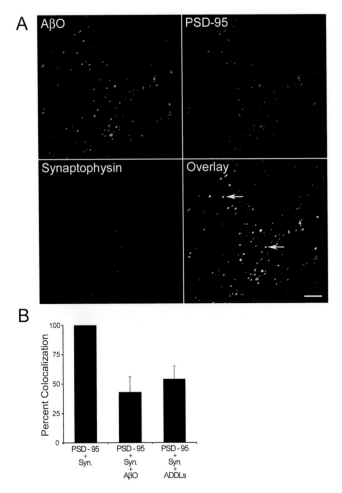

Figure 10.1. AßO colocalize with synaptic markers in HCN. (**A**) Triple immunofluorescence of 18 DIV HCN with anti-Aß oligomers (AßO; A11, green, 1:2500), anti-PSD-95 (red, 1:1000), and anti-synaptophysin (blue, 1:500). Cultures were incubated with 5μm AßO for 1 hr before fixation. The overlay image shows the co-localization of the three antibodies. Triple co-localization is observed as light yellow fluorescent spots (arrows). Scale bar = 5μm. (**B**) Quantification of the frequency of co-localization of AßO and ADDLs (antibody A11) with the synaptic markers PSD-95 and synaptophysin (PSD-95+Syn.+AßO, PSD-95+Syn.+ADDLs).

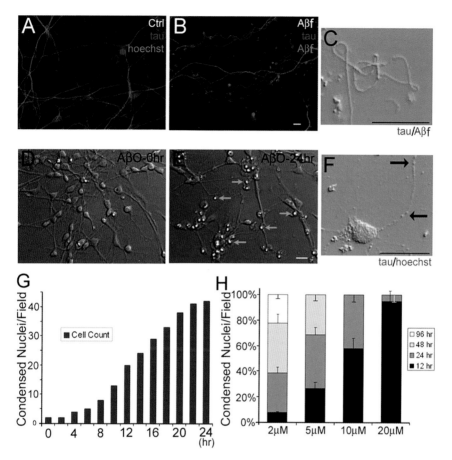

Figure 10.2. AßO cause rapid and massive neuronal death. Double immunofluorescence of 18 DIV HCN with anti-tau (red, 1:500) and anti-Aß (blue). (**A**) Neuronal processes in vehicle-treated HCN exhibit considerable development and a normal, smooth appearance (Ctrl). (**B**) After 10 days of treatment with 20μm Aßf, neuronal processes display aberrant morphologies, including tortuosity and irregular neuritic caliber. (**C**) Combined DIC/fluorescence at higher magnification illustrates a neuronal process exhibiting loops and sharp turns close to Aßf deposits (blue). (**D–F**) DIC images of living HCN cultures treated with 5μm AßO. Immediately after AßO addition the culture exhibits normal appearance (**D**); after 24 hr extensive cell death is indicated by retraction and disintegration of processes, and by nuclear condensation (arrows, **E**). At higher magnification, the beading and disintegration of neuronal processes is clearly observed (arrows, **F**). Scale bars = 20μm. (**G**) Quantification of condensed nuclei/field over the 24 hr period of AßO treatment. The graph illustrates one representative field. At least 20 different fields were analyzed with similar results. (**H**) Bar graph illustrating the increase in condensed nuclei in HCN cultures treated with increasing concentrations of AßO. The number of condensed nuclei was scored at the indicated time points. Similar results were obtained in 5 independent experiments.

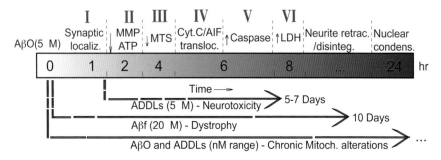

Figure 10.3. Timeline of neurodegenerative events induced by Aß toxic species. Progression of AßO- and ADDL-induced neurotoxicity: (**I**) synaptic localization of AßO and ADDLs; (**II**) reduced mitochondrial membrane potential (MMP) and ATP levels; (**III**) reduced mitochondrial oxidoreductase activity (MTS); (**IV**) cyt C and AIF translocation from the mitochondrial matrix to the cytosol; (**V**) increase caspase activity; (**VI**) increased LDH levels in culture medium, massive neuritic retraction and disintegration, and nuclear condensation. The timeline for AßO is 24 hr. ADDLs are already detected at synaptic sites by 1 hr, but progression of similar alterations takes 96 hr. Aßf (20μm) requires 10 days to induce generalized neuronal dystrophy and modest cell death. Lower concentrations (nM range) of AßO and ADDLs lead to chronic mitochondrial dysfunction and minimal cell death over time.

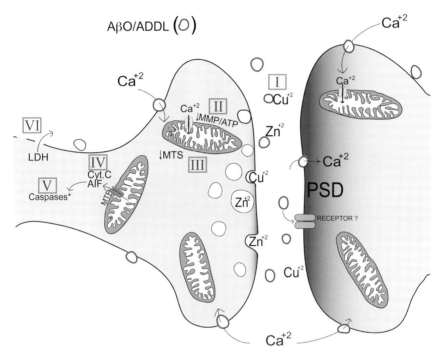

Figure 10.4. Proposed model of Aβ soluble species neurotoxicity. The alterations included in the timeline in Fig. 10.3 (**I–VI**) are illustrated taking place at a synapse. AβO or ADDLs (red circles) are recruited to synaptic sites, where they associate with metal ions (Cu^{+2} and Zn^{+2}) or bind post-synaptic receptors (**I**). The pore-/channel-forming activity of Aβ soluble species causes massive calcium influx, general destabilization of ion homeostasis, and mitochondrial alterations (**II**, reduced MMP and ATP; **III**, reduced MTS), leading to the opening of the mitochondrial transition pore (MTP) and cyt C and AIF translocation (**IV**), caspase activation (**V**), and cell death evidenced by LDH release (**VI**). PSD, post-synaptic density.

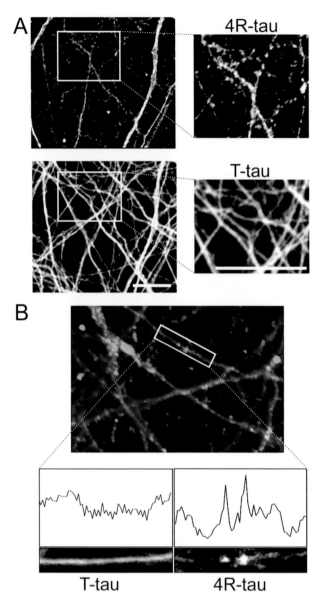

Figure 10.5. Differential distribution of 3R and 4R tau in HCN. (**A**) Double immunofluorescence analysis of HCN at 20 days in culture with anti-4R tau (clone 4RT) and polyclonal anti-total tau antibodies illustrate the stippled appearance of 4R immunoreactivity along axonal processes in sharp contrast with the smooth-textured appearance of total tau immunoreactivity. Insets in the left panels correspond to regions magnified in the right panels. (**B**) Densitometric analysis of immunofluorescence signal intensity along axonal processes revealed significantly larger peaks and valleys in the 4R tau densitometric profile compared to that of total tau. The images correspond to the same microscopic field. Scale bars = 20μm.

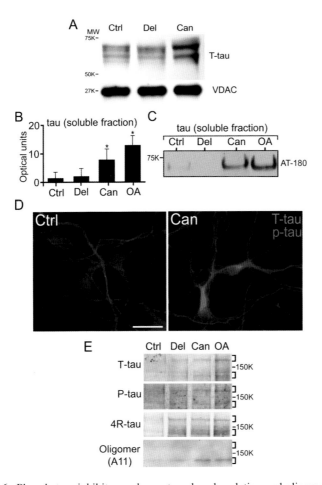

Figure 10.6. Phosphatase inhibitors enhance tau phosphorylation and oligomerization in HCN. (**A**) Western blot of HCN treated with 40 pM deltamethrin (Del) and 10 nM cantharidin (Can) for 10 days, homogenized, and probed with polyclonal anti-tau (T-tau) and anti-VDAC antibodies. All treatments were initiated at day 20 in culture. Note the change in the profile of tau isoforms after cantharidin treatment. (**B**) Dot blot quantification of total tau in the soluble fraction of cytoskeletal preparations after treatment with deltamethrin and cantharidin at the concentrations indicated above, and 5 nM okadaic acid (OA). (**C**) There is a significant increase in soluble tau after treatment with cantharidin and okadaic acid, which was accompanied by a marked elevation in phosphorylated tau in the soluble fraction, as shown after blotting with antibody AT-180, which recognizes tau phosphorylated at Thr231. (**D**) Double immunofluorescence analysis with polyclonal anti-tau (T-tau, blue channel) and PHF-1 (phosphorylated tau at Ser 396/404, red channel) illustrates both the increase in phosphorylated tau immunoreactivity and its translocation to the somatodendritic compartment after cantharidin (Can) treatment. PHF-1 immunoreactivity was negative in nontreated cells (Ctrl). (**E**) Western blot of HCN treated with cantharidin (Can) and okadaic acid (OA) showed induction of ~140–170 kD tau multimers, which labeled positive with an antibody that recognizes all tau isoforms (T-tau). Anti-phosphorylated tau antibody AT-180 preferentially labeled the ~170kD bands (P-tau). The multimers were also strongly labeled by anti-4R tau antibody (clone 4RT). Lower MW multimers (~140 kD) were detected by the conformation-dependent antibody A11, which recognizes oligomeric structures regardless of the protein sequence (A11). Scale bar = 20μm.

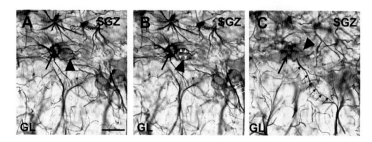

Figure 12.1. Light photomicrographs of double-labeled preparations showing DCX-positive cells (brown) and GFAP-positive astrocytes (purple) in the subgranular zone (SGZ). **A–C** show a through-focus series of a DCX-labeled cell (black arrowheads) that has a rudimentary process. A GFAP-immunolabeled astrocyte (large black arrows) is adjacent to this cell, and its fine GFAP-immunolabeled bundles (white arrowheads in **B**) wrap around the DCX-labeled cell. Note that this astrocyte has a radial process (small black arrows) extending through the GL in panel **C**. Another GFAP-positive radial process (white arrows in **B**) is adjacent to an apical dendrite of a DCX-labeled cell in the granule cell layer (GL). Scale bar = 10μm. Reprinted with permission from Shapiro et al. (2005).

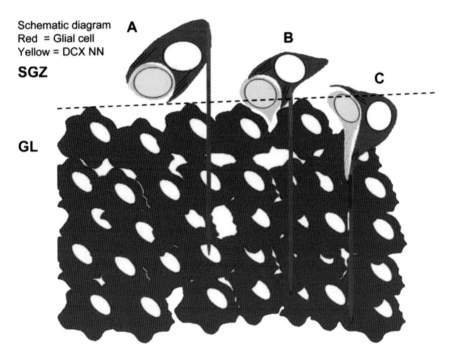

Figure 12.4. A schematic diagram shows the described one-to-one relationship in the adult dentate gyrus between a GFAP-expressing radial glia-like cell (red) and the DCX-labeled newly generated neuron (NN) (yellow). In **A**, an NN in the subgranular zone (SGZ) is cradled by the nonradial processes of a radial astrocyte. Note that the NN lacks processes and the majority of its surface is enveloped by this astrocyte that also sends a radial process through the granule cell layer (GL). In **B**, the NN displays a rudimentary apical process that projects into the GL. Note that the NN is still apposed by some of the nonradial processes of the GFAP-expressing radial glia-like cell. **C** shows a later stage in the development of an NN, where its apical dendrite extends into the GL. Note that this apical dendrite is apposed to the radial process of a radial astrocyte and this radial process provides a scaffold for the apical dendrite to extend. The blue cells represent mature granule cells in the GL. Reprinted with permission from Shapiro et al. (2005).

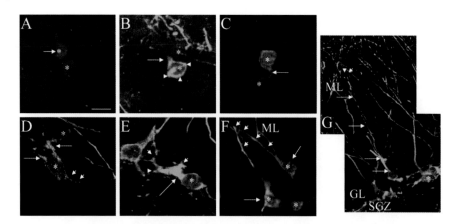

Figure 12.6. Confocal micrographs of BrdU-immunolabeled and DCX/BrdU double-immunolabeled cells at 4–96 hr after a single BrdU injection in adult rat dentate gyrus. In **A**, a pair of BrdU-labeled cells (asterisks) is shown at the 4 hr time point at the base of the granule cell layer. Note that the double-labeled cell (arrow) has a rudimentary DCX-labeled apical process. In **B**, another pair of BrdU-labeled cells (asterisks) at the base of the granule cell layer is shown at 12 hr after BrdU injection. Note the thin shell of DCX-labeled perikaryal cytoplasm (arrowheads) and a rudimentary DCX-labeled apical process (arrow). In **C** and **D**, pairs of BrdU-labeled cells are shown (asterisks) from the 24 hr time point. In each case, one of the BrdU-labeled cells is double-labeled for DCX (arrow), whereas the other cell is not. In **C**, the double-labeled cell has a basal dendrite, but no apical dendrite is observed. In **D**, the double-labeled cell has two apical dendrites extending into the granule cell layer (arrows) and a basal process (arrowheads) that is curving toward the granule cell layer, as described for recurrent basal dendrites (Ribak et al., 2000). In **E**, a double-labeled cell (asterisk) is shown lying horizontally at the base of the granule cell layer from the 48 hr time point. Note that this cell has a thick apical process (arrow) with several branches displaying growth cones (arrowheads). In **F**, 3 BrdU-labeled cells (asterisks) are shown from the 72 hr time point, 2 of which are double-labeled with DCX (arrows) and the third that has a DCX-labeled process adjacent to it. Note that the 2 double-labeled cells have apical dendrites (arrowheads) that extend through the granule cell layer and into the molecular layer (ML) at this time point. In **G**, a BrdU/DCX double-labeled cell is shown from the 96 hr time point in the granule cell layer with its apical dendrite (arrows) extending into the ML and a terminal branching (arrowheads). Also, note that there is a second double-labeled cell (asterisk) located at the base of the granule cell layer (GL) adjacent to the subgranular zone (SGZ). Scale bar in **A** = 10μm for **A–E**, 15μm for **F**, and 20μm for **G**. Reprinted with permission from Shapiro et al. (2007b).

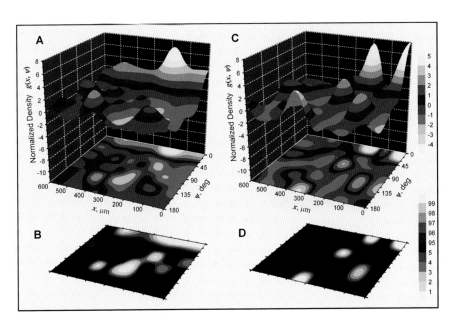

Figure 13.2. Neuronal density fields computed for two mutually orthogonal dimensions: perpendicular (**A,B**) and parallel (**C,D**) to the cortical surface. **A** and **C**, 3D landscape of the density $g(x, \psi)$ of pairs of cells recorded at a spatial distance x and showing an angular deviation ψ between their PDs. **B** and **D**, 2D contour map showing the probability $p(x, \psi)$ that the neuronal density field, produced by a uniformly random sample, was less than the density field generated from actual penetrations. Color scales are shown to the right. Modified from Amirikian and Georgopoulos (2003).

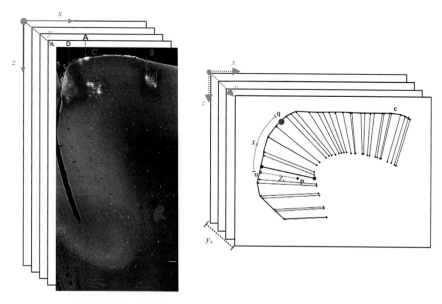

Figure 13.3. Left panel: electrode trajectory parameters are measured using fluorescence imaging: grayscale image of a sagittal section through the CS. Axes of the extrinsic coordinate system used to express recording site coordinates are depicted as blue arrows labeled x, y, and z. Black borders surrounding the image indicate its position within a stack of similar images. Marks made by dye-coated electrodes from several penetrations appear as bright white blobs. **A**: insertion point for an electrode. **B**: marks made by 2 coated electrodes at the corners of the same array. **C**: red circles show intersection of the current slice and all 16 reconstructed electrode trajectories from a single penetration. **D**: in some cases, diffusion of the fluorescent dye away from corner electrodes outlined the full region covered by the 16-electrode array. Scale bar = 0.5mm.

Right panel: unfolded coordinates are derived from measurements taken in each Nissl slice: unfolded coordinates of each recording site are a function of the measurements (X_N, Y_N, Z_N) shown here with dashed lines. The black diamond–labeled p indicates the position within a slice of a single recording site. The dashed line segment extending from the recording site is parallel to the nearest labeled anatomical column (thick black line; other columns shown by thin black lines). The small black dot labeled u is the intersection of this line segment with the cortical surface c. X_N measures the distance along c between u and q, the crown of the CS (large red dot). Z_N measures the distance between u and p within the plane of section. Y_N measures the distance from the most medial sagittal slice. For comparison, axes of the extrinsic coordinate system are shown as blue arrows labeled x, y, and z. Used with permission and modified from Naselaris et al. (2005).

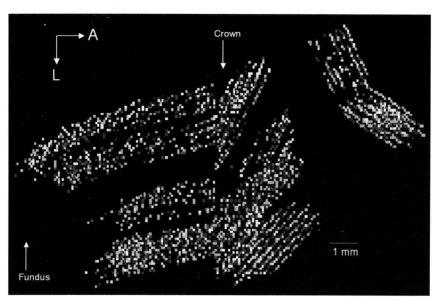

Figure 13.4. Location on the flattened motor cortical surface of the preferred directions of directionally tuned sites. The octant of the unit sphere to which a preferred direction belongs is color-coded depending on the sign of the directional cosines [*x, y, z*]. (Modified from Georgopoulos et al. 2007.) A, anterior; L, lateral.

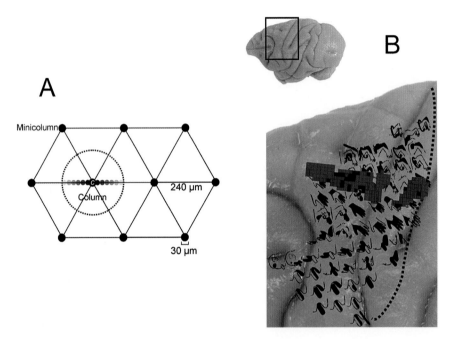

Figure 13.6. (**A**) Schematic model of short-range tangential organization of preferred directions in the motor cortex. The letter c inside a black circle denotes a minicolumn at the center of a 240μm column, depicted as a dashed circle. Inside the column there is a gradient (in gray scale) of minicolumns, whose PDs become farther and farther away from the PD in c. The other black circles are minicolumns with the same preferred direction. (**B**) Model of the motor cortical hypercolumns with a surface area of 3 mm², with bimodial (red), unimodal (blue), or uniform (black) local PD distribution superimposed on the somatotopic organization of the primary motor cortex, taken from the original maps of Woolsey et al. (1952).

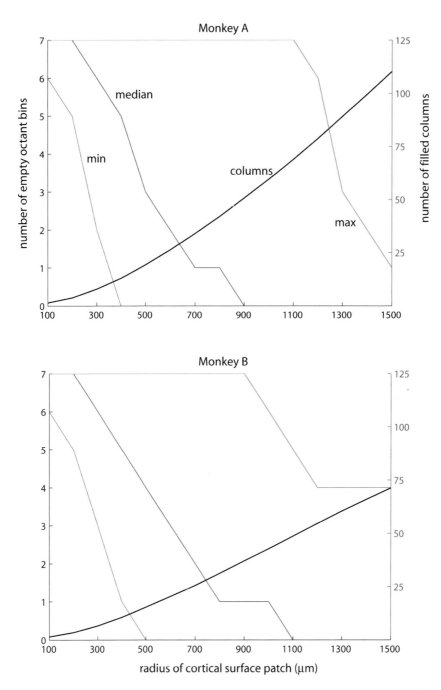

Figure 13.7. Spatial scale of PD dispersion. The number of empty octants was counted for the set of PDs within a circular region of a given radius (abscissa) centered at each recording site. Minimum, median, and maximum number of empty octants (left axis) as a function of radius is shown by the green, blue, and red lines, respectively. Black line shows the average number of column-sized (80μm diameter) patches within each circular region that contained a recording site (right axis). Used with permission and modified from Naselaris et al. (2006b).

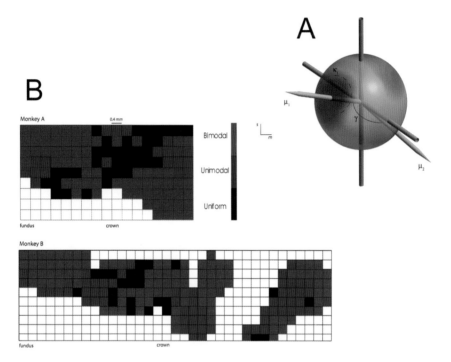

Figure 13.8. (**A**) 3D representation of the distribution of PDs. The sphere is rotated so that the forward pole appears in the foreground. The perspective is that of an observer facing the monkey; thus the hemisphere to the viewer's right of the blue meridian corresponds to reaching directions to the monkey's left. Gray cylinders extend from the up/down and left/right poles. Green arrows extending from the surface show the direction of the two modes (μ_1 and μ_2), the dashed circle surrounding the forward mode is the corresponding dispersion (κ_1), and γ is the angle between the two modes. These values were obtained from a mixture model for the global distribution of PDs (modified from Naselaris et al. 2006a). (**B**) Surface maps of local PD distributions. This map was constructed by partitioning the cortical surface into overlapping squares spaced at 400μm intervals with a side of 1.6mm. The distribution of PDs in each region is classified as uniform (black), unimodal (blue), or bimodal (red). Used with permission and modified from Naselaris et al. (2006b).

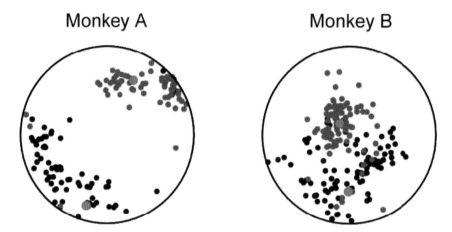

Figure 13.9. Distribution of local primary directions. A mixture model was fitted to the distribution of PDs in each local region defined as nonuniform. Primary directions from each of these local regions are shown under an equal-area projection, where red dots indicate the forward hemisphere and black dots the backward hemisphere. Primary directions for the global distribution are shown as large green dots. Used with permission and modified from Naselaris et al. (2006b).

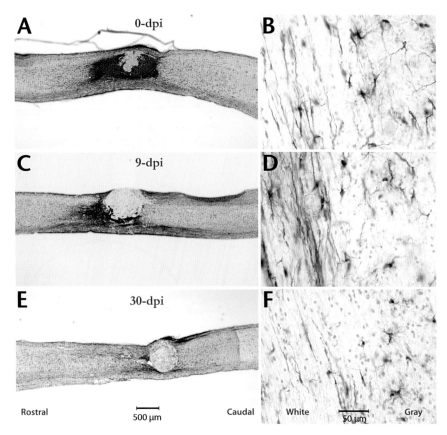

A 0-dpi

B

C 9-dpi

D

E 30-dpi

F

Rostral   500 μm   Caudal   White   50 μm   Gray

Figure 15.1. (**A–F**): Survival, migration, and site-specific differentiation of HuCNS-SCs in the injured mouse spinal cord. Photomicrographs of spinal cord 12 weeks (0-dpi) or 16 weeks (9-dpi and 30-pdi) post-transplantation immunostained for a human cytoplasmic marker (SC121, brown DAB, StemCells, Inc.) and counterstained with methyl green to reveal host mouse cells. Scale bar for **A, C,** and **E** = 500μm; scale bar for **B, D,** and **E** = 50μm. All images are orientated the same as indicated in **E** or **F** (**A, C, E,** rostral to the left; **B, D, F,** white matter to the left). (**A**) Low-power parasagittal image from an acute (0-dpi) transplant demonstrating many SC121 immunopositive human cells (brown) migrated toward the lesion epicenter as well as rostral and caudal from the injection sites. Human cells within the epicenter were predominantly GFAP-positive astrocytes (not shown). (**B**) High-power image of SC121 immunopositive human cells (brown) at a site distal to the lesion demonstrates that human cells were morphologically distinct depending on locus within either white matter or gray matter in an acute transplant. (**C**) Low-power parasagittal image demonstrating SC121 immunopositive cells (brown) migrated away from the lesion epicenter in a subacute (9-dpi) transplant. (**D**) High-power image of SC121 immunopositive human cells (brown) with the morphological appearance of oligodendrocytes in white matter and neuronal phenotypes in gray matter in a subacute transplant. (**E**) Low-power parasagittal image demonstrating SC121 immunopositive human cells (brown) migrated away from the lesion epicenter in a chronic (30-dpi) transplant. (**F**) High-power image of SC121 immunopositive human cells (brown) with the morphological appearance of oligodendrocytes in white matter and neuronal phenotypes in gray matter.

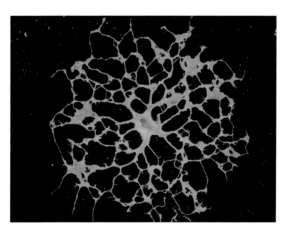

Figure 16.1 Photomicrograph of galactocerebroside-immunostained oligodendrocyte derived from human embryonic stem cell cultures.

Wiltse J. Mode of action: inhibition of histone deacetylase, altering WNT-dependent gene expression, and regulation of beta-catenin-developmental effects of valproic acid. *Crit Rev Toxicol* 2005; 35(8–9):727–38.

Wlodarczyk B, Tang L, Triplett A, Aleman F, Finnell RH. Spontaneous neural tube defects in splotch mice supplemented with selected micronutrients. *Toxicol Appl Pharmacol* 2006; 213:55–63.

Ybot-Gonzalez P, Copp AJ. Bending of the neural plate during mouse spinal neurulation is independent of actin microfilaments. *Dev Dyn* 1999; 215:273–83.

Yoshizawa J, Sbragia L, Paek BW, Sydorak RM, Yamazaki Y, Harrison MR, Farmer DL. Fetal surgery for repair of myelomeningocele allows normal development of anal sphincter muscles in sheep. *Pediatr Surg Int* 2004; 20:14–8.

Zhang L, Chang Y, Barker J, Hu Q, Zhang L, Maric D, Li B and Rubinow D. Testosterone and estrogen affect neuronal differentiation but not proliferation in early embryonic cortex of the rat: the possible roles of androgen and estrogen receptors. *Neuroscience Letters* 2000; 281(1):57–60.

Chapter Six

Quantitative Electroencephalography in the Normal and Abnormal Developing Human Brain

Thalía Harmony, Alfonso Alba, José Luis Marroquín,
Antonio Fernández-Bouzas, Gloria Avecilla,
Josefina Ricardo-Garcell, Efraín Santiago-Rodríguez,
Gloria Otero, Eneida Porras-Kattz, and Thalía Fernández

INTRODUCTION

Electroencephalographic (EEG) waves recorded from the scalp are integrated excitatory and inhibitory postsynaptic potentials of neuronal membranes. They reflect extracellular currents caused by synchronized neural activity within the local brain volume. Oscillations in the EEG indicate periodic activity of large populations of synchronized neurons, usually called neuronal assemblies, a term coined by Hebb (1949). It has been proposed that such distributed network formation is involved in a variety of cognitive operations: sensory integration, object representation, selective attention, memory encoding and retrieval, and language comprehension (Mesulam 1990; Bastiaansen and Hagoort 2003). Synchronization of neural activities is widely known to occur in individual neural firing and among the local field potentials of cortical regions; consequently it is thought to be a potentially powerful temporal structuring strategy that links anatomically and functionally related regions of the brain (Freeman 1991; Singer and Gray 1995; Varela et al. 2001).

According to Lopes da Silva and Van Rotterdam (2005) two kinds of factors determine the properties of EEG oscillations: (1) the intrinsic membrane properties of the neurons (depolarizing or hyperpolarizing currents) and the dynamics of synaptic processes (excitatory and inhibitory postsynaptic potentials, dendritic events as calcium action potentials), and (2) the strength and extent of interconnections between the network elements producing synchrony on neuronal activity. The main factor that produces synchrony is of a structural nature. Neuronal masses are, in general, organized as combinations of interlocked excitatory and inhibitory populations. The interlocking takes place by way of recurrent collaterals forming different type of synapses that possibly include dendrodendritic synapses and even gap junctions. Synchrony at a larger scale is most often produced by thalamo-cortical or cortico-cortical feedback loops, either at short or long distances.

The human brain undergoes complex organizational changes during development in- and ex utero. Pathogenic events affecting the developing brain cause abnormalities or lesions, the patterns of which depend on the stage of brain development. During the first and second trimester, cortical neurogenesis takes place predominantly, characterized by proliferation, migration, and organization of neuronal cells. Brain pathology is characterized by maldevelopments. During the third trimester, growth and differentiation events prevail and persist into postnatal life. Disturbances of brain development during this period cause mainly lesions. During the early third trimester, periventricular white matter is especially affected, whereas toward the end of the third trimester, gray matter—either cortical or deep gray matter—appears to be more vulnerable (Volpe 2001; Bhutta and Anand 2002). By around the time of birth in humans, the sulci and gyri of the cerebral cortex are visible, though relatively immature in terms of inter- and intraregional connectivity. There is a rapid increase in synaptogenesis around the time of birth for all cortical areas studied; the most rapid burst of synapse formation and the peak density of synapses occurs at different ages in different areas. In the visual cortex there is a rapid burst of synapse formation between 3 months and 4 months (corrected age), and the maximum density—about 150% of the adult level—is reached between 4 months and 12 months (corrected age). Synaptogenesis starts at the same time in the prefrontal cortex, but the density of synapses increases much more slowly and does not reach its peak until well after the first year (Johnson 2001; Krageloh-Mann 2004). Myelination seems to begin at birth in the pons and cerebellar peduncles, and by 3 months has extended to the optic radiation and splenium of the corpus callosum. At around 8–12 months of age, the white matter associated with the frontal, parietal, and occipital lobes becomes apparent (Paus 2001).

Much of the research on neural and behavioral development has related the anatomical maturation of a specific region of the brain to newly emerging sensory, motor, and cognitive functions. However, it is important to consider that postnatal functional brain development—at least within the cerebral cortex—involves a process of organization of inter-regional interactions. In the study of brain development it is becoming evident that new cognitive functions during infancy and childhood may be the result of emerging patterns of interactions between different regions (Johnson 2001).

In this chapter we will give an overview of the normal and abnormal development of the EEG during the first year after birth. An extensive review of EEG characteristics at different weeks of gestation has been made by Niedermeyer (2005). The origins of the different EEG oscillations in the newborn are unknown. At birth the baby already has the functional organization for the sleep-wakefulness cycle. The EEG and polygraphic characteristics may identify quiet and active sleep cycles (Otero 2005). During the first 3 months of life the EEG and polygraphic data indicate sleep onset with active (REM) sleep in neonates and gradual evolution of sleep onset with quiet (non-REM) sleep during the ensuing weeks. The "slow" sleep of the infant is dominated by diffuse delta (0.7–3 Hz) activity, with a maximum of amplitude over the occipital areas. There are some intermixed theta (4–7 Hz), alpha (8–13 Hz), and beta (14–30 Hz) frequencies of smaller amplitudes. Spindles appear usually during the second month of life, and the spindle frequency ranges from 12–15 Hz, with 14 Hz preponderance. Throughout infancy, spindles are maximal over central and parietal areas. Spindles are originated by reticular thalamic-cortical loops (Steriade et al. 1993). Vertex waves and K complexes are usually seen around the age of 5 months, although rudiments may be seen much earlier. The delay in the appearance of these features is considered abnormal.

These observations have been made by visual inspection of EEG records; hence EEG background activity of higher frequencies has been difficult to describe. The Goteborg group headed by Ingemar Petersén was the first to describe quantitative variables for EEG maturation and create the first quantitative EEG (qEEG) norms from 1 year to 20 years old. They used analog filters to describe power in different bands: delta, theta, alpha 1, alpha 2, beta 1, and beta 2 (Matousek and Petersén 1973). Hagne et al. (1973), of the same school, used the Fast Fourier Transform for EEG analysis in 20 children recorded every 2 months of age, between birth and 1 year old. They studied only frequencies from 1 Hz to 12.5 Hz and reported the decrease in delta power and the increase in mean frequencies. Other authors have made qEEG analysis from delta to beta frequencies in healthy full-term newborns (Willekens et al. 1984) and prematures (Victor et al. 2005), as well as comparisons between premature and full-term newborns (Scher et al. 1994; Joseph et al. 1976). However, the studies evaluating brain maturation by qEEG analysis are scarce (Thatcher 1999).

NORMAL AND ABNORMAL EEG MATURATION

In this chapter we report the evolution of EEG power and synchrony between each pair of electrodes during the first year of age. In this study we analyzed the differences in power and synchrony of EEG background activity between 3 months and 12 months of age in 3 groups of infants. Infants of the three groups had periodic clinical and psychological evaluations up to 18 months. The results of these evaluations at this age and the magnetic resonance imaging results in the first month of age were used for the classification into groups:

1. Normal infants (n = 23)
2. Infants with leukomalacia (*diffuse cerebral white matter injury*) with a normal outcome at 18 months (n = 9),
3. Infants with leukomalacia with an abnormal outcome and neurological sequels at 18 months (n = 8)

EEG recordings were obtained at 1–3 months and 10–12 months (corrected age). The EEG was recorded in the 10/20 International System during quiet sleep or sleep phase II. EEG segments, lasting 2.56 seconds with no artifacts or vertex responses, sleep spindles, and synchronous runs of slow activity were obtained. The first step of the analysis consisted in passing these EEG signals through a bank of quadrature band-pass filters to extract amplitude and phase information for each signal. In particular, we used sinusoidal quadrature filters (SQFs) (Guerrero et al. 2005), which provide more reliable phase estimates at low tuning frequencies than the typical Gabor filters (for a detailed description, see Alba et al. 2006). In the case of induced changes in amplitude and synchronization, the analysis is commonly performed by first subtracting a baseline level from the measure of interest (amplitude or synchrony). Typically, this baseline level is obtained as the average of the measure across a time segment corresponding to a neutral condition. This is done to estimate relative changes of the measure with respect to the neutral condition. However, when analyzing the EEG at rest, there is not necessarily a neutral condition against which a comparison can be made; thus the baseline level is unknown. One way to overcome this problem consists in using the relative amplitude $R_{\omega,j,e}(t)$ and relative synchrony $\mu_{\omega,j,e}(t)$ instead, that is, the amplitude or synchrony at each frequency band divided by the sum of amplitude or synchrony, respectively, across all frequency bands.

For the comparison of EEG relative power (RP) or relative synchrony (RS) at 3 months and 12 months, as well as among groups, differences were assessed by nonparametric statistics at $p < 0.01$ (see Appendix). The results of the comparisons of EEG RP and RS between 3 months and 12 months for each group are shown in Figure 6.1.

In the normal group, power and synchrony increased from 6 Hz to 9 Hz in all regions and from 10 Hz to 12 Hz in frontal regions. Power also increased from 25 Hz to 40 Hz mainly in the left hemisphere. Synchronization increases were also present at 4 Hz and 5 Hz.

In the group with total improvement (TI), power and synchrony increased from 4 Hz to 8 Hz in all regions. Synchrony also increased from 1 Hz to 3 Hz in all regions and from 9 Hz to 13 Hz; at these last frequencies central increases in power were found. Power increased also from 28 Hz to 40 Hz.

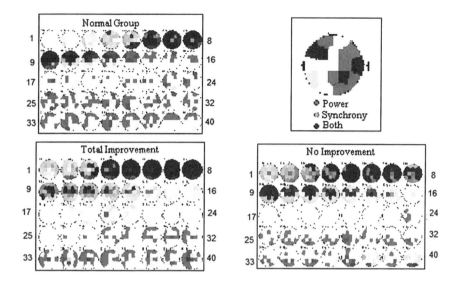

Figure 6.1. Display of significant (p < 0.01) increases in power and synchrony from 3 months to 12 months old in the different groups. Each circle corresponds to a head (front in the upper portion) at different frequencies from 1 Hz to 40 Hz. Magenta color indicates a significant (p < 0.01) increase in power. Cyan color corresponds to a significant (p < 0.01) increase in synchrony. Blue stands for common increases in power and synchrony. (See color Figure 6.1)

The group with no improvement (NI) showed power and synchrony increases in all regions from 5 Hz to 8 Hz and at 9–11 Hz only in frontal regions. In addition, increased synchrony at 1–4 Hz and increased power from 25 Hz to 40 Hz were also observed.

The comparison between the groups at 3 months old showed inconsistent results. However, at 12 months old, clear differences appeared:

1. At 12 months, infants with TI showed more theta power than normal infants, whereas infants with NI exhibited more delta power than normal infants. Evidence indicates that increased delta activity is related to cortical deafferentation (Gloor et al. 1977), suggesting that infants with NI have a myelination delay. An increase in theta activity in childhood has been reported in children with learning (Harmony et al. 1990, 1995; Chabot et al. 2001) and attention deficit (Chabot et al. 2001; Ricardo-Garcell 2004) disorders, suggesting underlying delayed brain maturation in these children. We do not know whether the presence of more theta at 1 year old is the precedence for a possible cognitive disorder later in development. The follow-up of these children may give an answer to this question. If this were the case, EEG recordings at 1 year old in those infants with such biological risk antecedents as prematurity, low birth weight, and asphyxia,

may be of great importance in order to begin with sensory and attentional early stimulation. There are several reports relating prematurity and low birth weight to deficits in performance in cognitive tests at 8 years old and older (Marlow et al., 1993; Rickards et al. 2001).

2. Normal infants showed more alpha, beta, and gamma power than the other two groups, indicating more advanced brain maturation.

3. The normal and TI groups showed higher synchrony at 25–40 Hz than the NI group. Synchronization of gamma frequencies has been related to several cognitive processes, including visual perception, attention, learning, and memory (for a review, see Kaiser and Lutzenberger 2005), and even consciousness (Melloni et al. 2007). Thus, the lower synchrony in the NI group may be related to cognitive deficiencies. We have found no antecedent in relation to the evaluation of EEG synchrony during the first year of life.

4. The NI group exhibited higher synchrony from 1 Hz to 15 Hz than TI and normal groups. This result is difficult to explain. An increase in synchronization above normality may be due to an inadequate balance between inhibition and excitation; this could be one of the mechanisms producing the failure in development.

From these results we may conclude that:

1. In all groups delta power decreases, whereas theta, alpha, high beta, and gamma RP increases from 3 months to 12 months. These results confirm what is already known: infants during the first year of life experience a power decrease in delta frequencies and an increase in frequencies within the theta and alpha bands (Niedermeyer 2005).

2. In all groups synchrony increased from 4 Hz to 12 Hz. This increase in synchrony during the first year of life could be related to the development of connections between cortical regions. The frequencies on which these increases were observed have been mainly associated with mnemonic and attention processes (Gevins et al. 1997; Klimesch 1999; Bastiaansen and Hagoort 2003; Deiber et al. 2007), which are known to develop rapidly during the first year.

3. In the normal group the increase in power at high alpha, low and high beta, and gamma frequencies was greater than in the other groups, indicating that maturation of these oscillations is delayed in infants with white matter lesions. To our knowledge, this is the first report of an increase in gamma activity during the first year of life.

4. Enhanced synchrony in the low frequencies (1–3 Hz) among all regions was observed both in TI and NI. These increases have been related to connections between distant regions (Buszáki 2006). We cannot provide an interpretation of this result, though it could be an indication of plastic changes in the injured cerebral white matter.

5. We may conclude that there is a clear relationship between maturation of EEG oscillations at different frequencies of EEG background activity at 1 year old and motor and cognitive development at 18 months.

EVENT-INDUCED EEG ACTIVITY DURING SPEECH PROCESSING IN 6-WEEK-OLD INFANTS

Recently, increasing interest in electroencephalogram synchronization and desynchronization has developed, because these states may provide a window into the dynamics of cell assembly formation, by which spatially distributed brain areas become linked together in dynamic networks (Varela et al. 2001). Changes in power of cortical oscillatory activity time-locked—but not phase-locked—to the event have been called event-related synchronization (Pfurtscheller 1992) and event-related desynchronization (Pfurtscheller 1977), which consists in either increases or decreases, respectively, in power at given frequency bands. These changes have been considered as increases or decreases in synchrony of the underlying neuronal populations, respectively (Pfurtscheller and Lopes da Silva 1999). When changes in power are not time-locked to the stimuli, it is referred to as event-induced synchronization or desynchronization. However, it has been shown that power alone is an insufficient marker for synchronous activity among different cortical areas (Lachaux et al. 1999; Miltner et al. 1999). These authors suggest that phase synchrony between pairs of electrodes, independent of amplitude, provides a better measure of synchronized neural activity establishing a cell assembly. Nevertheless, Rodríguez et al. (1999) demonstrated that desynchronization co-exists with periods of above-average gamma power. Therefore, changes in spectral power should not be interpreted simply as phase synchrony.

In this part of the chapter we present a study in normal infants and infants with leukomalacia at 6 weeks of age. Event-induced EEG power and synchrony were obtained from two different stimuli: phonemes (*ba*, *pa*) and tones (1000 Hz, 1250 Hz) with similar physical characteristics. The analysis pathway is shown in Figure 6.2. It is known that the ability to distinguish phonemes and syllables is an essential prerequisite for speech perception and language and that this remarkable sensitivity to phonetic units develops mainly during the first year of life (Eimas et al. 1971; for a review see Werker and Vouloumanos 2001; Kuhl 2004). Our goal was to develop a procedure for the early detection of language disorders, because premature children with leukomalacia frequently present delayed language acquisition (Miller et al. 2005).

The questions we want to pose are:

1. Do different auditory events (tones and phonemes) produce characteristic patterns of increased and decreased induced amplitude and synchrony in healthy 6-week-old babies?

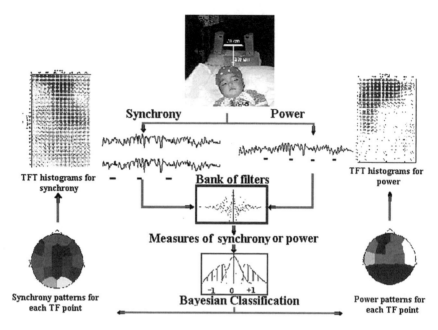

Figure 6.2. Analysis pathway. Selected EEG recordings (one channel for computation of power, two channels for the calculation of phase synchrony) are passed through a bank of band-pass filters (SQFs) centered at 1 Hz intervals (from 1 Hz to 40 Hz). Power analysis is performed by taking the log-power of each filtered signal and subtracting the pre-stimulus average. Phase-synchrony is obtained by estimating the mean phase difference, baseline-corrected by subtracting its pre-stimulus average. Baseline log-power and synchrony values are classified using a Bayesian estimation procedure, indicating significantly ($p < 0.01$) higher (+1), equal (0), or lower (-1) values than pre-stimulus values. In this way, maps for increasing or decreasing values are constructed (not shown in the diagram). For each frequency and time it is possible to display a simple head diagram. In this illustration significant ($p < 0.01$) increasing values for both power and synchrony were selected. However, differential colors indicate the stimulus condition, magenta for syllables, cyan for tones, and blue when in both conditions values increased in relation to baseline. A time-frequency topography (TFT) or multitoscopic display is obtained by dividing the time-frequency plane into cells for each Hz and every 50 ms. Thus, a representative head diagram at each cell (the mode of all class values within the cell) is produced. (See color Figure 6.2)

2. Do babies of the same age with leukomalacia have the same induced patterns as normal babies?

Figure 6.3 shows the results obtained in relation to induced power to tones and phonemes in both groups. In normal babies, induced power was greater for syllables than for tones. Changes induced by syllables were observed between 200 ms and 450 ms at frequencies from 1 Hz to 25 Hz. However, in infants with leukomalacia, induced power was smaller for syllables than for tones and with

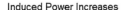

Induced Power Increases

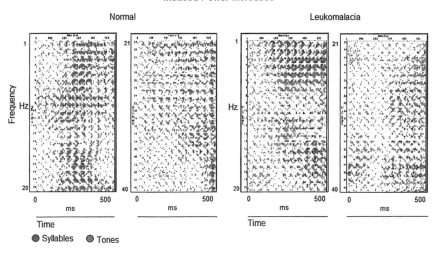

Normal   Leukomalacia

● Syllables   ○ Tones

Figure 6.3. Multitoposcopic display of significant (p < 0.01) increases in power. Time is plotted in the x-axis and frequency in the y-axis. Magenta color indicates an increase in power only in the syllables condition. Cyan color corresponds to an increase in power only in the tones condition. Blue indicates common increases in power. (See color Figure 6.3)

Induced Synchrony Increases

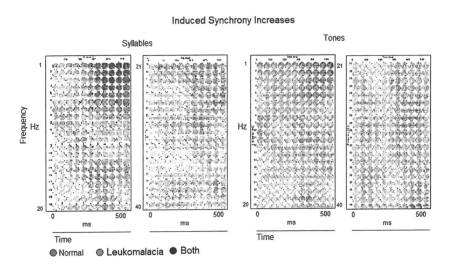

Syllables   Tones

● Normal   ● Leukomalacia   ● Both

Figure 6.4. Multitoposcopic display of significant (p < 0.01) increases in synchrony. Time is plotted in the x-axis and frequency in the y-axis. Magenta color indicates an increase in synchrony only in the syllables condition. Cyan color corresponds to an increase in synchrony only in the tones condition. Blue indicates common increases in synchrony. (See color Figure 6.4)

different topography in relation to normal infants. Changes were in the frequencies of 3–7 Hz.

Figure 6.4 illustrates the results obtained in relation to induced synchrony in both groups. Patterns of increases in synchrony were very different for tones and syllables in both groups; however, important differences were found between groups. Synchrony increases in the normal group were not only greater to syllables than to tones, but they also had shorter latencies. Conversely, the group with leukomalacia exhibited larger induced synchrony values for tones than for syllables; these changes were markedly prolonged.

These results suggest an abnormal cortical auditory processing of speech in the group with white-matter lesions, and an increased risk to develop delays or language impairments. The procedure presented may be useful for the early discrimination of language disorders.

In conclusion, power and synchrony of background EEG oscillations provide important information in relation to normal and abnormal brain development. Gamma activity increases during the first year of age in normal infants more than in infants with leukomalacia, which may be related to cognitive development. On the other hand, the study of auditory- and speech-induced EEG oscillations may be useful for the early evaluation of infants at risk of language disorders.

ACKNOWLEDGMENTS

The authors acknowledge the technical participation of engineer Héctor Belmont Tamayo, technician David Avila Acosta, librarians Pilar Galarza Barrios and Rafael Silva Cruz, and Dr. Marcela Sanchez for revision of the English version of the manuscript.

REFERENCES

Alba A, Marroquin JL, Peña J, Harmony T, González-Frankenberger B. 2006. Exploration of event-induced EEG phase synchronization patterns in cognitive tasks using Time-Frequency-Topography-Visualization system. *J Neurosci Methods* 161: 166–82.
Bastiaansen M, Hagoort P. 2003. Event-induced theta responses as a window of the dynamics of memory. *Cortex* 39:967–92.
Buszáki, G. 2006. Rhythms of the brain. Oxford University Press, New York.
Butta AT, Anand KJS. 2002. Vulnerability of the developing brain. *Clin Perinatol* 29:357–72.
Chabot RJ, Di Michelle F, Prichep L, John ER. 2001. The clinical role of computerized EEG in the evaluation and treatment of learning and attention disorders in children and adolescents. *J Neuropsychiatry Clin Neurosci* 13:171–86.

Csibra G, Davis G, Spratling W, Johnson MN. 2000. Gamma oscillations and object processing in the infant brain. *Science* 290:1582–5.

Deiber MP, Missonier P, Bertrand O, Gold G, Fazio-Costa L, Ibanez V, Giannakopoulos P. 2007. Distinction between perceptual and attentional processing in working memory tasks: a study of phase-locked and induced oscillatory brain dynamics. *J Cogn Neurosci* 19: 158–72.

Eimas PD, Siqueland ER, Jusczyk PW, Vigorito J. 1971. Speech perception in humans. *Science* 171:303–6.

Freeman WJ. 1991. The physiology of perception. *Sci Am* 264:78–85.

Gevins A, Smith M, McEvoy L, Yu D. 1997. High-resolution EEG mapping of cortical activation related to working memory: effects of task difficulty, type of processing, and practice. *Cereb Cortex* 7: 374–85.

Gloor P, Ball G, Schaul N. 1977. Brain lesions that produce delta waves in the EEG. *Neurology* 27:326–33.

Guerrero JA, Marroquin JL, Rivera M, Quiroga JA. 2005. Adaptive monogenic filtering and normalization of ESPI fringe patterns. *Opt Lett* 22: 3018–20.

Hagne I, Persson J, Magnusson R, Petersén I. 1973. Spectral analysis via Fast Fourier Transform of waking EEG in normal infants. In Kellaway P and Petersén I. (Eds.) Automation of Clinical Electroencehalography, Raven Press, New York, p. 103–44.

Harmony T, Hinojosa G, Marosi E, Becker J, Fernández Harmony T, Rodríguez M, Reyes A, Rocha C. 1990. Correlation between EEG spectral parameters and an educational evaluation. *Int J Neuroscience* 54: 147–55.

Harmony T, Marosi E, Becker J, Rodríguez M, Reyes A, Fernández T, Silva J, Bernal J. 1995. Longitudinal quantitative EEG study of children with different performances on a reading-writing test. *Electroenceph Clin Neurophysiol* 95:426–33.

Hebb DO. 1949. The Organization of Behaviour, Wiley, New York.

Johnson MH. 2001. Functional brain development in humans. *Nature Reviews Neuroscience* 2:475–83.

Joseph JP, Lesevre N, Dreyfus-Brisac C. 1976. Spatiotemporal organization of EEG in premature infants and full-term new-borns. *Electroenceph Clin Neurophysiol* 40:153–68.

Klimesch, W. 1999. EEG alpha and theta oscillations reflect cognitive and memory performance: a review and analysis. *Brain Res Rev* 29: 169–95.

Kuhl P. 2004. Early language acquisition: Cracking the speech code. *Nature Reviews Neuroscience* 5: 831–43.

Lachaux JP, Rodríguez E, Martinerie J, Varela FJ. 1999. Measuring phase synchrony in brain signals. *Hum Brain Mapp* 8: 194–208.

Lopes da Silva F, Van Rotterdam A. 2005. Biophysical aspects of EEG and Magnetoencephalogram generation. In Niedermeyer Z. and Lopes da Silva, FH. (Eds.) 2005. Electroencephalography: Basic principle, clinical applications and related fields. 5th edition. Williams and Wilkins, Baltimore MD, pp. 93–109.

Marlow N, Roberts L, Cooke R. 1993. Outcome at 8 years for children with birth weights of 1250 g or less. *Arch Dis Child* 68:286–90.

Matousek M, Petersén I. 1973. Frequency analysis of the EEG in normal children and adolescents. In Kellaway, P. and Petersén, I. (Eds.) Automation of Clinical Electroencehalography, Raven Press, New York, p. 75–102.

Melloni L, Molina C, Pena M, Torres D, Singer W, Rodríguez E. 2007. Synchronization of neural activity across cortical areas correlates with conscious perception. *J Neurosci* 27:2858–65.

Mesulam MM. 1990. Large-scale neurocognitive networks and distributed processing for attention, language, and memory. *Ann Neurol* 28, 597–613.

Miller S, Ferriero D, Leonard C, Piecuch E, Glidden D, Partridge C, Perez M, Mukherjee P, Vigneron D, Barkovich J. 2005. Early brain injury in premature newborns detected with magnetic resonance imaging is associated with adverse early neurodevelopmental outcome. *J Pediatrics* 147: 609–16.

Miltner WHR, Braun C, Arnold M, Witte H, Taub E. 1999. Coherence of gamma-band activity as a basis for associative learning. *Nature* 397: 434–6.

Niedermeyer Z. Maturation of the EEG: Development of waking and sleep patterns. In Niedermeyer Z, Lopes da Silva, FH. (Eds.) 2005. Electroencephalography: Basic principle, clinical applications and related fields. 5th edition. Williams and Wilkins, Baltimore MD, pp. 189–214.

Otero G. 2001. Ontogenia y maduración del electroencefalograma. In Alcaraz VM and Guma E. (Eds) Texto de neurociencias cognitivas. Manual Moderno, México DF, pp. 371–94.

Pfurtscheller G. 1977. Graphical display and statistical evaluation of event-related desynchronization (ERD). *Electroenceph Clin Neurophysiol* 43: 757–60.

Pfurtscheller G. 1992. Event-related synchronization: an electrophysiological correlate of cortical areas at rest. *Electroenceph Clin Neurophysiol* 83: 62–9.

Pfurtscheller G, Lopes da Silva FH. 1999. Event-related EEG/MEG synchronization and desynchronization: basic principles. *Clinical Neurophysiol* 110: 1842–57.

Ricardo-Garcell J. 2004. Aportes del electroencefalograma convencional y el análisis de frecuencias para el estudio del trastorno por déficit de la atención. *Salud Mental* 27:22–7.

Rickards AL, Nelly EA, Doyle LW, Callanan C. 2001. Cognition, academic progress, behavior and self-concept at 14 years of low weight children. *J Dev Behav Pediat* 22:11–8.

Rodríguez E, George N, Lachaux JP, Martinerie J, Renault B, Varela FJ. 1999. Perception's shadow: Long-distance synchronization of human brain activity. *Nature* 3885: 430–3.

Scher MS, Sun M, Steppe DA, Guthrie RD, Sclabassi RJ. 1994. Comparisons of EEG spectral and correlation measures between healthy term and preterm infants. *Pediatr Neurol* 10:104–8.

Singer W, Gray CM. 1995. Visual feature integration and the temporal correlation hypothesis. *Annu Rev Neurosci* 8:555–86.

Steriade M, Contreras D, Curro Dossi R, Nuñez A. 1993. The slow (<1Hz) oscillation in reticular thalamic and thalamocortical neurons: Scenario of sleep rhythm generation in interacting thalamic and neocortical networks. *J Neurosci* 13:3266–83.

Thatcher RW. 1999. EEG database-Guided Neurotherapy. In Evans JR. and Abarbanel A. (Eds.) *Introduction to quantitative EEG and neurofeedback.* Academic Press, New York, pp. 29–64.

Varela F, Lachaux JP, Rodriguez E, Martinerie J. 2001. The brainweb: phase synhronization and large scale integration. *Nat Rev Neurosci* 2: 229–39.

Victor S, Appleton RE, Beirne M, Marson AG, Weindling AM. 2005. Spectral analysis of electroencephalography in premature newborn infants: normal ranges. *Pediatr Res* 57:336–41.

Volpe JJ. 2001. Hypoxic ischemic encephalopathy: Clinical aspects. In Volpe J.J. editor. *Neurology of the newborn.* 4th ed. Philadelphia. W.B. Saunders, pp. 331–40.

Volpe JJ. 2003. Cerebral white matter injury of the premature infant- More common than you think. *Pediatrics* 112:176–80.

Werker JF, Vouloumanos A. 2001.Speech and language processing in infancy: A neuro-cognitive approach. In Nelson CA. and Luciana M. (Eds) Handbook of Developmental Cognitive Neuroscience. MIT Press, Cambridge, MA, pp. 269–80.

Willekens H, Dumermuth G, Duc G, Mieth D. 1984. EEG spectral power and coherence analysis in healthy full-term neonates. *Neuropediatrics* 15:180–90.

APPENDIX

Methodology

The methodology described here is designed to estimate the significance of the differences in amplitude and synchronization between narrow-band EEG signals corresponding to two conditions at rest. Artifact-free segments with a constant length of 2.56 s (512 samples), called *episodes*, were extracted from raw EEG recordings, resulting in a set of time series $V_{j,e}(t)$ for each condition, where j is the episode index, e represents the electrode, and t is the time index. The first step of the analysis consists in passing these EEG signals through a bank of quadrature band-pass filters in order to extract amplitude and phase information for each signal. In particular, we use sinusoidal quadrature filters (SQFs) (Guerrero et al. 2005), which provide more reliable phase estimates at low tuning frequencies than the typical Gabor filters (for a detailed comparison, see Alba et al. 2007). The frequency response of SQFs is given by:

$$G_{\omega_n,h}(\omega) = \begin{cases} \frac{1}{2}[1+\cos((\omega-\omega_n)\pi/h_n)] & \text{if } \omega \in [\omega_n-h_n,\omega_n], \\ \frac{1}{2}[1+\cos((\omega-\omega_n)\pi/h)] & \text{if } \omega \in [\omega_n,\omega_n+h], \\ 0 & \text{otherwise.} \end{cases}$$

where ω_n is the tuning frequency, h is the bandwidth, and $h_n = \min\{h, \omega_n\}$. We have chosen a set of filters tuned at each Hz from 1 to $N_\omega = 40$Hz, with a bandwidth $h = 5.3$ Hz (equivalent to around 1.76 Hz within 3 db attenuation). Filtering is performed by convoluting the input signal with the complex filter kernel, which can be obtained as the inverse Fourier transform $g_{w_k,h}(t)$ of $G_{\omega_k,h}$. This yields a new set of filtered signals $F_{\omega,j,e}(t)$ given by:

$$F_{\omega,j,e}(t) = V_{j,e}(t) * g_{w_k,h}(t),$$

from which amplitude and phase information can be directly obtained.

Synchronization between pairs of electrode signals is estimated with the mean phase difference (MPD) measure proposed in Alba et al.(2007), given by:

$$MPD_{j,\omega,e_1,e_2}(t) = 1 - \frac{1}{\pi}\left|wrap(\phi_{j,\omega,e_1}(t) - \phi_{j,\omega,e_2}(t))\right|,$$

where $\phi_{j,\omega,e}(t)$ is the argument of $F_{\omega,j,e}(t)$, and wrap(ϕ) returns the angle ϕ wrapped into the interval $[-\pi, \pi]$.

In the case of induced changes in amplitude and synchronization, the analysis is commonly performed by first subtracting a baseline level from the measure of interest (amplitude or synchrony). Typically, this baseline level is obtained as the average of the measure across a time segment corresponding to a neutral condition. This is done to estimate relative changes of the measure with respect to the neutral condition. However, when analyzing the EEG at rest, one does not necessarily have a neutral condition against which one can make a comparison. Thus, the baseline level is unknown. One way to overcome this problem is to use the relative amplitude $R_{\omega,j,e}(t)$ and relative synchrony $\mu_{\omega,j,e}(t)$ instead, that is, the amplitude or synchrony at each frequency band divided by the sum of amplitude or synchrony, respectively, across all frequency bands. These parameters are respectively given by:

$$R_{\omega_n,j,e}(t) = \frac{\left|F_{\omega_n,j,e}(t)\right|}{\sum_{m=1}^{N\omega}\left|F_{\omega_m,j,e}(t)\right|},$$

and

$$\mu_{\omega_n,j,e}(t) = \frac{MPD_{\omega_n,j,e}(t)}{\sum_{m=1}^{N\omega}MPD_{\omega_m,j,e}(t)}.$$

To test for significant differences in amplitude between two conditions $k = 1,2$, we perform the following analysis for each frequency of interest ω, and each electrode e:

1. Let R_j^k be the average relative amplitude of the signal observed at site e and frequency ω for episode $j \in \{1,...,N_k\}$ corresponding to condition $k \in \{1, 2\}$, with N_k the number of episodes in condition k. This average can be estimated across the time segment corresponding to the episode as follows:

$$R_j^k = \frac{1}{N_t}\sum_{t=1}^{N_t}R_{\omega,j,e}(t),$$

where N_i is the length of the episode.

2. Choose N episodes $\{i_1,...,i_N\}$ for condition $k = 1$, and N episodes $\{j_1,...,j_N\}$ for condition $k = 2$. Compute the comparison statistics $\gamma^{1,2}$ given by:

$$\gamma^{1,2} = \frac{1}{N}\sum_{n=1}^{N} R^1_{j_n} - R^1_{i_n}.$$

3. To test the significance of $\gamma^{1,2}$ against the null hypothesis (that the distribution of the relative amplitude does not depend on the condition), one can generate a population $\{\gamma^{1,1}_{(q)}\}$, for $q = 1,...,N_q$, where each element $\gamma^{1,1}_{(q)}$ is obtained by randomly choosing N pairs of episodes (i_n, j_n), $n = 1,...,N$, and computing the average

$$\gamma^{1,1}_{(q)} = \frac{1}{N}\sum_{n=1}^{N} R^1_{j_n} - R^1_{i_n}.$$

4. Estimate the distribution P_γ of $\{\gamma^{1,1}_{(q)}\}$ (i.e., the null distribution) using the kernel density estimation [Silverman 1995].

5. Estimate the significance index S of $\gamma^{1,2}$ under P_γ given by:

$$S = \begin{cases} \dfrac{(P_\gamma(\gamma^{1,2}) - P_\gamma(0))}{(1 - P_\gamma(0))} & \text{if } P_\gamma(\gamma^{1,2}) > 0, \\[2em] \dfrac{(P_\gamma(\gamma^{1,2}) - P_\gamma(0))}{P_\gamma(0)} & \text{if } P_\gamma(\gamma^{1,2}) > 0, \end{cases}$$

The sign of the significance index S indicates whether the relative amplitude in condition $k = 2$ is greater ($S > 0$) or smaller ($S < 0$) than the amplitude in condition $k = 1$. The absolute value of S represents the significance of these differences, thus one can display only those sites where $|S|$ is higher than some confidence level, which we have chosen to be 0.99.

Synchrony analysis is performed in a similar manner, by replacing the relative amplitude with the relative synchrony measure, and computing the results for each electrode pair instead of for each single electrode.

Part 3

Degenerative Brain Diseases

Chapter Seven

The Nigro-Striatal DA Neurons and Mechanisms of Their Degeneration in Parkinson's Disease

Kjell Fuxe, Daniel Marcellino, Tiziana Antonelli,
Giuseppa Mudó, Paul Manger, Susanna Genedani,
Luca Ferraro, Natale Belluardo, Sergio Tanganelli,
and Luigi F. Agnati

INTRODUCTION

The nigral dopamine (DA) nerve cells were first discovered in 1964 in the rat substantia nigra (Dahlström and Fuxe 1964a) using the Falck-Hillarp technique to determine the cellular localization of monoamines (Falck et al. 1962). In the same year, the nigro-striatal DA pathway extending to the caudate-putamen was mapped (Anden et al. 1964) through a method that was developed to visualize monoamine axonal pathways containing very low concentrations of monoamines (Dahlström and Fuxe 1964b); for recent reviews see Fuxe et al. (2006 and 2007a). These discoveries made it clear for the first time that the motor deficits found in Parkinson's disease (PD)—including hypokinesia, rigidity, and resting tremor—were caused by the degeneration of the nigro-striatal DA pathway, taking into consideration the large reductions of nigral DA levels reported in postmortem brains from patients with PD (Hornykiewicz 1963).

Research on familial forms of PD has identified several genes responsible for the degeneration of nigro-striatal DA neurons that also may be involved in their degeneration in sporadic PD (see Mizuno et al. 2006; Sulzer 2007). As a matter of fact, based on new genetic research, many types of PD now appear to exist from different pathogenetic mechanisms that all result in the degeneration of nigral DA nerve cells. There also exists genetic evidence for the involvement of mitochondrial dysfunction in PD (Heutink 2006; Fukae et al. 2007). The PD gene products PINK-1 (mitochondrial kinase) and DJ-1 (antioxidant and redox-sensor role) have been identified based on loss-of-function mutations within these genes present in autosomal recessive young onset familial PD (PARK6 and PARK7), and they play an important cellular role in protection against mitochondrial dysfunction and oxidative stress (Figure 7.1). In fact, these PD genes encode mitochondrial proteins like LRRK2/dardarin, a gene that encodes a kinase associated with the outer mitochondrial membrane (Fig. 7.1), where its mutation causes autosomal dominant PD (PARK8) (Kwong et al. 2006). Another mitochondrial protein involved in PD is OMI/HTRA2, a serine protease that operates as an enhancer of apoptosis upon its release into the cytoplasm (see Kwong et al. 2006).

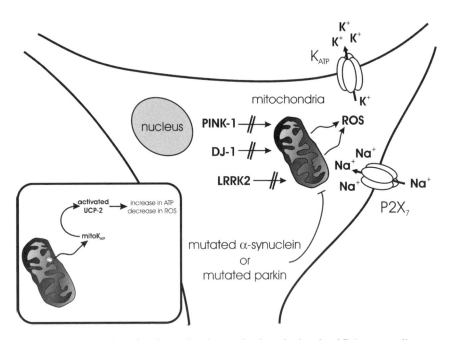

Figure 7.1. Illustration of major molecular mechanisms in the nigral DA nerve cells contributing to the pathogenesis of PD. The genetic evidence suggests that mutated Pink-1, DJ-1, and LRRK2 mitochondrial proteins gives rise to mitochondrial dysfunction, as do the mutated cytoplasmic proteins α-synuclein and parkin underlining the role of mitochondria in PD development. Activation of the mitoK$_{ATP}$ channels probably spurring increases in UCP-2 activity leads to increased ATP synthesis and reduced ROS formation and represents important neuroprotective mechanisms and targets for treatment of PD. Persistent and progressive increases in ROS formation with age have serious consequences by, e.g., activating the plasma membrane K$_{ATP}$ channels with silencing of the nigral DA neurons and reduced neurotrophic support. Also, ROS together with high ATP concentrations in the extracellular space from dying DA cells may activate the P2X$_7$ receptors on the DA cells with influx of Na$^+$ ions through the cation channels causing depolarization, excitotoxicity, and DA cell death (see Fuxe et al. 2006).

Furthermore, environmental evidence also exists based on neurotoxins, like 1-methyl-4-phenyl-1,2,3,6-tetrahydropyridine (MPTP), with regard to mitochondrial dysfunction in PD as well as mtDNA mutations that may also play a role in the pathogenesis of PD (see Kwong et al. 2006; Fukae et al. 2007).

This chapter will focus on the link between correct mitochondrial function and the function of the plasma membrane ion channels and receptors (Figures 7.1 and 7.2), especially K_{ATP} channels (Liss et al. 2005), $P2x_7$ channels (North 2002; Fuxe et al. 2006; Burnstock 2007), and Ca_v 1.3 Ca^{2+} channels (see Chan et al. 2007; Surmeier 2007) that control the firing of the nigral DA cells and consequently their survival. The roles of the nicotinic (Mudo et al. 2007), adenosine A_{2A} (Fuxe et al. 2006; Schwarzschild et al. 2006; Fuxe et al. 2007b; Fuxe et al. 2007c), and neurotensin (Antonelli et al. 2007) receptors in these neurodegenerative processes will also be discussed (Figures 7.2 and 7.3). Furthermore, how an understanding of these molecular mechanisms may lead to the development

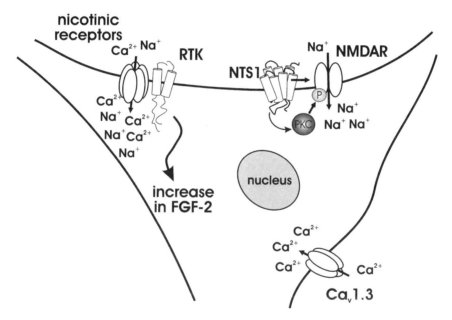

Figure 7.2. The Ca_v1.3 Ca^{2+} channels represent the adult pace-making mechanism in the nigral DA cells, and the calcium influx will cause an age-dependent rise of mitochondrial stress. The nicotinic receptors exert neuroprotective actions by activation of FGF-2 mechanisms and other neurotrophic effects that may involve the transactivation of receptor tyrosine kinases (RTK), and their chronic activation by nicotine agonists may therefore increase DA cell survival with reduction of burst firing and of energy demands as an additional factor due to their partial desensitization. Other excitatory mechanisms are the NMDA and the interacting neurotensin NTS1 receptors on the DA nerve cells that may cause excitotoxity also due to excitatory NTS1/NMDA receptor interactions involving PKC. NTS1 receptor antagonists have been shown to protect against glutamate neurotoxicity and may be novel neuroprotective drugs against PD.

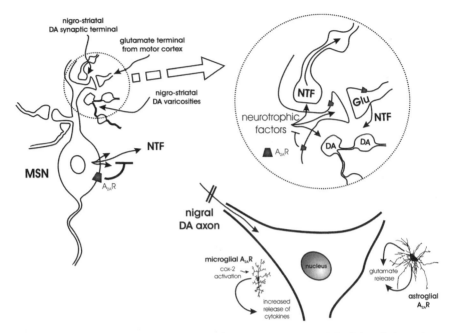

Figure 7.3. A_{2A} receptors appear to accelerate the degeneration of the DA cells by reducing trophic retrograde signaling in the nigro-striatal DA neurons by striatal neurotrophic factors (NTF), via increases in astroglial glutamate release, and by microglia-mediated neuroinflammation (COX-2 activation, increased release of cytokines) in the substantia nigra.

of novel neuroprotective strategies or to differential treatment for the various types of PD due to their partially overlapping pathogenetic mechanisms will also be addressed. Nevertheless, it is important to be aware of the spatio-temporal sequence of the events leading to degeneration to understand how the intracellular progression of the pathological phenomena occurs (Conforti et al. 2007). Although highly relevant, it is not required to begin to understand the pathogenetic mechanisms, because the site of degeneration is not a reliable indicator of where the initial defect occurred (Conforti et al. 2007) and will not be addressed in this chapter.

NEURODEGENERATION AND NEUROTROPHISM: MITOCHONDRIAL DYSFUNCTION AND ITS IMPACT ON ION CHANNEL REGULATION IN THE NIGRO-STRIATAL DA NEURONS—RELEVANCE FOR NEUROPROTECTIVE THERAPY IN PD

It should be considered that not only mutant mitochondrial proteins (see Introduction) but also mutated α-synuclein, the origin of the autosomal dominant familial PD (PARK1), are located in the cytoplasm and produce mitochondrial dysfunction

(Fig. 7.1) and nigral DA cell degeneration (Kwong et al. 2006; Mizuno et al. 2006). Moreover, parkin, in its mutated form, can cause autosomal recessive juvenile PD (PARK2) and is capable of directly altering mitochondrial function through mechanisms unrelated to its ubiquitin E3 ligase activity (Fig. 7.1). Through the investigation of inherited PD, clear indications exist that mitochondrial dysfunction is most likely a major factor among the multiple causes of sporadic PD.

In line with this view, it has been found that conditional knock-out mice that lack the gene for mitochondrial transcription factor A, specifically in DA neurons, are associated with respiratory chain deficiency and demonstrate progressive Parkinsonism (Ekstrand et al. 2007). Mitochondria-dependent DA neurodegeneration in experimental PD is initiated via two molecular pathways (Perier et al. 2007). One involves the transcriptional induction of the pro-apoptotic Bcl-2 family member Bax mediated through the tumor suppressor p53. The other involves the mitochondrial translocation of Bax that primarily occurs via a JNK-dependent activation of the "BH3-only" protein Bim that in turn results in the post-translational activation of Bax (Perier et al. 2007). It has also been demonstrated that the deletion of Bax prevents nigral DA neuron degeneration in the MPTP mouse model of PD (Vila et al. 2001). The impact that mitochondrial dysfunction has on ion channel and receptor function in the plasma membrane of nigral DA nerve cells and any reciprocal action will follow.

Mitochondrial ATP-Sensitive Potassium Channels (mitoK$_{ATP}$)

MitoK$_{ATP}$ channels (Fig. 7.1) are located on the inner mitochondrial membrane and, although not completely characterized, are assumed to be structured similar to plasmalemmal K$_{ATP}$ channels, comprised of inwardly rectifying potassium subunits (Kir) and sulfonylurea receptor subunits (SUR) (Bajgar et al. 2001). These channels are activated upon mitochondrial dysfunction due to the reduction of the ATP levels. This leads to the depolarization of the mitochondria and is associated with neuroprotection against both anoxic and chemical stresses in the central nervous system (CNS) (Busija et al. 2004). In fact, the selective mitoK$_{ATP}$ channel opener BMS-191095 protects against transient focal cerebral ischemia without the generation of radical oxygen species (ROS) (Mayanagi et al. 2007). The proposed mechanism behind this protection is one in which the opening of the mitoK$_{ATP}$ channels leads to mitochondrial depolarization thereby producing the activation of ATP synthesis where ATP subsequently acts as an intra- and intermitochondrial signal (Fuxe et al. 2006).

Uncoupling Protein-2 (UCP-2)

It seems possible that the likely presence of mitochondrial dysfunction in several types of PD leads to an activation of the mitoK$_{ATP}$ channels in order to counteract the progressive degeneration of the DA nerve cell. The hypothesis is that mito-K_{ATP} channel activation leads to a postulated increase in ATP synthesis and neuroprotection through the depolarization-induced activation of UCP-2 (Fig. 7.1). Activated UCP-2 has a potential to prevent the development of PD and other neurological diseases (Diano et al. 2003; Andrews et al. 2005a). As previously reported (Andrews et al. 2006), UCP-2 activation allows protons to enter the mitochondrial matrix without reaching the ATP synthase. In this manner, it leads to a partial uncoupling of respiration from ATP synthesis. This activation will reduce mitochondrial ROS production and, importantly, promote ATP synthesis via a compensatory increase in mitochondrial biogenesis (Diano et al. 2003; Andrews et al. 2005a).

In fact, UCP-2 promotes nigro-striatal DA neuronal function and counteracts MPTP-induced loss of DA nerve cells (Andrews et al. 2005b; Andrews et al. 2006) demonstrated through the use of UCP-2 knock-out mice. Also the majority of the nigral DA nerve cells show strong UCP-2 like immunoreactivity (see Andrews et al. 2005b; Fuxe et al. 2005; Rivera et al. 2006). Therefore, it is possible that a reduction in the expression of mitoK$_{ATP}$ channels and/or UCP-2 may predispose individuals to PD. Potentially, elective mitoK$_{ATP}$ channel openers such as BMS-191095 will offer a new strategy for a neuroprotective therapy early in PD (see Fuxe et al. 2006) relying on the fact that the activation of UCP-2 plays a major role in neuroprotection through a compensatory increase of ATP formation (Fig. 7.1). However, nigral DA cells with low UCP-2–like immunoreactivity may be more vulnerable to degeneration in PD.

Plasma Membrane K$_{ATP}$ Channels

Similar to mitoK$_{ATP}$ channels, the plasma membrane K$_{ATP}$ channels also open during mitochondrial dysfunction and in conditions of metabolic stress (Fig. 7.1). This results in the hyperpolarization and loss of firing of nigral DA cells due to the development of an outward potassium current (Liss and Roeper 2001). In an acute state, this is an appropriate survival response function to maintain an energy balance during conditions of high metabolic demands (Liss and Roeper 2001; Fuxe et al. 2006). The plasma membrane K$_{ATP}$ channels are comprised of four Kir6.2 channels and four regulatory SUR. Alternative SUR subtype expression defines the metabolic sensitivity of K$_{ATP}$ channels in nigral DA cells in which K$_{ATP}$ channels formed by SUR1/Kir6.2 demonstrate the highest metabolic sensitivity (Liss et al. 1999a).

Interestingly, in the genetic model of DA cell degeneration (the *weaver* mouse with mutated GIRK2 channels exhibiting a chronic depolarizing sodium current), nigral DA cells that express SUR2B subunits were no longer observed (Liss et al. 1999b). This discovery indicates a possible neuroprotective role of the SUR1/Kir6.2 K$_{ATP}$ channels through the silencing of calbindin-positive nigral DA neurons by reducing ATP consumption in these cells (see Liss and Roeper 2001). The widespread distribution of these channels in the brain also indicates a universal neuroprotective role in multiple neuronal cell types (Dunn-Meynell et al. 1998).

In addition, ROS can activate these channels and thereby silence nigral DA neurons even when ATP levels are only moderately affected (Fig. 7.1) (Avshalumov and Rice 2003; Avshalumov et al. 2005; Bao et al. 2005). Such results help explain why the unexpected activation of K_{ATP} channels has been found to enhance the degeneration of nigral DA neurons in animal models of PD (Liss et al. 2005). The genetic inactivation of the Kir6.2 subunit results in a selective protection of nigral DA cells in the MPTP model and a partial protection in the *weaver* mouse model. Early ROS formation in nigral DA cells exposed to stress leads to the silencing of these neurons by the activation of plasma membrane K_{ATP} channels and enhanced DA cell death. In agreement with this view, it has been demonstrated that midbrain DA neurons in vitro can be rescued by veratridine-induced stimulation of voltage-gated sodium channels introducing electrical activity and counteracting apoptosis (Salthun-Lassalle et al. 2004).

However, because the DA neurodegeneration in the *weaver* model is only partially protected, this indicates that a chronic depolarizing sodium influx may not be effectively counteracted by the inactivation of the plasma membrane K_{ATP} channels, channels closed during depolarization (Bryan et al. 2004). According to these results, it follows that certain state blockers of plasma membrane SUR1/Kir6.2 K_{ATP} channels—but not mitoK_{ATP} channels—particularly when combined with activators of UCP-2 (see above), will reduce ROS formation and may provide neuroprotection against nigral DA cell degeneration (see, among others, Deutch and Winder 2006). Neuronal pace-making activity may in this manner be crucial for the long-term survival of nigral DA neurons by, possibly, maintenance of gene expression for neuronal trophism, although the reduction of acute firing may be neuroprotective by reducing energy loss through the firing of the DA neuron (Liss et al. 2005; Fuxe et al. 2006).

An additional mechanism may also be considered based on the fact that acute axotomy of the nigro-striatal DA pathway produces a rapid (within 15 minutes) and long-lasting rise of DA levels in striatal—but to a lesser extent in accumbal—DA nerve terminal networks (Anden et al. 1972). Silencing of the nigro-striatal DA neurons appears to markedly increase DA synthesis. This may also be the case after the activation of the plasma membrane K_{ATP} channels in the nigro-striatal DA neurons leading to hyperpolarization and prevention of action potential formation in these neurons (Liss et al. 2005). Therefore, an increase in cytosolic DA levels may develop and its oxidation may lead to increased ROS formation, thereby increasing damage to the DA cells and contributing to their progressive degeneration (Greenamyre and Hastings 2004).

In line with this view, it has been found that α-synuclein/DAT protein complexes are formed that enhance DA uptake and DA-induced toxicity (Lee et al.

2001). Parkin has been reported to disrupt this interaction and also protect against DA-induced toxicity (Moszczynska et al. 2007), in addition to its protective role in the nigro-striatal DA neurons through the ubiquination of several proteins (Mizuno et al. 2006).

Contrary to this proposal, it may be argued that L-dopa treatment does not lead to an increased rate of PD progression (Fahn 2005) or in pathological cytoplasmic levels of DA; rather, it only produces a temporary cessation in the firing of nigro-striatal DA neurons from the activation of D_2 autoreceptors coupled to GIRK channels. This latter mechanism remains to be considered and is attractive because it contributes to our understanding of why the nigro-striatal DA neurons are especially vulnerable to degeneration in PD.

ATP P2X Receptors

Seven types of P2X receptors ($P2X_{1-7}$) exist, each monomer consisting of two transmembrane domains and an interconnecting extracellular loop (see North 2002). These channels, permeable to small monovalent cations, are formed by the assembly of several monomer subtypes and are comprised of either homomeric or heteromeric P2X receptors. P2X receptor subtypes are present not only on neurons but also on astrocytes, microglia, and oligodendrocytes. ATP has a major role in neuron-glia interactions (see Burnstock 2007) and represents not only a wiring transmission signal but also an important volume transmission signal (Fuxe et al. 2006).

It is of substantial interest to mention that there are indications that certain types of P2X receptors may be activated by ROS through studies on vagal lung afferents (Ruan et al. 2005) similar to plasma membrane K_{ATP} channels (see above). It is therefore postulated that these receptors may exist and especially appear on nigral DA nerve cells during progressive degeneration in PD and where ROS-activated P2X receptor subtypes may contribute to further degeneration (Fuxe et al. 2006).

Particular focus should be placed on the $P2X_7$ receptor subtype because it does not desensitize upon activation (Fig. 7.1) (North 2002). Thereby, these receptors lead to a persistent influx of sodium ions and subsequent depolarization due to ATP depletion with a failure of Na^+/K^+ ATPase maintenance of ion gradients in DA cells. Also, a prolonged activation of $P2X_7$ leads to membrane blebbing and microvesiculation as well as the formation of large pores permeable to large organic cations and chloride ions that produce apoptotic cell death (North 2002; Tsukimoto et al. 2005).

An important aspect of mitochondrial dysfunction in many forms of PD is the generation of ROS. ROS may not only activate hyperpolarizing plasma membrane K_{ATP} channels but also $P2X_7$ receptors on DA cells that produce a depolarizing influx of sodium ions and further enhance the degenerative process (Fig. 7.1)

(Fuxe et al. 2006). In addition, release of ATP from the surrounding neurons and glia within the nigral environment may also contribute to their activation as well as the activation of glial $P2X_7$ receptors that may further increase ATP release (Suadicani et al. 2006) and other P2X receptor subtypes in the nigral microglial and astroglial networks to modulate a neuroinflammatory response (Burnstock 2007).

In support of the present hypothesis, evidence has been obtained that $P2X_7$ receptor activation may contribute to trauma-induced degeneration of spinal cord neurons by an enhancement of excitotoxicity (Wang et al. 2004; Burnstock 2007). When discussing the $P2X_7$ hypothesis, it should also be mentioned that extracellular ATP released from injured tissue may lead to necrotic cell swelling and cell death in SN4741 DA neurons by activating their $P2X_7$ receptors (Jun et al. 2007). Furthermore, DA cell degeneration based on increases in extracellular ATP was blocked by the knock-down of $P2X_7$ receptors through small interfering RNAs (siRNA) or by prior treatment of cells with the $P2X_7$ receptor antagonist KN62. Clearly, taken together, these results indicate that $P2X_7$ receptor antagonists may represent a new strategy for treatment of PD.

It is of substantial interest to note that rapid-onset dystonia Parkinsonism is produced after mis-sense mutations in the Na^+/K^+-ATPase-3 gene, mutations that lead to persistent hyperexcitability (de Carvalho Aguiar et al. 2004). Based on the $P2X_7$ hypothesis and from the results in the *weaver* mouse model, degeneration of the nigral DA cells is expected to take place under these conditions, but definitive studies on this issue are still warranted (see Michel et al. 2007).

ATP acting at other P2X receptor subtypes instead may give rise to more complex responses that include neuroprotective actions (Volonte et al. 2003; Burnstock 2007). It has also been shown that parkin and ubiquitin carboxy-terminal hydrolase L1 can enhance ATP-induced currents over P2X receptors (Manago et al. 2005; Sato et al. 2006). This is of particular interest because the "loss of function" mutations of these two proteins leads to PARK2 and PARK5 (Mizuno et al. 2006). Thus, maintenance of excitability and of neuronal activity in the physiological range in the DA cells may have a survival value (Liss et al. 2005; Michel et al. 2007). Therefore, neurotrophism in the nigral DA neurons may be dependent on their pace-making activity.

$Ca_v1.3$ Ca^{2+} Channels

Recently, Surmeier and colleagues (Chan et al. 2007) elegantly demonstrated that the nigro-striatal DA neurons rely on $Ca_v1.3$ Ca^{2+} channels for their pace-making activity and also discovered that their blockade produces a rejuvenation of the adult nigral DA nerve cells through the reversal of the pace-making mechanism into a juvenile form using Na^+/HCN channels, where HCN stands for hyperpolarization-activated and cyclic nucleotide–gated cation channels (Fig. 7.2).

This rejuvenation was found to protect the nigral DA cells in models of PD (Chan et al. 2007) and introduced a new strategy for treatment, namely $Ca_v1.3$ Ca^{2+} channel antagonists. In the present absence of such selective drugs, dihydropyridine isradipine has been proposed because it is currently used for treatment of cardiovascular disease (discussed in detail by Surmeier 2007). This mechanism also provides an understanding of why nigral DA cells with calcium-buffering proteins like calbinidin-D28K are relatively spared in PD (Yamada et al. 1990).

Of particular interest for a focus on mitochondria/ion channel interactions is the fact that the frequent influx of Ca^{2+} into the DA cells through these channels must be pumped out. This will consume ATP stores provided by the mitochondria. Ca^{2+} is also sequestered into the endoplasmic reticulum and the mitochondrial matrix, the latter producing a further loss of ATP because the electrochemical gradient generated by the respiratory chain necessary for ATP synthesis is reduced (Surmeier 2007). With various degrees of mitochondrial dysfunction— including "damaging" polymorphisms of mtDNA, high rates of mtDNA mutations due to the actions of ROS, and genetic mutations as discussed above, all of which increase with age—DA nerve cell degeneration will appear sooner or later. This is especially dependent on the combined impact of mitochondrial dysfunction with its interaction with plasma membrane K_{ATP} channels, $P2X_7$ channels, and/or $Ca_v1.3$ Ca^{2+} channels that may determine the onset of degeneration of the DA cells and the onset of PD.

NEURODEGENERATION AND NEUROTROPHISM: FGF-2 MECHANISMS IN THE NIGRO-STRIATAL DA NEURONS AND THEIR MODULATION BY NICOTINIC RECEPTORS

In 1988 it was discovered that chronic nicotine treatment counteracts the degeneration of the nigro-striatal DA neurons after either partial hemitransection in the rat or treatment with MPTP in the mouse (Janson et al. 1988; Fuxe et al. 1990). Many years later, in 2006, it was further shown that chronic nicotine treatment could counteract MPTP-induced degeneration of DA nerve terminals in the primate model (Quik et al. 2006). These results are in agreement with epidemiological evidence for a negative association between cigarette smoking and PD (Baron 1986; Quik 2004) and with high densities of high-affinity nicotinic receptors found in the nigro-striatal DA neurons (see Klink et al. 2001). It is likely that partially desensitized nicotinic receptors were mediating the neuroprotective actions of nicotine following chronic exposure to nicotine (see Mudo et al. 2007). This receptor desensitization would in fact reduce the influx of cations through the nicotinic receptor subtypes located on the nigral DA cells as well as through the voltage-gated calcium channels through a reduction in nicotinic receptor–induced depolarization of the DA cell (Fig. 7.2) (see Mudo et al. 2007). Indeed, chronic nicotine treatment leads to a reduction in the burst firing in the surviving DA cells after partial hemitransection at the meso-diencephalic junction (Grenhoff et al. 1991). As a result, metabolic stress on the mitochondria would be reduced because the pumping out of calcium ions and/or their sequestration into the mitochondria—both energy-dependent processes leading to loss of ATP—is reduced (see above).

It should be noted, however, that a chronic inactivation of the nicotinic receptor is probably not responsible for neuroprotective action of nicotine, because the chronic and continuous infusion of nicotine via Alzet minipumps caused a dose-dependent increase in MPTP-induced degeneration of nigral DA cells in the higher dose range (Janson et al. 1991). Such a result may be explained on the basis discussed above under plasma membrane K_{ATP} channels, namely that such a complete nicotine receptor inactivation may have led to a silencing of the nigro-striatal DA neurons with a loss of activity-dependent neurotrophism.

In fact, in 1996 we obtained additional evidence that chronic and continuous infusion of nicotine via minipumps resulted in a reduction of basic fibroblast growth factor (FGF-2) mRNA levels in the ventral midbrain (Blum et al. 1996). In contrast, after an acute intermittent treatment with nicotine, a marked increase in FGF-2 mRNA and protein levels were observed in the substantia nigra and other brain regions including the striatum, the hippocampus, and the cerebral cortex (Fig. 7.2) (Belluardo et al. 1998, 2000). Similar results have also been observed after acute treatment with different types of nicotinic agonists, including one with preferential activation of α4/β2 nicotinic receptors (Belluardo et al. 1999, 2000). This rise of FGF-2 mRNA levels after acute activation of nicotinic receptors is also preserved in the aged brain (Belluardo et al. 2004) and underlies the relevance of nicotinic receptor subtype–specific agonists for treatment of PD. It is possible that the increase in FGF-2 within the striatum mainly reduces the MPTP-induced degeneration of the striatal DA terminals whereas its rise in the substantia nigra contributes to the survival of the entire nigral DA neuron.

The molecular mechanism for the nicotinic receptor–induced rise of FGF-2 mRNA levels and protein may involve a CREB site on the promotor of the FGF-2 gene. Nicotinic-receptor activation and subsequent increases in intracellular calcium are known to activate CREB signaling and the ERK/MAPK signaling cascades (Mudo et al. 2007). Another important molecular mechanism may be a nicotinic receptor–induced transactivation of receptor tyrosine kinases (RTK) in the DA cell membrane (Fig. 7.2) that also leads to the activation of the ERK/MAPK signaling pathways. It is also possible that the nicotinic receptors form a receptor mosaic with RTK at the plasma membrane (Fuxe et al. 2007a), which may allow an efficient activation of the ERK/MAPK system, thus contributing to the activation of CREB and thereby increasing FGF-2 gene expression (Fig. 7.2).

It seems possible that subtypes of high-affinity nicotinic receptors on nigral DA nerve cells have the unique ability to activate neurotrophic mechanisms within these cells, particularly the FGF-2 neurotrophic system, providing protection of the DA nerve cells from MPTP injury (Chadi et al. 1993). Therefore, treatment with nicotinic receptor agonists, using the $\alpha4/\beta2$ subtype as the major target, remains an important strategy to be evaluated further as a neuroprotective treatment of PD, especially with treatment of activators of mitoK$_{ATP}$ channels to reduce the mitochondrial dysfunction (see above).

NEURODEGENERATION AND NEUROTROPHISM: EXCITOTOXIC MECHANISMS IN THE NIGRO-STRIATAL DA NEURONS AND THE CONTRIBUTION OF NEUROTENSIN PEPTIDES

High densities of neurotensin receptor 1 (NTS1) exist on the nigral DA cell bodies and their striatal axon terminals (Palacios and Kuhar 1981; Boudin et al. 1998). NTS1 signals mainly via activation of phospholipase C, which leads to increases in intracellular Ca^{2+} and protein kinase C activity (Fig. 7.2) (Antonelli et al. 2007; Ferraro et al. 2008). It is of substantial interest that neurotensin (NT) via NTS1 receptors can increase glutamate release in the substantia nigra, the striatum, and cortical areas of the living brain (Ferraro et al. 1995; Ferraro et al. 1998; Ferraro et al. 2001; Antonelli et al. 2007), providing evidence for NTS1 as an important modulator of glutamate transmission in the brain. This view was strengthened by the demonstration of the existence of facilitatory NTS1/NMDA receptor interactions in primary rat cortical cultures that control the release of glutamate (Antonelli et al. 2004). The phosphorylation of NMDA receptors by PKC may play an important role in this interaction because glutamate release was blocked by the PKC inhibitor calphostin C (Fig. 7.2).

These neurochemical signaling events were found to be correlated with an NT enhancement of glutamate toxicity of rat cortical neurons and rat mesencephalic DA neurons in primary cultures (Antonelli et al. 2002; Antonelli et al. 2004). The NTS1 receptor antagonist SR48692 blocked the glutamate-induced toxic changes in morphology and biochemistry, including apoptotic neuronal death, thereby indicating the involvement of NTS1 receptors in excitotoxic cell death. Excessive glutamate receptor signaling, particularly via NMDA receptors, contribute to neuronal cell death in PD and other neurodegenerative disorders (Sonsalla et al. 1998). In fact, it is well known that NMDA receptor antagonists are able to block the neurodegeneration of nigral DA nerve cells in models of PD (Zeevalk et al. 2000). This is probably related to the fact that nigral DA cells are metabolically compromised in these PD models via mitochondrial dysfunction, as emphasized in this chapter. Thus, the dysfunctional mitochondria can no longer maintain critical ionic gradients during the increased burst firing brought about by increased glutamate and neurotensin signaling (Antonelli et al. 2007; Ferraro et al. 2008). It should also be considered that the antagonistic NTS1/D_2 autoreceptor interaction in nigral DA cells will also block the ability of the D_2 autoreceptor to activate G protein–gated inwardly rectifying K^+ channels (GIRK) and will contribute to an increase in DA cell firing and increased energy demands (Tanganelli et al. 1989; Shi and Bunney 1990; Antonelli et al. 2007). Also, long-asting increases in NTS1 and NMDA signaling associated with increases in calcium signaling and PKC activation may cause a chronic activation of ERK that may trigger programmed DA cell death (Colucci-D'Amato et al. 2003; Antonelli et al. 2007).

This research clearly indicates that NTS1 receptor antagonists may have neuroprotective actions in early PD and represent an important novel strategy for treatment. Recent evidence for this view has been demonstrated by Tanganelli and colleagues in the unilateral 6-OHDA rat model of PD. Chronic treatment with the NTS1 antagonist SR48692 resulted in a reduction of apomorphine-induced contralateral turning in this model and in the protection of striatal glutamatergic inputs as determined biochemically (Ferraro et al. 2008). Neuroprotective treatment with NTS1 antagonists may be combined, for example, with activators of mitochondrial function in the compromised DA cells, such as specific openers of mitoK_{ATP} channels together with antioxidants to reduce the damaging effects of ROS.

NEURODEGENERATION AND NEUROTROPHISM: OTHER MECHANISMS OF IMPORTANCE FOR THE SURVIVAL OF THE NIGRO-STRIATAL DA NEURONS AND THEIR MODULATION BY A_{2A} RECEPTORS

In recent years, evidence has been obtained that A_{2A} antagonists may represent neuroprotective drugs in treatment of PD (Ross et al. 2000; Chen et al. 2001; Xu et al. 2005; Schwarzschild et al. 2006; Chen et al. 2007). People who drink coffee exhibit a reduced risk of developing PD, most likely related to the A_{2A} receptor–blocking activity of caffeine. Futhermore, selective A_{2A} antagonists protect from nigral DA cell degeneration in models of PD including the mouse MPTP model. Neuroprotective actions of A_{2A} antagonists have also been observed in ischemic and excitotoxic injuries as well as injuries produced by mitochondrial toxins (Alfinito et al. 2003); however, the specific mechanism of action behind this neuroprotective effect against various types of injuries is unknown. A_{2A} receptors are not present on the DA neurons themselves and therefore indirect effects must be considered. Multiple sites of action have been proposed, including a counteraction of A_{2A}-induced glutamate release from glutamate terminals and astroglia, A_{2A}-induced activation of cyclooxygenase-2 (COX-2) in microglia within the substantia nigra, and the enhancement of D_2 receptor–mediated neuroprotection (Fig. 7.3) (Schwarzschild et al. 2006; Chen et al. 2007; Fuxe et al. 2007c). An interesting proposal is that an important mechanism of action of A_{2A} antagonists may be to enhance retrograde neurotrophic support of the nigral DA cells. By blocking striatal A_{2A} receptors, which exist in high densities on the striato-pallidal GABA neurons as well as on the striatal glutamate axon terminals, retrograde transport of neurotrophic factors are increased (Fig. 7.3) (Fuxe et al. 2007c). Glial cell line–derived neurotrophic factor (GDNF) could be one such neurotrophic factor, although other neurotrophic factors may also contribute (Burke 2006). It is also important that Popoli and colleagues have observed in normal mouse hippocampus that A_{2A} receptors are required for normal BDNF levels, as well as for the BDNF-induced enhancement of synaptic transmission (Tebano et al. 2008). There is little doubt that multiple actions of A_{2A} antagonists exist to produce their neuroprotective actions on the nigral DA cells that, as all cells in the brain, are part of a trophic unit of cells to assist in the survival of one another (Agnati et al. 1995; Fuxe et al. 1996, 2007c). The increased survival of the DA cells within trophic units of the substantia nigra is observed after A_{2A} antagonist treatment and is dependent on the integrated effects of blocking A_{2A} receptors located on the various cellular elements of these units. These include the microglia, astroglia, bone marrow–derived cells, and ependymal cells, as well as the striatal A_{2A} receptors controlling the retrograde trophism to nigral DA nerve cells. The outcome may vary depending on the trophic state found after different types of injuries or PD gene mutations of the nigral trophic units. In fact, A_{2A} agonists in combination with L-dopa have also been found to produce protective effects on the nigral DA cells after 6-OHDA induced lesions of the nigro-striatal DA neurons (Agnati et al. 2004).

Future work will clarify the major action and mechanism for the protective effects produced by A_{2A} antagonists in PD.

CONCLUSIONS

This chapter serves to illustrate the crucial importance of the balance between neurodegeneration and neurotrophism for the survival of the nigro-striatal DA neurons in order to delay the onset of PD (Figure 7.4). The research on familial forms of PD has underscored the importance of mitochondrial dysfunction for the development of familial and sporadic forms of the disease. This has been achieved through the demonstration that mitochondrial proteins encoded by PINK-1, DJ-1, and DRRK2/dardarin genes are neuroprotective and that mutated cytoplasmatic proteins, like α-synuclein and parkin, disrupt mitochondrial function.

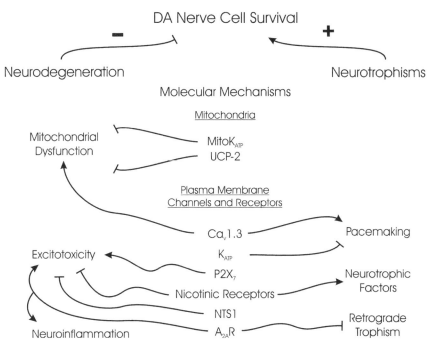

Figure 7.4. Schematic representation of certain molecular mechanisms regulating nigral DA nerve cell survival via modulation of neurodegeneration and neurotrophism. It is illustrated how mitochondrial proteins like mitoK$_{ATP}$ channels and UCP-2 can improve mitochondrial dysfunction whereas plasma membrane Ca$_v$1.3 Ca^{2+} channels may enhance it. Activation of ATP P2X$_7$ receptors and neurotensin NTS1 receptors can enhance excitotoxicity, which may be true also for A$_{2A}$ receptor, whereas chronic activation of nicotinic receptors by partial desensitization can reduce excitotoxicity. Nicotinic receptors can also increase neurotrophism by promoting FGF-2 formation in nigral DA cells, whereas A$_{2A}$ receptors may bring down retrograde trophic signaling in the nigro-striatal DA neurons. Ca$_v$1.3 Ca^{2+} channels can enhance neurotrophism by maintaining pace-making, whereas activation of plasma membrane K$_{ATP}$ channels stops pace-making and reduces neurotrophism. Finally, microglia A$_{2A}$ receptors may increase neuroinflammation in the substantia nigra.

This chapter emphasizes that activation of mitoK$_{ATP}$ channels occurs after ATP depletion and is likely followed by the activation of uncoupling proteins that lead to a reduction of ROS production and promotion of ATP synthesis through an increase in mitochondrial biogenesis (Fig. 7.4). A therapeutic approach targeting the mitochondrial K$_{ATP}$ channels therefore represents one promising and novel neuroprotective strategy for treatment of PD.

The opening of plasma membrane K$_{ATP}$ channels by ROS (Fig. 7.4) may have an acute survival value by a hyperpolarization-induced silencing of the nigro-striatal DA neurons. However, chronically, it leads to reduced neurotrophism and increased DA cell degeneration via several possible mechanisms, including the disappearance of pace-making–induced neurotrophism, essential for the activation of RTK in DA cells. As a result, pace-making activity may exist as a mechanism for the survival of the nigro-striatal DA neurons with both its silencing (reduced neurotrophism) and exaggerated burst firing (energy loss; excitotoxicity) contributing to neurodegeneration. The modulation of these mechanisms is exemplified below (see Fig. 7.4).

1. The hypothesis has been introduced that ROS-activated $P2X_7$ receptors located on nigral DA cells will lead to a massive influx of cations, depolarization, and loss of energy gradients due to ATP depletion and can produce DA cell death (excitotoxicity), strongly contributing to the development of PD (Fig. 7.4) (Fuxe et al. 2006). Therefore, $P2X_7$ antagonists may represent novel and important drugs for neuroprotective treatment of PD.

2. Surmeier and colleagues have introduced a new strategy for PD treatment, namely $Ca_v 1.3$ Ca^{2+} channel antagonists that will bring aged DA neurons into a juvenile pace-maker mechanism via Na^+/HCN channels. In this way, calcium stress on mitochondria (mitochondrial dysfunction) will be reduced and will lead to neuroprotection (Fig. 7.4).

3. Nicotinic receptor agonists appear to be neuroprotective drugs by producing a partial desensitization of nicotinic receptor subtypes on the nigral DA cells, leading to reduced burst firing and excitotoxicity and by activating a neurotrophic mechanism in the DA cells, namely FGF-2 (Fig. 7.4). This gives nicotinic receptors a special value in the neuroprotective treatment of PD by increasing neurotrophism as well as reducing excitotoxicity.

4. NTS1 receptor antagonists, by blocking NTS1 receptors on the nigral DA cells, appear to have neuroprotective properties mainly by reducing excitotoxicity through counteraction of glutamate and NMDA toxicity on the DA cells (Fig. 7.4). The mechanisms involve the blockade of facilitatory NTS1/NMDA receptor interactions and antagonistic NTS1/D_2 autoreceptor interactions. Thus, burst firing and excitotoxicity is reduced, as is the calcium stress on the mitochondria (reduced mitochondrial dysfunction) (Fig. 7.4).

5. The neuroprotective effects of A_{2A} antagonists on the DA cells may instead mainly involve increased retrograde trophic signaling from the striatal DA terminal networks to the nigral DA cells, as well as reduced damaging influences from the DA nerve cell containing nigral trophic units in terms of astroglial glutamate release and release of cytokines from and COX-2 activation in microglia (Fig. 7.4).

Many strategies for neuroprotective treatments are being developed through animal research. Several of them should be combined, based on pharmacological grounds in view of complementary mechanisms, in order to enhance the neuroprotective outcome. One hopes it will be soon that clinical trials can be initiated to test the value of the strategies outlined in this chapter.

ACKNOWLEDGMENTS

This work has been supported by grants from the Swedish Research Council, the Marianne and Marcus Wallenberg Foundation, the Knut and Alice Wallenberg Foundation, and a rapid innovation award from the Michael J. Fox Foundation.

REFERENCES

Agnati, L. F., Cortelli, P., Pettersson, R. and Fuxe, K. (1995). "The concept of trophic units in the central nervous system." *Prog Neurobiol* 46(6): 561–74.

Agnati, L. F., Leo, G., Vergoni, A. V., Martinez, E., Hockemeyer, J., Lluis, C., Franco, R., Fuxe, K. and Ferre, S. (2004). "Neuroprotective effect of L-DOPA co-administered with the adenosine A2A receptor agonist CGS 21680 in an animal model of Parkinson's disease." *Brain Res Bull* 64(2): 155–64.

Alfinito, P. D., Wang, S. P., Manzino, L., Rijhsinghani, S., Zeevalk, G. D. and Sonsalla, P. K. (2003). "Adenosinergic protection of dopaminergic and GABAergic neurons against mitochondrial inhibition through receptors located in the substantia nigra and striatum, respectively." *J Neurosci* 23(34): 10982–7.

Anden, N. E., Bedard, P., Fuxe, K. and Ungerstedt, U. (1972). "Early and selective increase in brain dopamine levels after axotomy." *Experientia* 28(3): 300–2.

Anden, N. E., Carlsson, A., Dahlstroem, A., Fuxe, K., Hillarp, N. A. and Larsson, K. (1964). "Demonstration and Mapping Out of Nigro-Neostriatal Dopamine Neurons." *Life Sci* 3: 523–30.

Andrews, Z. B., Diano, S. and Horvath, T. L. (2005a). "Mitochondrial uncoupling proteins in the CNS: in support of function and survival." *Nat Rev Neurosci* 6(11): 829–40.

Andrews, Z. B., Horvath, B., Barnstable, C. J., Elsworth, J., Yang, L., Beal, M. F., Roth, R. H., Matthews, R. T. and Horvath, T. L. (2005b). "Uncoupling protein-2 is critical for nigral dopamine cell survival in a mouse model of Parkinson's disease." *J Neurosci* 25(1): 184–91.

Andrews, Z. B., Rivera, A., Elsworth, J. D., Roth, R. H., Agnati, L., Gago, B., Abizaid, A., Schwartz, M., Fuxe, K. and Horvath, T. L. (2006). "Uncoupling protein-2 promotes nigro-striatal dopamine neuronal function." *Eur J Neurosci* 24(1): 32–6.

Antonelli, T., Ferraro, L., Fuxe, K., Finetti, S., Fournier, J., Tanganelli, S., De Mattei, M. and Tomasini, M. C. (2004). "Neurotensin enhances endogenous extracellular glutamate levels in primary cultures of rat cortical neurons: involvement of neurotensin receptor in NMDA induced excitotoxicity." *Cereb Cortex* 14(4): 466–73.

Antonelli, T., Fuxe, K., Tomasini, M. C., Mazzoni, E., Agnati, L. F., Tanganelli, S. and Ferraro, L. (2007). "Neurotensin receptor mechanisms and its modulation of glutamate transmission in the brain: relevance for neurodegenerative diseases and their treatment." *Prog Neurobiol* 83(2): 92–109.

Antonelli, T., Tomasini, M. C., Finetti, S., Giardino, L., Calza, L., Fuxe, K., Soubrie, P., Tanganelli, S. and Ferraro, L. (2002). "Neurotensin enhances glutamate excitotoxicity in mesencephalic neurons in primary culture." *J Neurosci Res* 70(6): 766–73.

Avshalumov, M. V., Chen, B. T., Koos, T., Tepper, J. M. and Rice, M. E. (2005). "Endogenous hydrogen peroxide regulates the excitability of midbrain dopamine neurons via ATP-sensitive potassium channels." *J Neurosci* 25(17): 4222–31.

Avshalumov, M. V. and Rice, M. E. (2003). "Activation of ATP-sensitive K+ (K(ATP)) channels by H2O2 underlies glutamate-dependent inhibition of striatal dopamine release." *Proc Natl Acad Sci U S A* 100(20): 11729–34.

Bajgar, R., Seetharaman, S., Kowaltowski, A. J., Garlid, K. D. and Paucek, P. (2001). "Identification and properties of a novel intracellular (mitochondrial) ATP-sensitive potassium channel in brain." *J Biol Chem* 276(36): 33369–74.

Bao, L., Avshalumov, M. V. and Rice, M. E. (2005). "Partial mitochondrial inhibition causes striatal dopamine release suppression and medium spiny neuron depolarization via H2O2 elevation, not ATP depletion." *J Neurosci* 25(43): 10029–40.

Baron, J. A. (1986). "Cigarette smoking and Parkinson's disease." *Neurology* 36(11): 1490–6.

Belluardo, N., Blum, M., Mudo, G., Andbjer, B. and Fuxe, K. (1998). "Acute intermittent nicotine treatment produces regional increases of basic fibroblast growth factor messenger RNA and protein in the tel- and diencephalon of the rat." *Neuroscience* 83(3): 723–40.

Belluardo, N., Mudo, G., Blum, M., Amato, G. and Fuxe, K. (2000). "Neurotrophic effects of central nicotinic receptor activation." *J Neural Transm Suppl*(60): 227–45.

Belluardo, N., Mudo, G., Blum, M., Itoh, N., Agnati, L. and Fuxe, K. (2004). "Nicotine-induced FGF-2 mRNA in rat brain is preserved during aging." *Neurobiol Aging* 25(10): 1333–42.

Belluardo, N., Mudo, G., Caniglia, G., Cheng, Q., Blum, M. and Fuxe, K. (1999). "The nicotinic acetylcholine receptor agonist ABT-594 increases FGF-2 expression in various rat brain regions." *Neuroreport* 10(18): 3909–13.

Blum, M., Wu, G., Mudo, G., Belluardo, N., Andersson, K., Agnati, L. F. and Fuxe, K. (1996). "Chronic continuous infusion of (-)nicotine reduces basic fibroblast growth factor messenger RNA levels in the ventral midbrain of the intact but not of the 6-hydroxydopamine-lesioned rat." *Neuroscience* 70(1): 169–77.

Boudin, H., Pelaprat, D., Rostene, W., Pickel, V. M. and Beaudet, A. (1998). "Correlative ultrastructural distribution of neurotensin receptor proteins and binding sites in the rat substantia nigra." *J Neurosci* 18(20): 8473–84.

Bryan, J., Vila-Carriles, W. H., Zhao, G., Babenko, A. P. and Aguilar-Bryan, L. (2004). "Toward linking structure with function in ATP-sensitive K+ channels." *Diabetes* 53 Suppl 3: S104–12.

Burke, R. E. (2006). "GDNF as a candidate striatal target-derived neurotrophic factor for the development of substantia nigra dopamine neurons." *J Neural Transm Suppl*(70): 41–5.

Burnstock, G. (2007). "Physiology and pathophysiology of purinergic neurotransmission." *Physiol Rev* 87(2): 659–797.

Busija, D. W., Lacza, Z., Rajapakse, N., Shimizu, K., Kis, B., Bari, F., Domoki, F. and Horiguchi, T. (2004). "Targeting mitochondrial ATP-sensitive potassium channels—a novel approach to neuroprotection." *Brain Res Brain Res Rev* 46(3): 282–94.

Chadi, G., Moller, A., Rosen, L., Janson, A. M., Agnati, L. A., Goldstein, M., Ogren, S. O., Pettersson, R. F. and Fuxe, K. (1993). "Protective actions of human recombinant basic fibroblast growth factor on MPTP-lesioned nigro-striatal dopamine neurons after intraventricular infusion." *Exp Brain Res* 97(1): 145–58.

Chan, C. S., Guzman, J. N., Ilijic, E., Mercer, J. N., Rick, C., Tkatch, T., Meredith, G. E. and Surmeier, D. J. (2007). "'Rejuvenation' protects neurons in mouse models of Parkinson's disease." *Nature* 447(7148): 1081–6.

Chen, J. F., Sonsalla, P. K., Pedata, F., Melani, A., Domenici, M. R., Popoli, P., Geiger, J., Lopes, L. V. and de Mendonca, A. (2007). "Adenosine A2A receptors and brain injury: broad spectrum of neuroprotection, multifaceted actions and "fine tuning" modulation." *Prog Neurobiol* 83(5): 310–31.

Chen, J. F., Xu, K., Petzer, J. P., Staal, R., Xu, Y. H., Beilstein, M., Sonsalla, P. K., Castagnoli, K., Castagnoli, N., Jr. and Schwarzschild, M. A. (2001). "Neuroprotection by caffeine and A(2A) adenosine receptor inactivation in a model of Parkinson's disease." *J Neurosci* 21(10): RC143.

Colucci-D'Amato, L., Perrone-Capano, C. and di Porzio, U. (2003). "Chronic activation of ERK and neurodegenerative diseases." *Bioessays* 25(11): 1085–95.

Conforti, L., Adalbert, R. and Coleman, M. P. (2007). "Neuronal death: where does the end begin?" *Trends Neurosci* 30(4): 159–66.

Dahlström, A. and Fuxe, K. (1964a). "Evidence for the existence of monoamine-containing neurons in the Central Nervous System. I. Demonstration of Monoamines in the Cell Bodies of Brain Stem Neurons." *Acta Physiol Scand* Suppl 232: 1–55.

Dahlström, A. and Fuxe, K. (1964b). "A method for the demonstration of monoamine-containing nerve fibers in the Central Nervous System." *Acta Physiol Scand* 60: 293–4.

de Carvalho Aguiar, P., Sweadner, K. J., Penniston, J. T., Zaremba, J., Liu, L., Caton, M., Linazasoro, G., Borg, M., Tijssen, M. A., Bressman, S. B., Dobyns, W. B., Brashear, A. and Ozelius, L. J. (2004). "Mutations in the Na+/K+ -ATPase alpha3 gene ATP1A3 are associated with rapid-onset dystonia parkinsonism." *Neuron* 43(2): 169–75.

Deutch, A. Y. and Winder, D. G. (2006). "A channel to neurodegeneration." *Nat Med* 12(1): 17–8.

Diano, S., Matthews, R. T., Patrylo, P., Yang, L., Beal, M. F., Barnstable, C. J. and Horvath, T. L. (2003). "Uncoupling protein 2 prevents neuronal death including that occurring during seizures: a mechanism for preconditioning." *Endocrinology* 144(11): 5014–21.

Dunn-Meynell, A. A., Rawson, N. E. and Levin, B. E. (1998). "Distribution and phenotype of neurons containing the ATP-sensitive K+ channel in rat brain." *Brain Res* 814(1–2): 41–54.

Ekstrand, M. I., Terzioglu, M., Galter, D., Zhu, S., Hofstetter, C., Lindqvist, E., Thams, S., Bergstrand, A., Hansson, F. S., Trifunovic, A., Hoffer, B., Cullheim, S., Mohammed, A. H., Olson, L. and Larsson, N. G. (2007). "Progressive parkinsonism in mice with respiratory-chain-deficient dopamine neurons." *Proc Natl Acad Sci U S A* 104(4): 1325–30.

Fahn, S. (2005). "Does levodopa slow or hasten the rate of progression of Parkinson's disease?" *J Neurol* 252 Suppl 4: IV37–IV42.

Falck, B., Hillarp, N. A., Thieme, G. and Torp, A. (1962). "Fluorescence of catecholamines and related compounds condensed with formaldehyde." *J Histochem Cytochem* 10: 348–354.

Ferraro, L., Antonelli, T., O'Connor, W. T., Fuxe, K., Soubrie, P. and Tanganelli, S. (1998). "The striatal neurotensin receptor modulates striatal and pallidal glutamate and GABA release: functional evidence for a pallidal glutamate-GABA interaction via the pallidal-subthalamic nucleus loop." *J Neurosci* 18(17): 6977–89.

Ferraro, L., Tanganelli, S., O'Connor, W. T., Bianchi, C., Ungerstedt, U. and Fuxe, K. (1995). "Neurotensin increases endogenous glutamate release in the neostriatum of the awake rat." *Synapse* 20(4): 362–4.

Ferraro, L., Tomasini, M. C., Fernandez, M., Bebe, B. W., O'Connor, W. T., Fuxe, K., Glennon, J. C., Tanganelli, S. and Antonelli, T. (2001). "Nigral neurotensin receptor regulation of nigral glutamate and nigroventral thalamic GABA transmission: a dual-probe microdialysis study in intact conscious rat brain." *Neuroscience* 102(1): 113–20.

Ferraro, L., Tomasini, M. C., Mazza, R., Fuxe, K., Fournier, J., Tanganelli, S. and Antonelli, T. (2008). "Neurotensin receptors as modulators of glutamatergic transmission." *Brain Res Rev* 58(2): 365–73.

Fukae, J., Mizuno, Y. and Hattori, N. (2007). "Mitochondrial dysfunction in Parkinson's disease." *Mitochondrion* 7(1–2): 58–62.

Fuxe, K., Dahlstrom, A., Hoistad, M., Marcellino, D., Jansson, A., Rivera, A., Diaz-Cabiale, Z., Jacobsen, K., Tinner-Staines, B., Hagman, B., Leo, G., Staines, W., Guidolin, D., Kehr, J., Genedani, S., Belluardo, N. and Agnati, L. F. (2007a). "From the Golgi-Cajal mapping to the transmitter-based characterization of the neuronal networks leading to two modes of brain communication: wiring and volume transmission." *Brain Res Rev* 55(1): 17–54.

Fuxe, K., Diaz, R., Cintra, A., Bhatnagar, M., Tinner, B., Gustafsson, J. A., Ogren, S. O. and Agnati, L. F. (1996). "On the role of glucocorticoid receptors in brain plasticity." *Cell Mol Neurobiol* 16(2): 239–58.

Fuxe, K., Ferre, S., Genedani, S., Franco, R. and Agnati, L. F. (2007b). "Adenosine receptor-dopamine receptor interactions in the basal ganglia and their relevance for brain function." *Physiol Behav* 92(1–2): 210–7.

Fuxe, K., Janson, A. M., Jansson, A., Andersson, K., Eneroth, P. and Agnati, L. F. (1990). "Chronic nicotine treatment increases dopamine levels and reduces dopamine utilization in substantia nigra and in surviving forebrain dopamine nerve terminal systems after a partial di-mesencephalic hemitransection." *Naunyn Schmiedebergs Arch Pharmacol* 341(3): 171–81.

Fuxe, K., Manger, P., Genedani, S. and Agnati, L. (2006). "The nigro-striatal DA pathway and Parkinson's disease." *J Neural Transm Suppl*(70): 71–83.

Fuxe, K., Marcellino, D., Genedani, S. and Agnati, L. (2007c). "Adenosine A(2A) receptors, dopamine D(2) receptors and their interactions in Parkinson's disease." *Mov Disord* 22(14): 1990–2017.

Fuxe, K., Rivera, A., Jacobsen, K. X., Hoistad, M., Leo, G., Horvath, T. L., Staines, W., De la Calle, A. and Agnati, L. F. (2005). "Dynamics of volume transmission in the brain. Focus on catecholamine and opioid peptide communication and the role of uncoupling protein 2." *J Neural Transm* 112(1): 65–76.

Greenamyre, J. T. and Hastings, T. G. (2004). "Biomedicine. Parkinson's—divergent causes, convergent mechanisms." *Science* 304(5674): 1120–2.

Grenhoff, J., Janson, A. M., Svensson, T. H. and Fuxe, K. (1991). "Chronic continuous nicotine treatment causes decreased burst firing of nigral dopamine neurons in rats partially hemitransected at the meso-diencephalic junction." *Brain Res* 562(2): 347–51.

Heutink, P. (2006). "PINK-1 and DJ-1--new genes for autosomal recessive Parkinson's disease." *J Neural Transm Suppl*(70): 215–9.

Hornykiewicz, O. (1963). "[The tropical localization and content of noradrenalin and dopamine (3-hydroxytyramine) in the substantia nigra of normal persons and patients with Parkinson's disease.]." *Wien Klin Wochenschr* 75: 309–12.

Janson, A. M., Fuxe, K., Agnati, L. F., Kitayama, I., Harfstrand, A., Andersson, K. and Goldstein, M. (1988). "Chronic nicotine treatment counteracts the disappearance of tyrosine-hydroxylase-immunoreactive nerve cell bodies, dendrites and terminals in the mesostriatal dopamine system of the male rat after partial hemitransection." *Brain Res* 455(2): 332–45.

Janson, A. M., Fuxe, K., Agnati, L. F., Sundström, E. and Goldstein, M. (1991). The effects of chronic nicotine treatment on 1-methyl-4-phenyl-1,2,3,6-tetrahydropyridine-induced degeneration of nigro-striatal dopamine neurons in the black mouse. *Advances in Pharmacological Sciences: Effects of Nicotine on Biological Systems*. F. Adlkofer and K. Thurau. Basel, Birkhäuser Verlag: 322–9.

Jun, D. J., Kim, J., Jung, S. Y., Song, R., Noh, J. H., Park, Y. S., Ryu, S. H., Kim, J. H., Kong, Y. Y., Chung, J. M. and Kim, K. T. (2007). "Extracellular ATP Mediates Necrotic Cell Swelling in SN4741 Dopaminergic Neurons through P2X7 Receptors." *J Biol Chem* 282(52): 37350–8.

Klink, R., de Kerchove d'Exaerde, A., Zoli, M. and Changeux, J. P. (2001). "Molecular and physiological diversity of nicotinic acetylcholine receptors in the midbrain dopaminergic nuclei." *J Neurosci* 21(5): 1452–63.

Kwong, J. Q., Beal, M. F. and Manfredi, G. (2006). "The role of mitochondria in inherited neurodegenerative diseases." *J Neurochem* 97(6): 1659–75.

Lee, F. J., Liu, F., Pristupa, Z. B. and Niznik, H. B. (2001). "Direct binding and functional coupling of alpha-synuclein to the dopamine transporters accelerate dopamine-induced apoptosis." *Faseb J* 15(6): 916–26.

Liss, B., Bruns, R. and Roeper, J. (1999a). "Alternative sulfonylurea receptor expression defines metabolic sensitivity of K-ATP channels in dopaminergic midbrain neurons." *Embo J* 18(4): 833–46.

Liss, B., Haeckel, O., Wildmann, J., Miki, T., Seino, S. and Roeper, J. (2005). "K-ATP channels promote the differential degeneration of dopaminergic midbrain neurons." *Nat Neurosci* 8(12): 1742–51.

Liss, B., Neu, A. and Roeper, J. (1999b). "The weaver mouse gain-of-function phenotype of dopaminergic midbrain neurons is determined by coactivation of wvGirk2 and K-ATP channels." *J Neurosci* 19(20): 8839–48.

Liss, B. and Roeper, J. (2001). "ATP-sensitive potassium channels in dopaminergic neurons: transducers of mitochondrial dysfunction." *News Physiol Sci* 16: 214–7.

Manago, Y., Kanahori, Y., Shimada, A., Sato, A., Amano, T., Sato-Sano, Y., Setsuie, R., Sakurai, M., Aoki, S., Wang, Y. L., Osaka, H., Wada, K. and Noda, M. (2005). "Potentiation of ATP-induced currents due to the activation of P2X receptors by ubiquitin carboxy-terminal hydrolase L1." *J Neurochem* 92(5): 1061–72.

Mayanagi, K., Gaspar, T., Katakam, P. V., Kis, B. and Busija, D. W. (2007). "The mitochondrial K(ATP) channel opener BMS-191095 reduces neuronal damage after transient focal cerebral ischemia in rats." *J Cereb Blood Flow Metab* 27(2): 348–55.

Michel, P. P., Alvarez-Fischer, D., Guerreiro, S., Hild, A., Hartmann, A. and Hirsch, E. C. (2007). "Role of activity-dependent mechanisms in the control of dopaminergic neuron survival." *J Neurochem* 101(2): 289–97.

Mizuno, Y., Hattori, N., Yoshino, H., Hatano, Y., Satoh, K., Tomiyama, H. and Li, Y. (2006). "Progress in familial Parkinson's disease." *J Neural Transm Suppl*(70): 191–204.

Moszczynska, A., Saleh, J., Zhang, H., Vukusic, B., Lee, F. J. and Liu, F. (2007). "Parkin disrupts the alpha-synuclein/dopamine transporter interaction: consequences toward dopamine-induced toxicity." *J Mol Neurosci* 32(3): 217–27.

Mudo, G., Belluardo, N. and Fuxe, K. (2007). "Nicotinic receptor agonists as neuroprotective/neurotrophic drugs. Progress in molecular mechanisms." *J Neural Transm* 114(1): 135–47.

North, R. A. (2002). "Molecular physiology of P2X receptors." *Physiol Rev* 82(4): 1013–67.

Palacios, J. M. and Kuhar, M. J. (1981). "Neurotensin receptors are located on dopamine-containing neurones in rat midbrain." *Nature* 294(5841): 587–9.

Perier, C., Bove, J., Wu, D. C., Dehay, B., Choi, D. K., Jackson-Lewis, V., Rathke-Hartlieb, S., Bouillet, P., Strasser, A., Schulz, J. B., Przedborski, S. and Vila, M. (2007). "Two molecular pathways initiate mitochondria-dependent dopaminergic neurodegeneration in experimental Parkinson's disease." *Proc Natl Acad Sci U S A* 104(19): 8161–6.

Quik, M. (2004). "Smoking, nicotine and Parkinson's disease." *Trends Neurosci* 27(9): 561–8.

Quik, M., Parameswaran, N., McCallum, S. E., Bordia, T., Bao, S., McCormack, A., Kim, A., Tyndale, R. F., Langston, J. W. and Di Monte, D. A. (2006). "Chronic oral nicotine treatment protects against striatal degeneration in MPTP-treated primates." *J Neurochem* 98(6): 1866–75.

Rivera, A., Agnati, L. F., Horvath, T. L., Valderrama, J. J., de La Calle, A. and Fuxe, K. (2006). "Uncoupling protein 2/3 immunoreactivity and the ascending dopaminergic and noradrenergic neuronal systems: relevance for volume transmission." *Neuroscience* 137(4): 1447–61.

Ross, G. W., Abbott, R. D., Petrovitch, H., White, L. R. and Tanner, C. M. (2000). "Relationship between caffeine intake and parkinson disease." *Jama* 284(11): 1378–9.

Ruan, T., Lin, Y. S., Lin, K. S. and Kou, Y. R. (2005). "Sensory transduction of pulmonary reactive oxygen species by capsaicin-sensitive vagal lung afferent fibres in rats." *J Physiol* 565(Pt 2): 563–78.

Salthun-Lassalle, B., Hirsch, E. C., Wolfart, J., Ruberg, M. and Michel, P. P. (2004). "Rescue of mesencephalic dopaminergic neurons in culture by low-level stimulation of voltage-gated sodium channels." *J Neurosci* 24(26): 5922–30.

Sato, A., Arimura, Y., Manago, Y., Nishikawa, K., Aoki, K., Wada, E., Suzuki, Y., Osaka, H., Setsuie, R., Sakurai, M., Amano, T., Aoki, S., Wada, K. and Noda, M. (2006). "Parkin potentiates ATP-induced currents due to activation of P2X receptors in PC12 cells." *J Cell Physiol* 209(1): 172–82.

Schwarzschild, M. A., Agnati, L., Fuxe, K., Chen, J. F. and Morelli, M. (2006). "Targeting adenosine A2A receptors in Parkinson's disease." *Trends Neurosci* 29(11): 647–54.

Shi, W. S. and Bunney, B. S. (1990). "Neurotensin attenuates dopamine D2 agonist quinpirole-induced inhibition of midbrain dopamine neurons." *Neuropharmacology* 29(11): 1095–7.

Sonsalla, P. K., Albers, D. S. and Zeevalk, G. D. (1998). "Role of glutamate in neurodegeneration of dopamine neurons in several animal models of parkinsonism." *Amino Acids* 14(1–3): 69–74.

Suadicani, S. O., Brosnan, C. F. and Scemes, E. (2006). "P2X7 receptors mediate ATP release and amplification of astrocytic intercellular Ca2+ signaling." *J Neurosci* 26(5): 1378–85.

Sulzer, D. (2007). "Multiple hit hypotheses for dopamine neuron loss in Parkinson's disease." *Trends Neurosci* 30(5): 244–50.

Surmeier, D. J. (2007). "Calcium, ageing, and neuronal vulnerability in Parkinson's disease." *Lancet Neurol* 6(10): 933–8.

Tanganelli, S., von Euler, G., Fuxe, K., Agnati, L. F. and Ungerstedt, U. (1989). "Neuro-tensin counteracts apomorphine-induced inhibition of dopamine release as studied by microdialysis in rat neostriatum." *Brain Res* 502(2): 319–24.

Tebano, M. T., Martire, A., Potenza, R. L., Gro, C., Pepponi, R., Armida, M., Domenici, M. R., Schwarzschild, M. A., Chen, J. F. and Popoli, P. (2008). "Adenosine A(2A) receptors are required for normal BDNF levels and BDNF-induced potentiation of synaptic transmission in the mouse hippocampus." *J Neurochem* 104(1): 279–86.

Tsukimoto, M., Harada, H., Ikari, A. and Takagi, K. (2005). "Involvement of chloride in apoptotic cell death induced by activation of ATP-sensitive P2X7 purinoceptor." *J Biol Chem* 280(4): 2653–8.

Vila, M., Jackson-Lewis, V., Vukosavic, S., Djaldetti, R., Liberatore, G., Offen, D., Kors-meyer, S. J. and Przedborski, S. (2001). "Bax ablation prevents dopaminergic neuro-degeneration in the 1-methyl- 4-phenyl-1,2,3,6-tetrahydropyridine mouse model of Parkinson's disease." *Proc Natl Acad Sci U S A* 98(5): 2837–42.

Volonte, C., Amadio, S., Cavaliere, F., D'Ambrosi, N., Vacca, F. and Bernardi, G. (2003). "Extracellular ATP and neurodegeneration." *Curr Drug Targets CNS Neurol Disord* 2(6): 403–12.

Wang, X., Arcuino, G., Takano, T., Lin, J., Peng, W. G., Wan, P., Li, P., Xu, Q., Liu, Q. S., Goldman, S. A. and Nedergaard, M. (2004). "P2X7 receptor inhibition improves recovery after spinal cord injury." *Nat Med* 10(8): 821–7.

Xu, K., Bastia, E. and Schwarzschild, M. (2005). "Therapeutic potential of adenosine A(2A) receptor antagonists in Parkinson's disease." *Pharmacol Ther* 105(3): 267–310.

Yamada, T., McGeer, P. L., Baimbridge, K. G. and McGeer, E. G. (1990). "Relative spar-ing in Parkinson's disease of substantia nigra dopamine neurons containing calbindin-D28K." *Brain Res* 526(2): 303–7.

Zeevalk, G. D., Manzino, L. and Sonsalla, P. K. (2000). "NMDA receptors modulate dopamine loss due to energy impairment in the substantia nigra but not striatum." *Exp Neurol* 161(2): 638–46.

Chapter Eight

Degeneration and Regeneration of Myelin in the Central Nervous System of the Aging Monkey

Alan Peters

Our studies have been carried out in the rhesus monkey, and their goal is to determine what happens to the central nervous system (CNS) during normal aging. The rhesus monkey is a good model in which to carry out such studies, because although these animals live to be as long as 35 years (Tigges et al. 1988), they do not develop Alzheimer's disease, which can be a confounding problem when trying to carry out studies of normal aging in older humans. Rhesus monkeys, like humans, exhibit cognitive decline as they age, and this decline can be assessed by using behavioral tests that are derived and adapted from ones used to assess cognitive decline and impairment in humans (see Bachevalier et al. 1991; Albert and Moss 1996; Herndon et al. 1997). On the basis of these behavioral tests a measure of their cognitive impairment, the cognitive impairment index (CII), is determined for each monkey, and after the cognitive status has been determined the brain can be properly prepared for a morphological analysis to ascertain what abnormal or pathological structural changes have occurred. Once the changes have been characterized, their extent can be quantified and a determination made of when the changes first occur, how they progress with age, and whether they correlate with the cognitive impairments displayed by aging monkeys. Taken together, these factors make the rhesus monkey an excellent model in which to study the effects of normal aging on the primate brain.

When our studies first began, the general consensus was that the cognitive impairment displayed by monkeys and humans occurs because there is an increasing loss of neurons from the cortex with age. But as more careful and better designed studies have been carried out, it has become evident that there is not a significant overall loss of cortical neurons during normal aging (see Morrison and Hof 1997; Peters et al. 1998a; Merrill et al. 1998). However, Smith et al. (2004) have recently claimed that when the prefrontal cortices of young and old monkeys are compared, it is found that there is a 32% loss of neurons from area 8A in old monkeys, even though there is no age-related loss of cortical neurons from adjacent area 46, as reported earlier by Peters et al. (1994). To date there have been no other studies of this type, but the important issue raised by Smith et al. (2004) needs further investigation.

Even though neurons may not be lost from most areas of the cortex, these cells are not unaffected by age, and one of the most obvious signs of aging is the accumulation of lipofuscin in neuronal cell bodies. In addition there is evidence that with age there is some pruning of the dendritic arbors of neurons, a situation that is very obvious in layer 1 of the cerebral cortex, which becomes much thinner with age and loses many of the branches of the apical tufts of pyramidal cells that largely occupy this layer (Peters et al. 1998b, 2001). There appears to be less of a loss of dendritic branches, dendritic spines, and their synapsing axon terminals in the deeper layers of the cortex (see Peters et al. 2007), and overall the synaptic input to cortical neurons is reduced by between 20% and 30% over the lifespan of the monkey (see Peters et al. 2007). If one wants to ascertain if a given section of cerebral cortex is from a young or an old monkey, it is also helpful to look at the neuroglial cells in both gray and white matter, because with age many of them come to contain extensive inclusions in their cytoplasm.

Other age-related changes—which are not too obvious in light microscopic preparations, but are very obvious in electron micrographs—are the profound alterations in myelinated nerve fibers of the CNS. This is the subject of this chapter.

NORMAL MYELIN SHEATHS

In the central nervous system myelin ensheaths many of the axons in both gray and white matter (Figures 8.1 and 8.2). The myelin is produced by oligodendrocytes and is laid down in segments that are referred to as internodal lengths or segments. There is very little data on the extent of these internodal segments, but in a recent study of the thoracic spinal cord of mice, Perrot et al. (2007) have determined that the internodal length is between 200µm and 800µm, with a mean length of about 393µm. Within the internodal lengths of mature myelin the lamellae that form the sheaths are wound around the enclosed axon in a compact spiral, formed by paired sheets of oligodendroglial plasma membrane that are apposed on their outer faces to form the intraperiod line of the myelin sheath. During development there is oligodendroglial cytoplasm between the turns of the spiral, but eventually this cytoplasm becomes excluded, so that the cytoplasmic faces of the membranes also become apposed to form the major dense line of the sheath. This line alternates with the intraperiod line.

At the two ends of each internodal length are the paranodal regions, where the spiraled lamellae of myelin gradually terminate and the major dense line of the sheath opens up to accommodate cytoplasm. Because of the gradual way in which the lamellae terminate, this cytoplasm is contained in a helical tunnel, which in longitudinal sections through paranodes appears as a series of pockets on each side of the axon. Another feature of the paranode is that the axolemma and the plasma membrane on the axonal side of the cytoplasmic pockets become apposed, to form a complex junction in which they are separated by a gap of only 3nm. This feature makes it very easy to recognize transverse sections through paranodes (Figs. 8.1 and 8.2). At the nodes of Ranvier, which are between adjacent internodal lengths of myelin, the axons are bare, but sections

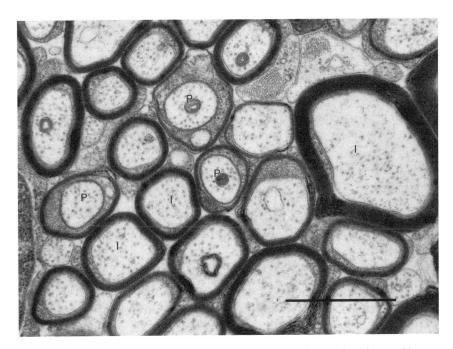

Figure 8.1. Myelinated nerve fibers from the anterior commissure of a 16-year-old monkey. At internodes (**I**) the myelin sheaths consist of tightly wrapped lamellae. At paranodes (**P**) the myelin lamellae gradually taper, and profiles of paranodes are easily recognized by the close apposition between the axolemma and the plasma membrane on the inside of the myelin sheath. Scale bar = 1 micron.

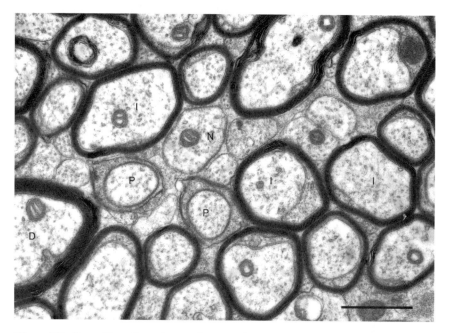

Figure 8.2. Nerve fibers from the anterior commissure of a 7-year-old monkey. The nerve fibers are sectioned at several levels, including internodes (**I**), paranodes (**P**), and nodes of Ranvier (**N**). At nodes the axon is bare, but profiles of nodes can be recognized by the presence of a dense undercoating of their plasma membrane. Scale bar = 1 micron.

through the nodal axon can be recognized by the distinctive electron-dense undercoating of the axolemma (Fig. 8.2). Much of this dense undercoating is due to the presence of complexes of cytoskeletal molecules and ankyrin, which are necessary for the concentration of sodium channels present at the nodes (e.g., Bennett and Lambert 1999). Another distinctive feature of nodes is that their axonal cytoplasm contains a higher concentration of microtubules than elsewhere in the axon.

LOSS OF NERVE FIBERS WITH AGE

The first hint that there are age-related alterations in myelin came from the study of Lintl and Braak (1982), who showed that in sections of human visual cortex stained with haemotoxylin, from the third decade of age onward there is a reduction in the intensity of staining of myelin in the line of Gennari. They suggested that this is due to a reduction in the amount of myelin in this intracortical plexus. Kemper (1994) also showed that there is an age-related decrease in the staining intensity of nerve fibers in the human cerebral cortex, and that this is most obvious in the association areas. These changes in staining intensity are probably a consequence of morphological changes in myelin, together with the loss of myelinated nerve fibers that occurs with age.

Magnetic resonance imaging (MRI) studies of both human (e.g., Albert 1993; Guttmann et al. 1998) and monkey (Lai et al. 1995) brains have indicated that there is a loss of white matter from the cerebral hemispheres with increasing age, especially from the frontal lobes. But in contrast to these studies, which emphasize white matter changes, there are other studies on humans (e.g., Pferrerbaum et al. 1994; Resnick et al. 2003; Sullivan et al. 2004) and monkeys (Andersen et al. 1999) that indicate that there is cortical thinning with age and that this thinning, and the consequent loss of gray matter, exceeds the white matter loss. However, as pointed out earlier, any loss of gray matter with age is unlikely to be due to an extensive loss of neurons, although there is some loss of dendritic branches, dendritic spines, and axon terminals with age (e.g., Peters et al. 2007). The problem associated with these MRI studies is that it is difficult to accurately define a white/gray matter boundary. Indeed, there is no distinct boundary, but a transition zone in which the concentration of myelinated nerve fibers gradually increases as the white matter is approached. That there is a loss of nerve fibers with age has been clearly demonstrated in a number of stereological studies of primate cerebral hemispheres.

Among the first of these stereological studies was that of Pakkenburg and Gundersen (1997), who examined a total of 94 normal human brains from individuals ranging from 20 to 95 years of age. As a result of their stereological analyses they concluded that there is a 28% decrease in the volume of white matter from the cortical hemispheres with age. In another publication, Tang et al. (1997) concluded that this white matter loss is due to an overall decrease of 27% in the total length of nerve fibers. Marner et al. (2003) later extended this study and concluded that the loss of white matter from the normally aging cerebral hemispheres is almost 23% between the ages of 20 and 80, and that the overall decrease of 45% in fiber length is the consequence of a loss of thinner nerve fibers, with a relative preservation of the large-diameter fibers. A similar loss of nerve fibers from the aging human brain has also been found by Meier-Ruge et al. (1992), who examined autopsied brains of a number of cognitively normal humans and concluded that there is a 16% loss of nerve fibers from the white matter of the precentral gyrus and a 10.5% loss of nerve fibers from the corpus callosum.

To ascertain if there is a loss of myelinated nerve fibers with age in the rhesus monkey, we have examined several fiber tracts in which the numbers of myelinated nerve fibers can be determined. The first fiber tract we examined was the optic nerve (Sandell and Peters 2001). In young monkeys of 4–10 years of age, the average number of myelinated nerve fibers in the optic nerve is 1.6×10^6, but in monkeys 25 years of age and older the average number of myelinated nerve fibers is reduced to an average of 9×10^5, which represents a 45% fiber loss. However, in extreme cases as many as 75% of the fibers can be lost, reducing the number of optic nerve fibers to as few as 4×10^5. In these extreme situations, the myelin sheaths of most of the nerve fibers show some defects; many fibers have degenerating axons; and in a number of cases the myelin sheaths are empty because the axon has completely disappeared (see Figure 8.3). This loss of nerve fibers is accompanied by alterations in the neuroglial cell population (Sandell and Peters 2002). Each of the neuroglial cell types develops inclusions in their cytoplasm; astrocytes hypertrophy to occupy much of the space created by the loss of nerve fibers and they become more filamentous. Also, both microglial cells and oligodendrocytes become more numerous with age, and the microglial cells become engorged by phagocytosed debris, much of which can be recognized as degenerating myelin. Cavalloti et al. (2001) have also reported an age-related loss of nerve fibers from the optic nerves of rats, accompanied by an increase in the numbers of astrocytes and in the GFAP labeling of these cells, which presumably reflects an increase in the number of astrocytic filaments and hypertrophy of the astrocytes, as occurs in the aging monkey optic nerve.

In the monkey, the anterior commissure also shows a loss of nerve fibers with age (Sandell and Peters 2003). Thus, in young monkeys the anterior commissure

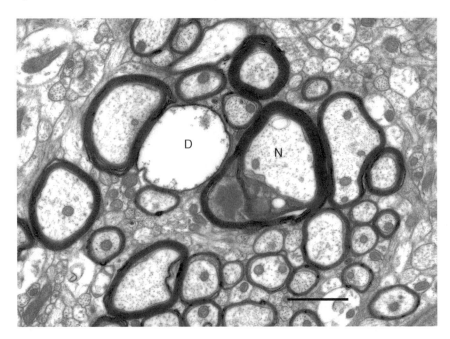

Figure 8.3. A nerve fiber bundle in layer 4 of the primary visual cortex of a 29-year-old monkey. One nerve fiber (**N**) shows an accumulation of dense cytoplasm between the lamellae of its sheath. The axon of an adjacent nerve fiber (**D**) has degenerated, leaving an empty myelin sheath. Other nerve fibers in this bundle are normal. Scale bar = 1 micron.

contains some 2.2×10^6 myelinated nerve fibers, and in monkeys 25 years of age and older, the mean number of nerve fibers is reduced to a mean of 1.2×10^6, representing a 45% loss of nerve fibers, which is similar to the fiber loss from the optic nerve. The anterior commissures of some middle-aged monkeys, 12–20 years old, were also examined, and it was found that in these monkeys the numbers of nerve fibers are similar to those of young monkeys, indicating that most of the nerve fiber loss occurs in old age. In the anterior commissure none of the three types of neuroglial cells show an increase in their total numbers, although as occurs throughout the brain, with increasing age each of the types acquires some inclusions in their perikarya.

Ongoing studies (unpublished data) on the splenium of the corpus callosum and on the fornix show that these structures also lose myelinated nerve fibers with age. When young and old monkeys are compared, it is found that the overall loss of myelinated nerve fibers from both of these fiber tracts is about 25%.

Thus, it appears that the loss of myelinated nerve fibers from white matter with age is ubiquitous, but in contrast there appears to be little loss of myelinated nerve fibers from gray matter. This became apparent in our study of the primary visual cortex in the monkey (Nielsen and Peters 2000). In this cortex there are very obvious vertically oriented bundles of myelinated nerve fibers that appear at the level of layer 4 and descend through the cortex to pass into the white matter. Using semi-thick plastic sections stained with toluidine blue, the numbers of transversely sectioned myelinated nerve fibers per mm^2 were determined at the level of layer 4β, in 16 monkeys ranging in age from 5 to 33 years. No significant change was found in the numbers of myelinated nerve fibers. Moreover, in electron microscopic evaluations, few degenerating myelinated nerve fibers were encountered, further indicating that there is little loss of myelinated nerve fibers from gray matter with age. Although no numerical studies have been carried out in area 46, we have also seen few signs of degenerating nerve fibers in the gray matter.

These data are summarized in Table 8.1, in which it is shown that there are strong correlations between age and the loss of myelinated nerve fibers from white matter. There are also good correlations between myelinated nerve fiber loss and cognitive impairment, as indicated by the CII values of the monkeys, for the anterior commissure and fornix. But there is no significant correlation between myelinated nerve fiber loss and cognitive impairment for the splenium of the corpus callosum. Whereas the anterior commissure appears to be involved in the interocular transfer of visual information and to facilitate transfer of visual information between the hemispheres (Sullivan and Hamilton 1973a, 1973b)— although its full function remains elusive (see Schmahmann and Pandya 2006)— sectioning of the corpus callosum has little effect on cognition (Innocenti 1986). In contrast, the fornix conveys hippocampal output to the mammillary bodies and the dorsomedial nucleus of the thalamus, and sectioning it severely affects

TABLE 8.1 Myelinated Nerve Fiber Loss with Age

Structure	Percent Loss	Correlation with Age	Behavioral Correlation with CII
Optic nerve	about 45%	p < 0.0001	no data
Anterior commissure	about 45%	p < 0.01	p < 0.01
Splenium of corpus callosum	about 25%	p < 0.0001	Not significant
Fornix	about 25%	p < 0.0002	p < 0.01
Cortical area 17	small	Not significant	Not significant
Cortical aera 46	small	Not signifcant	Not significant

cognition (e.g., Nilsson et al. 1987; Fletcher et al. 2006). But any loss of nerve fibers from white matter will result in some disconnection between various components of the CNS, and this can certainly be predicted to bring about some decline in cognition.

DEGENERATIVE ALTERATIONS IN MYELIN SHEATHS

The most common age-related degenerative alteration in myelin sheaths is the accumulation of dense cytoplasm in pockets produced by splits between myelin lamellae (e.g., Peters et al. 2000; Peters and Sethares 2002; Sandell and Peters 2003). These pockets are produced by splits of the major dense line, and because this line is formed by the apposition of the cytoplasmic faces of successive turns of the plasma membrane of the oligodendroglial cell forming the sheath, it can be concluded that the dense cytoplasm in the pockets is derived from the parent oligodendroglial cell. In transverse sections of sheaths sometimes only one pocket of dense cytoplasm is evident, but in other examples there may be several pockets in the same segment of the sheath (Figures 8.3 and 8.4). Also, the amount of dense cytoplasm is variable, and the amount determines the extent to which the sheath bulges out. Longitudinal sections show that these pockets of dense cytoplasm are localized, but there may be several loci of dense cytoplasm along the same internode. It is assumed that the accumulation of dense cytoplasm is a degenerative change because Cuprizone toxicity leads to the formation of dense cytoplasm in the inner tongue processes of degenerating sheaths (Ludwin 1978, 1995) and similar dense cytoplasm occurs in the sheaths of mice with a myelin-associated glycoprotein deficiency (e.g., Lassmann et al. 1997). Also, anti-ubiquitin antibodies immunolabel dense inclusions in focal swelling of myelin sheaths in white matter of old dogs (Uchida et al. 1992) and humans (Dickson et al. 1990), suggesting that the dense material in sheaths may be proteins that are not degraded by proteosomes.

Another less common, but more spectacular age-related alteration in myelin sheaths is the formation of balloons (e.g., Feldman and Peters 1998). These balloons

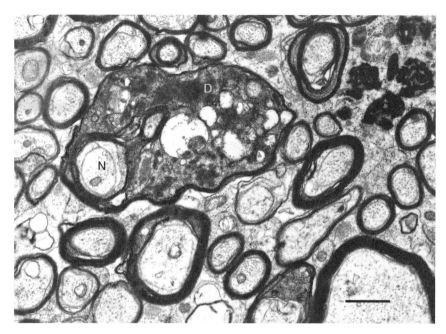

Figure 8.4. A degenerating myelin sheath in the anterior commissure of a 32-year-old monkey. The myelin sheath of the nerve fiber (**N**) has split to enclose an extensive mass of amorphous, dark and degenerating cytoplasm (**D**). Scale bar = 1 micron.

can be as large as 10μm in diameter and in light microscopic preparations they appear as holes in the neuropil. However, electron microscopic examination shows that these balloons are fluid-filled cavities produced by splits in the intra-period line of a sheath, and in sections through the largest balloons the axon is flattened against one side of the sheath, suggesting that the fluid in the balloon is under some pressure (Figure 8.5). In other sections through balloons no axon is visible, so the balloon appears as a large cavity surrounded by a thin layer of myelin. But it is now evident that such profiles are produced when sections pass to one side of the connection between the balloon and its parent sheath. The source of the fluid in balloons is not known, and it is interesting that even in the largest balloons there is no change in the thickness of the myelin lamellae sur-rounding the balloon (see Fig. 8.5). Consequently, the myelin is not elastic and the generation of these balloons must mean that the parent oligodendrocyte is generating a large amount of excess myelin. It should also be added that it is not uncommon to find some dense cytoplasm associated with balloons.

Myelin balloons have also been described in the anterior commissure of aging rodents (Sturrock 1987) and in the cochlear nucleus of aging gerbils (Faddis and McGinn 1997); they also can occur in severe diabetes (Tamura and Parry 1994) and in the early phases of Wallerian degeneration in the dorsal columns of the

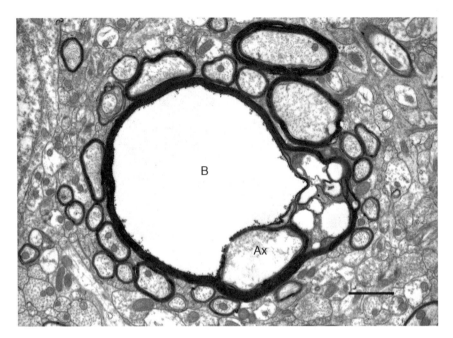

Figure 8.5. An altered myelin sheath in the primary visual cortex of a 29-year-old monkey. The myelin sheath has ballooned out (**B**) to enclose fluid. The balloon (**B**) is 5 microns in diameter and the fluid in the balloon has pushed the axon (**Ax**) to one side. Scale bar = 1 micron.

spinal cord induced by dorsal rhizotomy (Farnson and Ronnevi 1989). Balloons can also occur as a result of Cuprizone poisoning (Ludwin 1978), by toxicity produced by tetraethyl tin (Malamud and Hirano 1973), by lysolecithin (Blakemore 1978), and by chronic copper poisoning (Hull and Blakemore 1974). They can also occur in mutant mice that lack galactoproteins (Coetzee et al. 1996, 1998) and in mice that have a deficiency or an excess of proteolipid protein (Monuki and Lemke 1995). Consequently, there is little doubt that myelin balloons are a sign of age-related myelin sheath degeneration.

As shown in Table 8.2, there are strong correlations between age and the percentage of transversely sectioned myelin sheaths that contain either dense cytoplasm or balloons in area 17 (Peters et al. 2000), area 46 (Peters and Sethares 2002), splenium of the corpus callosum (Peters and Sethares 2002), anterior commissure (Sandell and Peters 2003), and fornix (unpublished data). Similar morphological alterations in myelin sheaths also occur in the aging optic nerve (Sandell and Peters 2001) and in the substantia nigra of rhesus monkeys (Siddiqi et al. 1999), so there is little doubt that these degenerative alterations in myelin sheaths are ubiquitous.

Except for area 17, these age-related alterations in the structure of myelin sheaths also correlate with the cognitive impairment (CII) shown by individual

TABLE 8.2 Altered Sheath Correlations

Structure	Correlation with Age	Behavioral Correlation with CII
Cortical area 17	$p < 0.0001$	$p = 0.29$
Cortical area 46	$p < 0.0001$	$p = 0.034$
Splenium of corpus callosum	$p < 0.0001$	$p = 0.06$
Fornix	$p < 0.001$	$p < 0.05$
Anterior commissure	$p < 0.001$	$p < 0.01$

monkeys (Table 8.2). This raises the question of what the basis is for this correlation, and it is likely that it has to do with the speed of conduction along nerve fibers. Myelin provides an insulation around nerve fibers and makes saltatory conduction possible, so it seems likely that alterations in the integrity of myelin sheaths will affect the conduction rate. This has not yet been determined in monkeys, but there are several studies in which the effects of age on conduction velocity have been examined. Aston-Jones et al. (1985) examined nerve fibers connecting nucleus basalis to the frontal cortex in rats and found a significant reduction of conduction rate in old animals. Morales et al. (1987) showed a similar age-related reduction in lumbar motor neurons of the spinal cord of cats, as did Xi et al. (1999) along the nerve fibers of the pyramidal tracts of old cats. There is also a reduction in conduction velocity as a result of demyelinating diseases (Waxman et al. 1995; Felts et al. 1997). Such reductions in conduction velocity would affect the timing in neuronal circuits and this, together with the disconnections produced by loss of nerve fibers from white matter with age, forms a likely basis for the age-related decline in cognition.

CONTINUED MYELIN FORMATION IN AGING

Although some myelin sheaths degenerate with age, myelin continues to be produced. This is shown by two other age-related types of morphological alterations in sheaths. One is the formation of sheaths in which the sheath is too large for the enclosed axon. Such redundant sheaths were first described by Rosenbluth (1966) in the cerebellum of the toad, whereas Sturrock (1976) encountered redundant sheaths in old mice. Interestingly, redundant sheaths generally surround small-diameter axons (see Figure 8.6). They are common in the optic nerves of metamorphosing toads, and Cullen and Webster (1979) suggest redundant sheaths are a sign that remodeling of sheaths is taking place and that the overproduction of myelin occurs to accommodate a subsequent increase in the size of the enclosed axon. However, the role that redundant sheaths play during aging is not known.

There is also an increase in the overall thickness of myelin sheaths with age. Thus, in a study of the primary visual cortex of the monkey, Peters et al. (2001b)

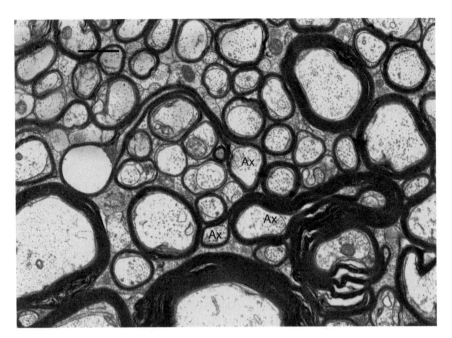

Figure 8.6. Axons (**Ax**) with redundant sheaths in the anterior commissure of a 25-year-old monkey. The sheaths are much too large for the enclosed axons and loop between the adjacent nerve fibers with normal sheaths. Scale bar = 1 micron.

showed that with age the mean numbers of lamellae in the sheaths of nerve fibers in the vertical bundles that pass through layer 4Cβ increase from 5.6 in young monkeys to 7.0 in old monkeys. Much of this increase in thickness is due to the fact that thick sheaths with more than ten lamellae are much more common in old, as compared with young, monkeys. In many cases these thicker sheaths show circumferential splitting, so that the sheaths appear to consist of an inner set of compact lamellae surrounded by an outer set. That there is new formation of myelin is also suggested by the overexpression of CNPase and myelin/oligodendrocyte-specific protein that occurs in old monkeys (Sloane et al. 2003).

The increase in the numbers of lamellae in some myelin sheaths affects the structure of the paranodes. Thus, whereas longitudinal sections of nerve fibers from young monkeys show the loops, or pockets, of cytoplasm at the paranodes to terminate in a regular sequence and to be in contact with the underlying membrane of the axon, in the thicker sheaths from older animals the paranodal loops pile up on one another and become disarrayed, so that only some of the loops are in contact with the axolemma (Hinman et al. 2006). Sugiyama et al. (2002) reported a similar situation in the thickened sheaths of nerve fibers in old rats, and it seems likely that this disruption of the paranodal region could compromise axonal conduction.

As far as can be determined, there have been no other studies of the effects of age on the thickness of myelin sheaths in primates. There have been studies made in rodents, but the results are inconclusive. For example, Godlewski et al. (1991) found the myelin sheaths in the optic nerves and corpus callosum of 2.5-year-old rats to be thicker than those of 4-month-old rats, but Sturrock (1976) found no change in the thickness of myelin sheaths in the anterior and posterior limbs of the anterior commissures of mice with increasing age.

In the monkey, at least, we conclude that the oligodendrocytes continue to produce myelin, even as they age. And indeed, as the next section will show, oligodendrocytes even undertake remyelination.

REMYELINATION IN AGING

As studies of the effects of aging on nerve fibers continued, it became evident that, in cross-sections of the vertical bundles of myelinated nerve fibers that pass through the deeper layers of both prefrontal and primary visual cortices, there is an age-related increase in the frequency of profiles of paranodes (Peters and Sethares 2003). As pointed out earlier, paranodes are the regions in which the myelin sheaths terminate, and profiles of paranodes are easily recognized by the presence of the junctional complex between the axolemma and the plasma membrane that bounds the axonal face of the paranodal loops (Figs. 8.1 and 8.2). When transverse sections of nerve fibers in young and old monkeys are compared, there is a 90% increase in the frequency of paranodal profiles from nerve fibers in prefrontal area 46 and a 57% increase in the primary visual cortex. However, there is only an 11% concomitant increase in the average lengths of paranodes with age, and this is obviously insufficient to account for the much larger percentage increase in the frequency of paranodal profiles. In our study of the anterior commissure (Sandell and Peters 2003), the increase in frequency of paranodal profiles was found to be about 60%, and it was considered that because some nerve fibers are lost with age, this increase in paranodal profiles might be due to a preferential loss of large-diameter fibers, which have the longest internodes. However, when the distribution of axon diameters was compared in the anterior commissures of young and old monkeys, no preferential loss of large-diameter fibers could be detected. Consequently, it can only be assumed that, with age, the increase in the number of paranodes is due to an increase in the number of internodal lengths of myelin. This would occur if there were remyelination taking place. In this situation some of the original long internodes of myelin that have degenerated would be replaced by shorter and thinner internodes (Figure 8.7). This is in concurrence with data that show that when remyelination takes place, either in experimental or natural conditions, the remyelinating axons display internodes that are inappropriately short for the diameter of the enclosed

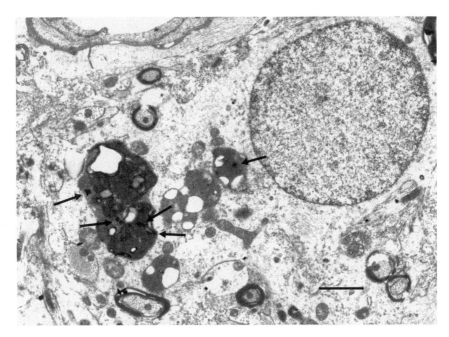

Figure 8.7. An astrocyte from layer 4 of primary visual cortex in a 25-year-old monkey. The dense inclusion body in the astrocyte has bound antibody to myelin basic protein, as indicated by the silver amplified particles of colloidal gold (arrows) overlying the inclusion. Consequently, some of the dense material in the inclusion must have come from myelin that the astrocyte has phagocytosed. Scale bar = 1 micron.

axon and sheaths that are inappropriately thin (e.g., Hirano 1989; Kreutzberg et al. 1997; Ludwin 1978, 1995; Pineas and McDonald 1997; Brück et al. 2003).

To support our contention that remyelination is taking place in normal aging, in the vertical bundles of myelinated nerve fibers in the deep layers of the primary visual cortex we have found short internodes that are 3μm to 8μm long (Fig. 8.7), and in a number of locations in old monkeys we have encountered sheaths that are inappropriately thin for the diameter of the enclosed axons (see Peters and Sethares 2003). We have not been able to identify bare lengths of demyelinated axons, but this is not surprising because it would not be possible to distinguish them from normal unmyelinated axons. However, in support of the concept that some myelin sheaths are degenerating with age, it has been found that some astrocytes in the cerebral cortices of old monkeys contain fragments of phagocytosed myelin, and that some of the amorphous phagocytosed material in astrocytes labels with antibodies to myelin basic protein (Figure 8.8; Peters and Sethares 2003).

As shown in Table 8.3, when the increases in the frequency of paranodal profiles are plotted against age, there are significant correlations in both white and gray matter. In contrast, when the cognitive impairment indices (CIIs) are

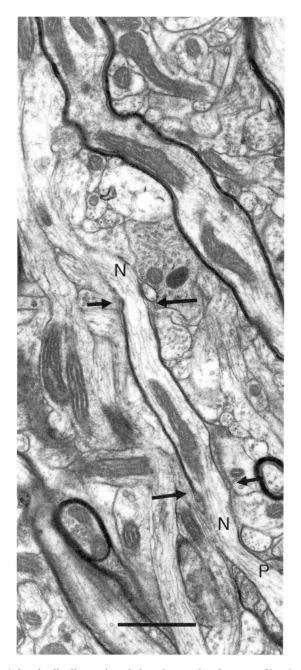

Figure 8.8. A longitudinally sectioned short internode of a nerve fiber in layer 4 of the primary visual cortex of a 25-year-old monkey. Arrows indicate the extent of the internode, which is 3 microns long. At the bottom of the field is the paranode (**P**) of the adjacent internode. The nodes of Ranvier at the ends of the short internode are indicated (**N**). Scale bar = 1 micron.

TABLE 8.3 Correlations of Increases in Paranodal Profiles

Structure	Correlation with aging	Correlation with CII
Cortical area 17	$p < 0.0001$	Not significant
Cortical area 46	$p < 0.0001$	$p < 0.01$
Splenium of corpus callosum	$p < 0.0001$	Not significant
Anterior commisure	$p < 0.01$	Not significant
Fornix	$p < 0.0002$	Not significant

considered, there is only a correlation between the two measures in area 46 of the prefrontal cortex ($p = 0.01$). There are no significant correlations between CIIs and paranodal frequency for either area 17 or any of the white matter tracts. How to interpret these data is not clear, unless it has to do with the role of the prefrontal cortex in cognition.

THE ROLE OF OLIGODENDROCYTES

Because oligodendrocytes form the myelin in the CNS, it is pertinent to inquire how they are affected by age. In preparations of monkey primary visual cortex and of area 46 stained by the Perl's reaction for ferric iron, the oligodendrocytes in young monkeys show only a few wispy processes, but in old monkeys bulbous swelling occurs along the processes (Figure 8.9). Some of these bulbous enlargements can be as large as 5µm in diameter, and they are filled with characteristic inclusions that resemble age pigment (Figure 8.10). Similar dense inclusions also occur in the cell bodies of oligodendrocytes from old monkeys (Figure 8.11) (Peters et al. 1991; Peters and Sethares 2004a). The origins of these inclusions are not yet known, but because they are not membrane-bound it is unlikely that they are phagocytic. It is more likely that they are derived from the degeneration of some of the components of myelin and are related to the dense material that occurs between some of the lamellae of degenerating sheaths (Figs. 8.3 and 8.4). Interestingly, it has been reported by LeVine and Torres (1992) that similar swellings along oligodendroglial processes occur in twitcher mice, which are a model for globoid cell leukodystrophy, and they suggest that the material in the swellings comes from components of myelin sheaths that are being turned over or replaced. In this situation the dense material would originate in the sheaths and then travel to the oligodendrocyte cell body. But at present this is speculation.

Another change is that with increasing age the frequency of oligodendrocytes that occur in pairs, groups, or rows increases (Fig. 8.11) (Peters and Sethares 2004a), suggesting that oligodendrocytes may be proliferating with age, and indeed, when a comparison is made between the mean numbers of oligodendrocytes in the primary visual cortex of young and old monkeys, the numbers of oligodendrocytes

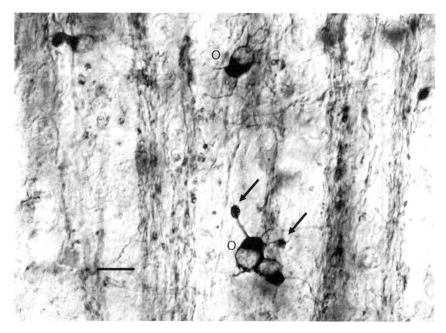

Figure 8.9. Light microscopic picture of oligodendrocytes (**O**) in area 17 of a 29-year-old monkey stained by Perl's reaction. One of the oligodendrocytes has processes with bulbous enlargements (arrows). In electron micrographs, as shown in Fig. 8.10, such bulbous enlargements are filled with dark inclusions. Scale bar = 10 microns.

appears to increase with age (Peters et al. 1991). Thus, in young monkeys oligodendrocytes comprise 35% of the neuroglial population, and in old monkeys their frequency increases to 40%. At the time of this study, few monkeys were available, but in a later study of layer 4C in the visual cortices of 22 monkeys a 50% increase in the numbers of oligodendrocytes was found when young (4–10 years of age) and old monkeys (25 years of age and older) were compared. This increase begins in middle age, but there appears to be no increase in the frequency of either astrocytes or microglial cells (Peters and Sethares 2004a). There is also an increase in the numbers of oligodendrocytes in the monkey optic nerve (Sandell and Peters 2002) but not in the anterior commissure (Sandell and Peters 2003).

When there is an age-related increase in the frequency of oligodendrocytes, as occurs in the cerebral cortex, two questions arise: Why are more oligodendrocytes needed, and where do they come from? They are probably needed to form the increased numbers of internodal lengths of myelin that occur with age (Peters and Sethares 2003). As to where they come from, the age-related increased frequency of occurrence of oligodendrocytes in pairs, groups, and rows could be taken to suggest that some oligodendrocytes are dividing, but the prevailing view is that there is little evidence that mature oligodendrocytes can divide (see Ludwin

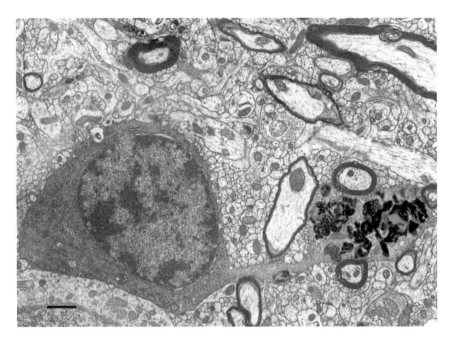

Figure 8.10. An oligodendrocyte in the primary visual cortex of a 35-year-old monkey. The process extending to the right from the perikaryon of the oligodendrocyte, expands into a bulbous enlargement, similar to those shown in Fig. 8.9, is filled with amorphous, dark inclusions that probably originate from the degeneration of the myelin sheath at the end of this oligodendroglial process. Scale bar = 1 micron.

1995; Norton 1996; Keirstead and Blakemore 1997), and in a recent study of newly generated cells in the adult monkey dentate gyrus using BrdU labeling, we encountered no labeled oligodendrocytes (Ngwenya et al. 2008). It is more likely that any increase in the numbers of oligodendrocytes originate from the oligodendroglial precursors (see Levine et al. 2001; Chen et al. 2002; Watanabe et al. 2002), which are labeled in the adult monkey dentate gyrus (Ngwenya et al. 2008). These cells, which can be visualized using antibodies to NG2 chondroitin proteoglycan, were earlier included in the population of cytoplasmic astrocytes, to which they bear many morphological resemblances (Fig. 8.11) (see Peters and Sethares 2004a, 2004b). Oligodendroglial precursors are relatively common in the CNS and can account for as many as 5% of the total neuroglial cell population (Levine et al. 2001).

Interestingly, Cerghet et al. (2006) have recently reported that in white matter of rodents the density of oligodendrocytes is 20–40% greater in males than in females, even though the degeneration of new glia, and the apoptosis of glia, is greater in the corpus callosum of females than males, indicating that the life-span of oligodendrocytes is shorter in females than in males. The frequency of

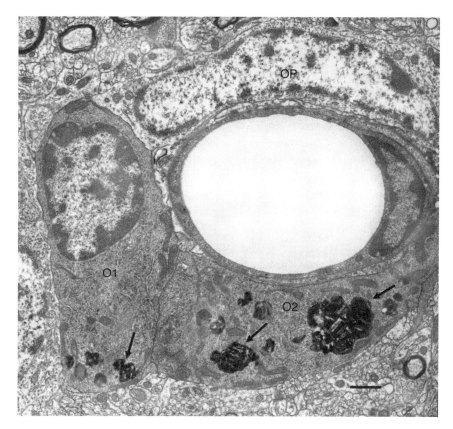

Figure 8.11. Two closely apposed oligodendrocytes (**O1** and **O2**) adjacent to a capillary in the primary visual cortex of a 28-year-old monkey. Both oligodendrocytes contain dense inclusions similar to those in the oligodendrocyte process shown in Fig. 8.10. On the other side of the capillary is an oligodendroglial precursor cell (**OP**), with a typical elongate and pale nucleus, surrounded by pale cytoplasm. These cells are similar in appearance to some astrocytes, but they do not have glial filaments in their cytoplasm. Scale bar = 1 micron.

oligodendrocytes in the anterior commissure (Sandell and Peters 2003) and cerebral cortex (Peters et al. 2008) seems not to be different in male and female monkeys, but there appears to be no information available about the turnover of oligodendrocytes with age in monkeys.

CONCLUSIONS

The effects of age on nerve fibers in the central nervous system are obviously complex. On the one hand there is some axonal degeneration with age, which results in a loss of nerve fibers. This loss is most pronounced in white matter tracts, because the loss of nerve fibers from the gray matter of cerebral cortex appears to be minimal. As axons degenerate, their ensheathing myelin degenerates, but there is also a progressive degeneration of sheaths around some axons that are not themselves degenerating. This degeneration of myelin sheaths is made evident by the age-related increased frequency of accumulations of dense material between myelin lamellae, and by the ballooning of other sheaths that accumulate fluid.

While this degeneration is occurring, myelin continues to form, so that with age the average number of lamellae in sheaths increases, and nerve fibers with thick sheaths become more common. In addition, there is an increase in the number of nerve fibers with redundant myelin, which is also taken to be a sign that myelin is continuing to form with age. Remyelination is also occurring, as shown by the age-related increase in the number of profiles of paranodes, by the existence of short internodes of myelin along some nerve fibers in old monkeys, and by the occurrence of sheaths that are inappropriately thin for the size of the enclosed axons. Both of these latter events are classical signs of remyelination.

The basic reason for this study is to determine whether any of these age-related alterations in nerve fibers can contribute to the decline in cognition that occurs in aging monkeys. Though there is a strong correlation between nerve fiber loss and age in the white matter tracts we have examined (see Table 8.1), only nerve fiber loss from the anterior commissure and the fornix showed correlations with cognitive decline; fiber loss from the splenium of the corpus callosum did not. The reason for this might be that loss of nerve fibers from the fornix (the main outflow from the hippocampus) and loss from the anterior commissure (a commissure of the frontal lobes of the cerebral hemispheres) can be expected to lead to some disconnection between structures that play a key role in cognition. The splenium is largely a commissure of the visual cortex, which is less likely to affect cognition. But in contrast to white matter, there appears to be little nerve fiber loss from the cerebral cortex.

Interestingly, the frequency of degenerative alterations in myelin sheaths correlates strongly with age, and as well with cognitive decline (see Table 8.2). Because myelin provides insulation around nerve fibers and makes saltatory conduction possible, it seems likely that any degenerative alterations in myelin sheaths will affect impulse conduction, as would an interposition of a number of short internodal lengths that occur in remyelination. Although we have no data of our own on this issue, as pointed out earlier, Aston-Jones (1985), Morales et al. (1987), and Xi et al. (1999) have all shown conduction velocity to be reduced in aged animals. A reduction in conduction velocity also occurs in demyelinating diseases (Waxman et al. 1995; Felts et al. 1997). Such a reduction in conduction velocity, together with any disconnection brought about by a loss of nerve fibers from white matter, would obviously affect the integrity and the timing of sequential events in neuronal circuits, and it is suggested that this is a strong contributing factor to age-related cognitive decline. In support of this suggestion, in a recent study of the visual system Wang et al. (2005) have shown that whereas neurons in layer 4 of the primary visual cortex have normal response latencies in old monkeys, in other parts of V1, and throughout V2, there is hyperactivity of neurons, so that they show increased firing frequency. This is accompanied by delays in both intracortical and intercortical transfer of information, such as would be brought about by alterations in myelin sheaths.

Finally, there is the question of the involvement of oligodendrocytes in the age-related myelin changes. Some nerve fibers degenerate with age, which leads to degeneration of their myelin sheaths, but how this affects the parent oligodendrocytes is not known. Other data suggest that, with age, there is also some oligodendrocytic death, and this would necessarily lead to the degeneration of the myelin sheaths they formed. Consequently, the axons dependent on those sheaths would become bare and it is presumed that it is these axons that eventually become remyelinated by new oligodendrocytes, which form shorter internodes of thin sheaths.

Clearly, the effects of age on nerve fibers and their sheaths are very complex and include both degenerative and regenerative changes, which probably play a significant role in age-related cognitive decline. The next phase of this study will be to determine what factors affect oligodendrocytes to bring about these degenerative alterations in myelin, and how the alterations may be retarded.

ACKNOWLEDGMENTS

Funded by National Institutes of Health, National Institute on Aging, Program Project Grant 1PO AG 00001.

REFERENCES

Albert, M. 1993 Neuropsychological and neurophysiological changes in healthy adult humans across the age range. *Neurobiol Aging* 14:623–5.

Albert, M. and Moss, M.B. 1996 Neuropsychology of aging; findings in humans and monkeys. In: *Handbook of the Biology of Aging*, 4th ed. (edited by Schneider, E., Rowe, J.W. and Morris, J.H.) pp 217–33. San Francisco: Academic Press.

Andersen, A.H., Zhang, Z., Gash, D.M. and Avison, M.J. 1999 Age-associated changes in CNS composition identified by MRI. *Brain Res* 829:90–8.

Aston-Jones, G., Rogers, J., Shaver, R.D., Dinan, T.G. and Moss, D.E. 1985 Age-impaired impulse flow from nucleus basalis to cortex. *Nature* 318:462–4.

Bachevalier, J., Landis, L.S., Walker, L.C., Brickso, M., Mishkin, M., and Price, D.L. 1991 Aging monkeys exhibit behavioral deficits indicative of widespread cerebral dysfunction. *Neurobiol Aging* 12:99–111.

Bennett, V. and Lambert, S. 1999 Physiological roles of axonal ankyrins in survival of premyelinated axons and localization of voltage-gated sodium channels. *J Neurocytol* 28:303–18.

Blakemore, W. F. 1978 Observations on remyelination in the rabbit spinal cord following demyelination induced by lysolecithin. *Neuropathol Appl Neurobiol* 4:47–59.

Brück, W., Kuhlmann, T. and Stadelmann, C. 2003 Remyelination in multiple sclerosis. *J Neurol Sci* 206:181–5.

Cavallotti, D., Cavallotti, C., Pescosolido, N., Iannetti, G.D. and Pacella, E.A. 2001 A morphometric study of age changes in the rat optic nerve. *Ophthalmologica* 215:366–71.

Cerghet, M., Skoff, R.P., Bessert, D., Zhang, Z., Mullins, C. and Ghandour. M.S. 2006 Proliferation and death of oligodendrocytes and myelin proteins are differentially regulated in male and female rodents. *J Neurosci* 26:1439–47.

Coetzee, T., Fujita, N., Dupree, J., Shi, R., Blight, A., Susuki, K. and Popko, B. 1996 Myelination in the absence of galatocerebroside and sulfatide: Normal structure with abnormal function and regional instability. *Cell* 86:209–19.

Coetzee, T., Susuki, K. and Popko, B. 1998 New perspectives on the function of myelin galactolipids. *Trends Neurosci* 21:126–30.

Cullen, M.J. and Webster, H.D. 1979 Remodelling of optic nerve sheaths and axons during metamorphosis in Xenopus laevis. *J Comp Neurol* 184:353–62.

Dhen, Z. J., Negra, M., Levine, A., Ughrin, Y. and Levine, J.M. 2002 Oligodendrocyte precursor cells: reactive cells that inhibit axon growth and regeneration. *J Neurocytol* 31:481–95.

Dickson, D.W., Crystal, H.A., Mattiace, L.A., Masur, D.M., Blau, A.D., Davies, P., Yen, S.H. and Aronson, M.K. 1992 Identification of normal and pathological aging in prospectively studied nondemented elderly humans. *Neurobiol Aging* 13:179–89.

Faddis, B.T. and McGinn, M.D. 1997 Spongiform degeneration of gerbil cochlear nucleus: An ultrastructural and immunohistochemical evaluation. *J Neurocytol* 26:625–35.

Feldman, M.L. and Peters, A. 1998 Ballooning of myelin sheaths in normally aged macaques. *J Neurocytol* 27:605–14.

Felts, P.A., Baker, R.A. and Smith, K.J. 1997 Conduction along segmentally demyelinated mammalian central axons. *J Neurosci* 17:7267–77.

Fletcher, B.R. Calhoun, M.E., Rapp, P.R. and Shapiro, M.L. 2006 Fornix lesions decouple the induction of hippocampal arc transcription from behavior but not plasticity. *J Neurosci* 26:1507–15.

Franson, P. and Ronnevi, L.-O. 1989 Myelin breakdown in the posterior funiculus of the kitten after dorsal rhizotomy: A qualitative light and electron microscopic study. *Anat Embryol* 180:273–80.

Godlweski, A. 1991 Morphometry of myelin fibers in corpus callosum and optic nerve of aging rats. *J Hirnforsch* 32:39–46.

Gutterman, C.R.G., Jolesz, F.A., Kikinis, R., Killiany, R.J., Moss, M.B., Sandor, T. and Albert, M.S. 1998 White matter changes with normal aging. *Neurology* 50:972–8.

Herndon, J., Moss, M.B., Killiany, R.J. and Rosene, D.L. 1997 Patterns of cognitive decline in early, advanced and oldest of the old aged rhesus monkeys. *Behav Res* 87:25–34.

Hinman, J.D., Peters, A., Cabral, H., Rosene, D.L., Hollander, W., Rasband, M.N. and Abraham, C.R. 2006 Age-related molecular reorganization at the node of Ranvier. *J Comp Neurol* 495:351–62.

Hirano, A. 1989 Review of the morphological aspects of remyelination. *Dev Neurosci* 11:112–7.

Innocenti, G.M. 1986 General organization of callosal connections in the cerebral cortex. In: Sensory-motor areas and aspects of cortical conectivity. *Cerebral Cortex,* vol 5. (edited by Jones, E.G. and Peters, A.) pp 291–354. New York: Plenum Press.

Kemper, T.L. 1998 Neuroanatomical and neuropathological changes during aging and dementia. In: *Clinical Neurology of Aging* (edited by Albert, M. and Knoefel, J.E.) pp 3–67. New York: Oxford University Press.

Kierstead, H.S., Levine, J.M. and Blakemore, W.F. 1998 Response of the oligodendrocyte progenitor cell population (defined by NG2 labeling) to demyelination of the adult spinal cord. *Glia* 22:161–70.

Kreutzeberg, G., Blakemore, W.F. and Graeber, M.B. 1997 Cellular pathology of the central nervous system. In: *Greenfield's Neuropathology.* 6th ed. (edited by Graham, D.I. and Lantos, P.L.) pp 85–156. London: Arnold.

Lai, Z.C., Rosene, D.L., Killiany, R.J., Pugliese, D., Albert, M.S. and Moss, M.B. 1995 Age-related changes in the brain of the rhesus monkey: MRI changes in white matter but not grey matter. *Soc Neurosci Abstracts* 21:1564.

Lassmann, H., Bartsch, U., Montag, D. and Schachner, M. 1997 Dying-back oligodendrogliopathy; A late sequel of myelin-associated glycoprotein deficiency. *Glia* 19:104–10.

Levine, J.M., Reynolds, R. and Fawcett, J.W. 2001 The oligodendrocyte precursor cell in health and disease. *Trends Neurosci* 24:39–47.

LeVine, S.M. and Torres, M.V. 1992 Morphological features of degenerating oligodendrocytes in twitcher mice. *Brain Res* 587:348–52.

Lintl, P. and Braak, H. 1983 Loss of intracortical myelinated fibers: a distinctive age-related alteration in the human striate area. *Acta Neuropathol* 61:178–82.

Ludwin, S.K. 1978 Central nervous system demyelination and remyelination in the mouse. An ultrastrructural study of cuprizone toxicity. *Lab Invest* 39:597–612.

Ludwin, S.K. 1995 Pathology of the myelin sheath. In: *The Axon: Structure, Function and Pathophysiology* (edited by Waxman, S, G., Kocsis, J. D. and Stys, P.K.) pp 412–437. New York: Oxford University Press.

Malamud, N. and Hirano, A. 1973 *Atlas of Neuropathology*. Berkeley: University of California Press.

Marner, L., Nyengaard, J. R., Tang, Y. and Pakkenberg. B. 2003 Marked loss of myelinated nerve fibers in the human brain with age. *J Comp Neurol* 462:144–52.

Meier-Ruge, A., Ulrich, J., Bruhlmann, M. and Meier, E. 1992 Age-related white matter atrophy in the human brain. *Ann NY Acad Sci* 673:260–9.

Merrill, D.A., Roberts, J.A.S. and Tuszyski, M.H. 2000 Conservation of neuron numbers and size in entorhinal cortex layers II, III, and V/VI of aged primates. *J Comp Neurol* 422:396–401.

Monuki, E.S. and Lemle, G. 1973 Molecular biology of myelination. In: *The Axon: Structure, Function and Pathophysiology* (edited by Waxman, S.G., Kocsis, J.D. and Stys, P.K.) pp 144–63. New York: Oxford Unversity Press.

Morales, F.R., Boxer, P.A., Fung, S.J. and Chase, M.H. 1987 Basic electrophysiological properties of spinal cord motoneurons during old age in the cat. *J Neurophysiol* 58:180–95.

Morrison, J.H. and Hof, P.R. 1997 Life and death of neurons in the aging brain. *Nature* 278:412–9.

Ngwenya, L.B., Rosene, D.L. and Peters, A. 2008 An ultrastructural study of the newly generated cells in the adult monkey dentate gyrus. *Hippocampus* 18:210–20.

Nielsen, K. and Peters, A. 2000 The effects of aging on the frequency of nerve fibers in rhesus monkey striate cortex. *Neurobiol Aging* 21:621–8.

Nilsson, O.G., Shapiro, M.L., Gage, F.H., Olton, D.S. and Bjorklund, A. 1987 Spatial learning and memory following fimbria-fornix transections and grafting of fetal septal neurons to the hippocampus. *Exptl Brain Res* 67:195–215.

Norton, W.T. 1996 Do oligodendrocytes divide? *Neurochem Res* 21:495–503.

Pakkenberg, B. and Gundersen, H.J.G. 1997 Neocortical neuron number in humans: Effects of sex and age. *J Comp Neurol* 384:312–20.

Perrot, R., Lonchampt, P., Peterson, A.C. and Eyer, J. 2007 Axonal neurofilaments control multiple fiber properties but do not influence structure or spacing of nodes of Ranvier. *J Neurosci* 27:9573–84.

Peters, A. 1996 Age-related changes in oligodendrocytes in monkey cerebral cortex. *J Comp Neurol* 371:153–63.

Peters, A. 2004 A fourth type of neuroglial cell in the adult central nervous system. *J Neurocytol* 33:345–57.

Peters, A., Josephson, K. and Vincent, S.L. 1991 Effects of aging on the neuroglial cells and pericytes with area 17 of the rhesus monkey cerebral cortex. *J Comp Neurol* 229:384–98.

Peters, A., Leahu, D., Moss, M.B. and McNally, K.J. 1994 The effects of aging on area 46 of the frontal cortex of the rhesus monkey. *Cerebr Cortex* 6:621–35.

Peters, A., Morrison, J.H., Rosene, D.L. and Hyman, B.T. 1998a Are neurons lost from the primate cerebral cortex during aging? *Cerebr Cortex* 8:295–300.

Peters, A., Moss, M.B. and Sethares, C. 2000 The effects of aging on myelinated nerve fibers in monkey primary visual cortex. *J Comp Neurol* 419:364–76.

Peters, A., Moss, M.B. and Sethares, C. 2001a The effects of aging on layer 1 of primary visual cortex in the rhesus monkey. *Cerebr Cortex* 11:93–103.

Peters, A. and Sethares, C. 2002 Aging and the myelinated fibers in prefrontal cortex and corpus callosum of the monkey. *J Comp Neurol* 442:277–91.

Peters, A. and Sethares, C. 2003 Is there remyelination during aging of the primate central nervous system? *J Comp Neurol* 460:238–54.

Peters, A. and Sethares, C. 2004 Oligodendrocytes, their progenitors and other neuroglial cells in the aging primate cerebral cortex. *Cerebr Cortex* 14:995–1007.

Peters, A., Sethares, C. and Killiany, R.J. 2001b Effects of age on the thickness of myelin sheaths in monkey primary visual cortex. *J Comp Neurol* 435:241–8.

Peters, A., Sethares, C. and Luebke, J.I. 2007 Synapses are lost during aging in the primate prefrontal cortex. *Neurosci* To be published.

Peters, A., Sethares, C. and Moss M.B. 1998b The effects of aging on layer 1 in area 46 of prefrontal cortex in rhesus monkey. *Cerebr Cortex* 8:671–84.

Peters, A., Verderosa, A. and Sethares, C. 2008 The neuroglial population in the primary visual cortex of the aging rhesus monkey. *Glia* 56:1151–61.

Pfefferbaum, A., Mathalon, D.H., Rawles, J.M., Zipursky, R.B. and Lim, K.O. 1994 A quantitative magnetic resonance study of changes in brain morphology from infancy to late adulthood. *Arch Neurol* 51:874–87.

Prineas, J.W. and McDonald, W.I. 1997 Demyelinating diseases. In: *Greenfield's Neuropathology*. 6th ed. (edited by Graham, D.I. and Lantos, P.L.) pp 813–96. London: Arnold.

Resnick, S.M., Pham, D.L., Kraut, M.A., Zonderman, A.B., and Davatzokos, C. 2003 Longitudinal magnetic resonance imaging studies of older adults: a shrinking brain. *J Neurosci* 23:3295–301.

Rosenbluth, J. 1966 Redundant myelin sheaths and other ultrastructural features of the toad cerebellum. *J Cell Biol* 28:73–93.

Sandell, J.H. and Peters, A. 2001 Effects of age on the nerve fibers in the rhesus monkey optic nerve. *J Comp Neurol* 429:541–53.

Sandell, J.H. and Peters, A. 2002 Effects of age on the glial cells in the rhesus monkey optic nerve. *J Comp Neurol* 445:13–28.

Sandell, J.H. and Peters, A. 2003 Disrupted myelin and axon loss in the anterior commissure of the aged rhesus monkey. *J Comp Neurol* 466:14–30.

Schmahmann, J.D. and Pandya, D.N. 2006 *Fiber pathways of the brain.* New York: Oxford University Press.

Siddiqi, Z.A. and Peters, A. 1999 The effect of aging on pars compacta of the substantia nigra in rhesus monkey. *J Neuropath Exptl Neurol* 58:903–20.

Sloane, J.S., Hinman, J.D., Lubonia, M., Hollander, W. and Abraham, C.R. 2003 Age-dependent myelin degeneration and proteolysis of oligodendrocyte proteins is associated with the activation of calpain-1 in the rhesus monkey. *J Neurochem* 84:157–68.

Smith, D.E., Rapp, P.R., McKay, H.M., Roberts, J.A. and Tuszynski, M.H. 2004 Memory impairment in aged primate is associated with focal death of cortical neurons and atrophy of subcortical neurons. *J Neurosci* 24:4373–81.

Sturrock, R.R. 1976 Changes in neuroglia and myelination in the white matter of aging mice. *J Gerontol* 31:513–22.

Sturrock, R.R. 1987 Age-related changes in the number of myelinated axons and glial cells in the anterior and posterior limbs of the mouse anterior commissure. *J Anat* 150:111–27.

Sugiyama, I., Tanaka, K., Akita, M., Yoshida, K., Kawase, T. and Asou, H. 2002 Ultrastructural analysis of the paranodal junction of myelinated fibers in 31-month-old rats. *J Neurosci Res* 7:309–17.

Sullivan, E.V., Rosenbloom, M., Serventi, K.L. and Pfefferbaum, A. 2004 Effects of age and sex on volume of the thalamus, pons, and cortex. *Neurobiol Aging* 25:185–92.

Sullivan, M.V. and Hamilton, C.R. 1973a Memory establishment via the anterior commissure of monkeys. *Physiol Behav* 11:873–9.

Sullivan, M.V. and Hamilton, C.R. 1973b Interocular transfer of reversed and nonreversed discrimination via the anterior commissure in monkeys. *Physiol Behav* 10:355–9.

Tamura, E. and Parry, G.J. 1994 Severe radicular pathology in rats with longstanding diabetes. *J Neurol Sci* 127:29–35.

Tang, Y., Nyengaard, J.R., Pakkenberg, B. and Gundersen, H.J.G. 1997 Age-induced white matter changes in the human brain: A stereological investigation. *Neurobiol Aging* 18:609–15.

Tigges, J., Gordon, T.P., Hall. H.M. and Peters, A. 1988 Survival rate and life span of the rhesus monkey. *Am J Primatol* 15:263–72.

Uchida, K. Nakayama, H., Tateyama, S. and Goto, N. 1992 Immuohistochemical analysis of constituents of senile plaques and cerebral-vascular amyloid in aged dogs. *J Vet Med Sci* 54:1023–9.

Wang, Y., Zhou, T., Ma, Y. and Leventhal, A.G. 2005 Degradation of signal timing in cortical area V1 and V2 of senescent monkeys. *Cerebr Cortex* 15:403–8.

Watanabe, M., Toyama, Y. and Nishiyama, A. 2002 Differentiation of proliferating NG2-positive glial progenitors cells in remyelinating lesions. *J Neurosci Res* 69:826–36.

Waxman, S.G., Kocsis, J.D. and Black, J.A. 1995 Pathophysiology of demyelinated axons. In: *The Axon: Structure, Function and Pathophysiology* (edited by Waxman, S.G., Kocsis, J.D. and Stys, P.K.) pp 438–61. New York: Oxford University Press.

Xi, M.-C., Liu, R.-H., Engelhardt, J.K., Morales, F.R. and Chase, M.H. 1999 Changes in the axonal conduction velocity of pyramidal tract neurons in the aged cat. *Neurosci* 92:219–25.

Chapter Nine
_____

Degeneration in Canine Brain Aging

Elizabeth Head

INTRODUCTION AND HISTORICAL PERSPECTIVE

Normal aging can be distinguished from pathological aging in the human brain by differences in the patterns of degeneration and the accumulation of specific types of neuropathology. The aged dog brain shows parallel age changes, with additional features that suggest similarities with early Alzheimer's disease (AD) or mild cognitive impairment in aging humans.

One of the first reports of age-associated neurodegeneration in dogs, abnormal pyramidal neuron sprouting, was described in 1914 (Lafora 1914). However, it was not until the 1950s that other types of neuropathology were reported in aged dog brain, including "Alzheimer-like" senile plaques (Braunmuhl 1956; Dahme 1962; Osetowska 1966; Dahme 1967, 1968). In 1970 H.M. Wisniewski was one of the first researchers to suggest that dogs would be a useful model of human brain aging (Wisniewski 1970). Aged dog brains display a number of morphological hallmarks that are similar to those observed in aged human brains, including cortical atrophy, white matter degeneration, neuron loss, the accumulation of pathological proteins (beta-amyloid and tau), cerebrovascular dysfunction, and oxidative damage. This chapter will summarize some of the neurobiological characteristics of the aging dog brain.

MACROSCOPIC STRUCTURAL BRAIN CHANGES

Changes in overall brain structure and volume can be seen using noninvasive techniques such as magnetic resonance imaging (MRI). Cross-sectional MRI studies in dogs reveal decreased brain volume, increased ventricular volume, lesions, and cortical atrophy of the gray and white matter that often correlate with increasing age and cognitive decline (Figure 9.1) (Su et al. 1998; Kimotsuki et al. 2005; Su et al. 2005).

Individual regions of the canine brain may have differing vulnerabilities to the aging process. An MRI study of beagles ranging from 3 months to 15 years revealed decreases in total brain volume in senior dogs 12 years and older, but frontal lobe atrophy began much earlier, at 8 years of age (Tapp et al. 2004). Similar frontal-dependent volumetric declines have been observed in human aging (Tisserand et al. 2002). Hippocampal atrophy is also observed in the aged dog brain, at later ages than in the prefrontal cortex and occurring after 11 years of age (Tapp et al. 2004). Interestingly, age-dependent atrophy in the aged dog brain is modified by sex. Using voxel-based morphometry, aged males showed larger losses in frontal volume than females, but temporal lobe atrophy was more pronounced in female beagles

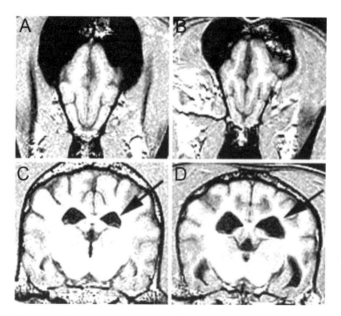

Figure 9.1. Age-associated structural changes in canine brain by magnetic resonance imaging. The prefrontal cortex of a young dog (**A**) compared with an aged dog (**B**) illustrates cortical atrophy present with aging. The lateral ventricles in an aged dog (**D**) are larger than that typically observed in young dogs (**C**) (arrows). (Images provided by Dr. Lydia Su at UCI.)

(Tapp et al. 2006). Gender differences similar to that reported in the dog have also been reported in aging humans (Coffey et al. 1998).

WHITE MATTER DEGENERATION

Although not as well explored as in the nonhuman primate (Chapter 8), the canine shows some evidence of white matter degeneration with age. Using T2-weighted imaging, white matter hyperintensities in the vicinity of the lateral ventricles are observed (Kimotsuki et al. 2005). Male and female dogs show differences in white matter aging. Aged males show larger volume losses in the internal capsule and cranial nerve bundles compared to females. In contrast, females show greater white matter atrophy in the alveus of the hippocampus than males (Tapp et al. 2006). At the microscopic level, white matter losses may be due to the accumulation of ubiquitinated granules along myelin fibers or within glial cells (Ferrer 1993). Degenerating axons, perivascular infiltration of macrophages, astrocytosis, and occasional small foci of hemorrhages or infarction may also contribute to white matter degeneration (Morita et al. 2005).

SELECTIVE NEURON LOSS IN THE AGING CANINE

Tissue volume losses observed in the prefrontal cortex and hippocampus by in vivo imaging methods may reflect neuron loss. In the human brain, neuron loss occurs within select brain regions and differences in the patterns and types of neurons affected differentiate normal from pathological aging. For example, normal aging is associated with hilar loss (37%) and subicular neuron loss (43%) in the hippocampus (West 1993, 1994), which can be differentiated from the additional losses noted in area CA1 (68%) and the entorhinal cortex (32–90%) in AD (West 1993, 1994; Gomez-Isla 1996). Neuron loss in the aged dog brain was initially reported by Morys and colleagues in the claustrum, who reported a 22% decrease (Morys 1994). In a recent unbiased stereology study, the number of neurons in the hippocampus and entorhinal cortex of young and aged dogs was estimated. Results suggest there is a 30% loss of neurons in the hilus of the hippocampus but no changes were observed in areas CA1–CA3, nor in the entorhinal cortex (Siwak-Tapp et al. 2008). Thus, to some extent, neuron loss in the canine hippocampus mimics some of the features of normal human brain aging, but interestingly, the same neuron losses are not observed in the rhesus monkey (Keuker et al. 2003).

A subset of neurons, in particular, may be vulnerable to aging based upon their location and phenotype in the aged dog brain. For example, there is a selective vulnerability of neurons expressing calcium-binding proteins, such as parvalbumin and calbindin, in the cerebellum (Siso et al. 2003). However, a different pattern is observed in the frontal cortex. Specifically, neurons expressing parvalbumin and calretinin were resistant to aging, but calbindin-positive GABAergic neurons were depleted (Pugliese et al. 2004). Further, a loss of gluatamic acid decarboxylase 67– positive GABA neurons is observed in area CA1 of the hippocampus of aged dogs, particularly those 10 years and older (Hwang et al. 2008b). However, as in the frontal cortex, parvalbumin positive neurons in the hippocampus do not change with age (Hwang et al. 2008a).

Bromodeoxyuridine (BrdU) administration is a useful tool to date the birth of the newly generated cells. In a study of 5 young and 5 aged dogs, the extent of neurogenesis was reduced substantially (90–96%) in the hippocampal subgranular zone in aged animals (Siwak-Tapp et al. 2007). In counts of doublecortin-positive neurons in the hippocampus, reflecting neurogenesis and neuronal differentiation, an 80% loss of neurons has been reported (Hwang et al. 2007). Loss of neurogenesis in aged dogs is similar to that reported in rodents (Kuhn 1996) and in nonhuman primates (Gould 1999).

β-AMYLOID DEPOSITION

One type of pathology of significant interest in the dog brain, and that may also contribute to neurodegeneration, is the accumulation of a protein fragment called β-amyloid (Aβ). Aβ contains 39 to 43 amino acids and is the primary constituent of amyloid plaques in the brains of patients with AD (Chapter 10). Aβ is toxic to neurons and is thought to play a causative role in the development of AD (Selkoe 2000).

Canines accumulate endogenous levels of human-type Aβ (Selkoe 1987; Johnstone et al. 1991) as they age (Wisniewski 1990; Cummings 1992; Hou 1997; Head et al. 2000). The canine β-amyloid precursor protein (APP), from which Aβ is produced, is virtually identical to human APP (~98% homology [http:// www.ensembl.org/Canis_familiaris/]). Most of the deposits in the canine brain are of the diffuse subtype, but they are fibrillar at the ultrastructural level, which models early plaque formation in humans (Figure 9.2) (Torp 2000a, 2000b; Torp et al. 2003). Aβ can also be observed along neuronal plasma membranes, particularly in the entorhinal cortex (Fig. 9.2) (Cummings 1993). Interestingly, there may be variability in Aβ deposition as a function of breed of dog, with beagles, boxers, and German shepherds being particularly vulnerable (Bobik 1994). Further, there is a high concordance rate among litter mates, with 15/16 litters showing congruence (Russell 1992).

Our work and the work of others demonstrate that specific canine brain regions show differential vulnerabilities to Aβ, paralleling the aged human brain (Wisniewski

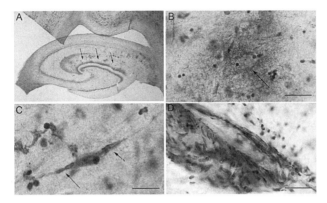

Figure 9.2. Aβ pathology in the aged canine brain. (**A**) Aβ accumulates as diffuse plaques and within the outer molecular layer in the hippocampus (arrows). (**B**) At higher magnification, Aβ within a diffuse plaque appears fibrillar but intact neurons (arrow) can be found within these deposits. (**C**) A subset of neurons in the entorhinal cortex show Aβ accumulation on dendrites (arrow). (**D**) Cerebrovascular Aβ can be observed in the walls of leptomeningeal blood vessels. All sections were immunolabeled with anti-Aβ1-42 after 90% formic acid pretreatment and counterstained with cresyl violet. Bars in B, C, D = 20μm. (See color Figure 9.2)

1970; Selkoe 1987; Giaccone 1990; Wisniewski 1990; Braak and Braak 1991; Ishihara 1991; Braak et al. 1993; Head et al. 2000; Thal et al. 2002). When cortical regions are sampled for Aβ deposition, each region shows a different age of Aβ onset (Head et al. 2000). Aβ deposition occurs earliest in the prefrontal cortex (similar observations have been reported in the AD brain [Thal et al. 2002]) and later in the temporal and occipital cortices. It is interesting to note that, by MRI, the prefrontal cortex also shows signs of early atrophy.

CEREBROVASCULAR Aβ PATHOLOGY IN CANINES

A common type of pathology observed in both normal human brain aging and particularly in AD is the accumulation of cerebrovascular Aβ angiopathy (CAA) (Attems 2005; Attems et al. 2005; Herzig et al. 2006). CAA may compromise the blood brain barrier (BBB), impair vascular function (constriction and dilation) (Prior 1996b), and cause microhemorrhages (Deane and Zlokovic 2007). Cerebrovascular Aβ in the canine brain was first observed by Braunmuhl as early as 1956 (Braunmuhl 1956) and was subsequently confirmed by Wisniewski and colleagues (Wisniewski 1990). Vascular and perivascular abnormalities and cerebrovascular Aβ pathology are frequently found in aged dogs (Fig. 9.2) (Giaccone 1990; Uchida et al. 1990; Ishihara 1991; Uchida et al. 1991; Shimada 1992; Uchida 1992a, 1992b, 1993; Yoshino 1996; Uchida 1997). Cultured vascular smooth muscle cells from the canine brain can mimic the pathological process that occurs in humans with AD and Down's syndrome (Frackowiak 1995; Prior 1995, 1996a, 1996b). Vascular Aβ is primarily the shorter 1–40 species, which is identical in dogs and humans (Wisniewski 1996).

There may be a direct link between vascular Aβ deposition and vessel wall integrity; leptomeninges obtained from old dogs affected by CAA showed segmental loss of vessel integrity at sites of Aβ deposition (Prior 1996b; Prior et al. 1996), suggesting that the presence of Aβ in old dogs causes disruption of the BBB and possibly cerebrovascular insufficiency. Using single photon emission tomography (SPET), a regional decrease in cerebral blood-flow was noted particularly in the fronto- and temporocortical regions (Peremans et al. 2002). Overall, canines are thought to be a good natural model for examining CAA and treatments for CAA (Walker 1997). Thus, cerebrovascular pathology may also be a significant contributor to neurodegeneration in the canine brain.

NEUROFIBRILLARY TANGLE PATHOLOGY

Neurofibrillary tangles are another feature of human brain aging and disease but are rare in other species. Tangles are composed of the abnormal accumulation of hyperphosorylated tau protein and can lead to impaired neuronal transport and degeneration (Goedert et al. 1989) (Chapter 10). Dogs do not develop neurofibrillary tangles (Ball 1983; Selkoe 1987; Giaccone 1990; Wisniewski et al. 1990; Cummings 1993). However, tau phosphorylation is a feature of the aged canine brain and can be classified into three stages, varying in degree from weak to strong (Wegiel 1998). Further, similar epitopes on the tau protein in canines are phosphorylated when compared with human tau (Papaioannou 2001; Head 2005; Pugliese et al. 2006). One of the possible reasons for the lack of development of tangles in dogs is that the sequence of the tau protein is different from that of humans; this in turn may affect the formation of paired helical filaments and subsequently neurofibrillary tangles.

OXIDATIVE DAMAGE

Progressive oxidative damage is a consistent feature of human and animal aging. Similarly, dog brains accumulate oxidative damage to proteins with age (Head et al. 2002; Skoumalova et al. 2003). In several studies, a relation between age and increased oxidative damage has been observed by measuring the amount of end-products of lipid peroxidation (oxidative damage to lipids), including the extent of 4-hydroxynonenal (Papaioannou et al. 2001; Rofina et al. 2004; Rofina et al. 2006), lipofuscin (Rofina et al. 2006), lipofuscin-like pigments (Papaioannou et al. 2001; Rofina et al. 2004), and malondialdehyde (Head et al. 2002). Last, there is evidence of increased oxidative damage to DNA or RNA (8OHdG) in the aged dog brain (Rofina et al. 2006). Further, reduced endogenous antioxidant enzymes such as glutamine synthetase activity and superoxide dismutase occur in parallel with increased protein damage (Kiatipattanasakul et al. 1997; Head et al. 2002). In combination, progressive protein, lipid, DNA, and RNA damage due to oxidative stress can also impair neuron function and lead to neurodegeneration.

SUMMARY

Aged canines develop signs of neuronal, white matter, and vascular degeneration as observed in human brain aging. Cortical atrophy, white matter degeneration, cerebrovascular dysfunction, and neuron loss may be due to progressive Aβ, tau phosphorylation, and oxidative damage accumulation. Neurodegeneration in the canine brain may form the basis for observations of cognitive decline in multiple domains, including learning and memory (Cummings 1996; Colle 2000; Head 2001).

REFERENCES

Attems J (2005) Sporadic cerebral amyloid angiopathy: pathology, clinical implications, and possible pathomechanisms. *Acta Neuropathol* 110:345–59.

Attems J, Jellinger KA, Lintner F (2005) Alzheimer's disease pathology influences severity and topographical distribution of cerebral amyloid angiopathy. *Acta Neuropathol* 110:222–31.

Ball MJ, MacGregor J, Fyfe IM, Rapoport SI, London E (1983) Paucity of morphological changes in the brains of ageing beagle dogs: Further evidence that Alzheimer lesions are unique for primate central nervous system. *Neurobiol Aging* 4:127–31.

Bobik M, Thompson T, Russell MJ (1994) Amyloid deposition in various breeds of dogs. *Abstr Soc Neurosci* 20:172.

Braak H, Braak E (1991) Neuropathological stageing of Alzheimer-related changes. *Acta Neuropathol* 82:239–59.

Braak H, Braak E, Bohl J (1993) Staging of Alzheimer-related cortical destruction. *Eur Neurol* 33:403–8.

Braunmuhl A (1956) Kongophile angiopathie und senile plaques bei greisen hunden. *Arch Psychiatr Nervenkr* 194:395–414.

Coffey CE, Lucke JF, Saxton JA, Ratcliff G, Unitas LJ, Billig B, Bryan RN (1998) Sex differences in brain aging: a quantitative magnetic resonance imaging study. *Arch Neurol* 55:169–79.

Colle M-A, Hauw J-J, Crespeau F, Uchiara T, Akiyama H, Checler F, Pageat P, Duykaerts C (2000) Vascular and parenchymal Aβ deposition in the aging dog: correlation with behavior. *Neurobiol Aging* 21:695–704.

Cummings BJ, Head E, Ruehl WW, Milgram NW, Cotman CW (1996) β-amyloid accumulation correlates with cognitive dysfunction in the aged canine. *Neurobiol Learn Mem* 66:11–23.

Cummings BJ, Su JH, Cotman CW, White R, Russell MJ (1992) BA4 accumulation in aged canine brain: An animal model of early plaque formation in Alzheimer's disease. *Abstr Soc Neurosci* 18:560.

Cummings BJ, Su JH, Cotman CW, White R, Russell MJ (1993) β-amyloid accumulation in aged canine brain: a model of plaque formation in Alzheimer's disease. *Neurobiol Aging* 14:547–60.

Dahme E (1962) Pathologische Befunde an den Hirngefeben bei Tieren: Die Verenderungen der Hirngefeben beim alten Hund. *Acta Neuropathol* (Suppl) 1:54–60.

Dahme E (1968) Aging changes in the brain of the animal. *Bulletin der Schweizerischen Akademie der Medizinischen Wissenschaften* 24:133–43.

Dahme E, Deutschlander N (1967) On the problem of the primary amyloid in meninx and cerebral cortex vessels in dogs. *Deutsche Tierarztliche Wochenschrift* 74:134–8.

Deane R, Zlokovic BV (2007) Role of the blood-brain barrier in the pathogenesis of Alzheimer's disease. *Curr Alzheimer Res* 4:191–7.

Ferrer I, Pumarola M, Rivera R, Zujar MJ, Cruz-Sanchez F, Vidal A (1993) Primary central white matter degeneration in old dogs. *Acta Neuropathol* 86:172–5.

Frackowiak J, Mazur-Kolecka B, Wisniewski HM, Potempska A, Carroll RT, Emmerling MR, Kim KS (1995) Secretion and accumulation of Alzheimer's β-protein by cultured vascular smooth muscle cells from old and young dogs. *Brain Res* 676:225–30.

Giaccone G, Verga L, Finazzi M, Pollo B, Tagliavini F, Frangione B, Bugiani O (1990) Cerebral preamyloid deposits and congophilic angiopathy in aged dogs. *Neurosci Letters* 114:178–83.

Goedert M, Spillantini MG, Jakes R, Rutherford D, Crowther RA (1989) Multiple isoforms of human microtubule-associated protein tau: sequences and localization in neurofibrillary tangles of Alzheimer's disease. *Neuron* 3:519–26.

Gomez-Isla T, Price JL, McKeel D, Morris JC, Growdon JH, Hyman BT (1996) Profound loss of layer II entorhinal cortex neurons occurs in very mild Alzheimer's disease. *J Neuroscience* 16:4491–500.

Gould E, Reeves AJ, Fallah M, Tanapat P, Gross CG, Fuchs, E (1999) Hippocampal neurogenesis in adult Old World primates. *Proc Natl Acad Sci USA* 96:5263–7.

Head E (2001) Brain aging in dogs: Parallels with human brain aging and Alzheimer's disease. *Vet Therapeutics* 2:247–60.

Head E, Liu J, Hagen TM, Muggenburg BA, Milgram NW, Ames BN, Cotman CW (2002) Oxidative damage increases with age in a canine model of human brain aging. *J Neurochem* 82:375–81.

Head E, McCleary R, Hahn FF, Milgram NW, Cotman CW (2000) Region-specific age at onset of β-amyloid in dogs. *Neurobiol Aging* 21:89–96.

Head EM, Moffat K, Das P, Sarsoza F, Poon WW, Landsberg G, Cotman CW, Murphy MP (2005) β-Amyloid deposition and tau phosphorylation in clinically characterized aged cats. *Neurobiol Aging* 26:749–63.

Herzig MC, Van Nostrand WE, Jucker M (2006) Mechanism of cerebral β-amyloid angiopathy: murine and cellular models. *Brain Pathol* 16:40–54.

Hou Y, White RG, Bobik M, Marks JS, Russell MJ (1997) Distribution of β-amyloid in the canine brain. *NeuroReport* 8:1009–12.

Hwang IK, Yoo KY, Li H, Choi JH, Kwon YG, Ahn Y, Lee IS, Won MH (2007) Differences in doublecortin immunoreactivity and protein levels in the hippocampal dentate gyrus between adult and aged dogs. *Neurochem Res* 32:1604–9.

Hwang IK, Li H, Yoo KY, Choi JH, Lee CH, Chung DW, Kim DW, Seong JK, Yoon YS, Lee IS, Won MH (2008b) Comparison of glutamic acid decarboxylase 67 immunoreactive neurons in the hippocampal CA1 region at various age stages in dogs. *Neurosci Lett* 431:251–5.

Hwang IK, Yoon YS, Yoo KY, Li H, Sun Y, Choi JH, Lee CH, Huh SO, Lee YL, Won MH (2008a) Sustained expression of parvalbumin immunoreactivity in the hippocampal CA1 region and dentate gyrus during aging in dogs. *Neurosci Lett* 434:99–103.

Ishihara T, Gondo T, Takahashi M, Uchino F, Ikeda S, Allsop D, Imai K (1991) Immuno-histochemical and immunoelectron microscopial characterization of cerebrovascular and senile plaque amyloid in aged dogs' brains. *Brain Res* 548:196–205.

Johnstone EM, Chaney MO, Norris FH, Pascual R, Little SP (1991) Conservation of the sequence of the Alzheimer's disease amyloid peptide in dog, polar bear and five other mammals by cross-species polymerase chain reaction analysis. *Brain Res Mol Brain Res* 10:299–305.

Keuker JI, Luiten PG, Fuchs E (2003) Preservation of hippocampal neuron numbers in aged rhesus monkeys. *Neurobiol Aging* 24:157–65.

Kiatipattanasakul W, Nakamura S, Kuroki K, Nakayama H, Doi K (1997) Immunohisto-chemical detection of anti-oxidative stress enzymes in the dog brain. *Neuropathology* 17:307–12.

Kimotsuki T, Nagaoka T, Yasuda M, Tamahara S, Matsuki N, Ono K (2005) Changes of magnetic resonance imaging on the brain in beagle dogs with aging. *J Vet Med Sci* 67:961–7.

Kuhn HG, Dickinson-Anson H, Gage FH (1996) Neurogenenisis in the dentate gyru of the adult rat: age-related decrease of neuronal progenitor proliferation. *J Neurosci* 16:2027–33.

Lafora G (1914) Neoformaciones dendriticas an las neuronas y alteraciones de la neurog-lia en el perro senil. *Trab del Lab de Investig Biol* 1.

Morita T, Mizutani Y, Sawada M, Shimada A (2005) Immunohistochemical and ultra-structural findings related to the blood—brain barrier in the blood vessels of the cere-bral white matter in aged dogs. *J Comp Pathol* 133:14–22.

Morys J, Narkiewicz O, Maciejewska B, Wegiel J, Wisniewski HM (1994) Amyloid deposits and loss of neurones in the claustrum of the aged dog. *NeuroReport* 5: 1825–8.

Osetowska E (1966) Morphologic changes in the brains of old dogs. *Neuropatologia Pol-ska* 4:97–110.

Papaioannou N, Tooten PC, van Ederen AM, Bohl JR, Rofina J, Tsangaris T, Gruys E (2001) Immunohistochemical investigation of the brain of aged dogs. I. Detection of neurofibrillary tangles and of 4-hydroxynonenal protein, an oxidative damage prod-uct, in senile plaques. *Amyloid: J Protein Folding Disord* 8:11–21.

Peremans K, Audenaert K, Blanckaert P, Jacobs F, Coopman F, Verschooten F, Van Bree H, Van Heeringen C, Mertens J, Slegers G, Dierckx R (2002) Effects of aging on brain perfusion and serotonin-2A receptor binding in the normal canine brain mea-sured with single photon emission tomography. *Prog Neuropsychopharmacol Biol Psychiatry* 26:1393–1404.

Prior R, D'Urso D, Frank R, Prikulis I, Pavloakovic G (1995) Experimental deposition of Alzheimer amyloid β-protein in canine leptomeningeal vessels. *NeuroReport* 6:1747–51.

Prior R, D'Urso D, Frank R, Prikulis I, Wihl G, Pavlakovic G (1996a) Canine leptomen-ingeal organ culture: a new experimental model for cerebrovascular β-amyloidosis. *J Neurosci Meth* 68:143–8.

Prior R, D'Urso D, Frank R, Prikulis I, Pavlakovic G (1996b) Loss of vessel wall viabil-ity in cerebral amyloid angiopathy. *NeuroReport* 7:562.

Pugliese M, Carrasco JL, Geloso MC, Mascort J, Michetti F, Mahy N (2004) Gamma-aminobutyric acidergic interneuron vulnerability to aging in canine prefrontal cortex. *J Neurosci Res* 77:913–20.

Pugliese M, Mascort J, Mahy N, Ferrer I (2006) Diffuse β-amyloid plaques and hyperphosphorylated tau are unrelated processes in aged dogs with behavioral deficits. *Acta Neuropathol* 112:175–83.

Rofina JE, Singh K, Skoumalova-Vesela A, van Ederen AM, van Asten AJ, Wilhelm J, Gruys E (2004) Histochemical accumulation of oxidative damage products is associated with Alzheimer-like pathology in the canine. *Amyloid: J Protein Folding Disord* 11:90–100.

Rofina JE, van Ederen AM, Toussaint MJ, Secreve M, van der Spek A, van der Meer I, Van Eerdenburg FJ, Gruys E (2006) Cognitive disturbances in old dogs suffering from the canine counterpart of Alzheimer's disease. *Brain Res* 1069:216–26.

Russell MJ, White R, Patel E, Markesbery WR, Watson CR, Geddes JW (1992) Familial influence on plaque formation in the beagle brain. *NeuroReport* 3:1093–6.

Selkoe DJ, Bell DS, Podlisny MB, Price DL, Cork LC (1987) Conservation of brain amyloid proteins in aged mammals and humans with Alzheimer's disease. *Science* 235:873–7.

Shimada A, Kuwamura M, Akawkura T, Umemura T, Takada K, Ohama E, Itakura C (1992) Topographic relationship between senile plaques and cerebrovascular amyloidosis in the brain of aged dogs. *J Vet Med Sci* 54:137–44.

Siso S, Tort S, Aparici C, Perez L, Vidal E, Pumarola M (2003) Abnormal neuronal expression of the calcium-binding proteins, parvalbumin and calbindin D-28k, in aged dogs. *J Comp Pathol* 128:9–14.

Siwak-Tapp CT, Head E, Muggenburg BA, Milgram NW, Cotman CW (2007) Neurogenesis decreases with age in the canine hippocampus and correlates with cognitive function. *Neurobiol Learn Mem* 88:249–59.

Siwak-Tapp CT, Head E, Muggenburg BA, Milgram NW, Cotman CW (2008) Region specific neuron loss in the aged canine hippocampus is reduced by enrichment. *Neurobiol Aging* 29:521–8.

Skoumalova A, Rofina J, Schwippelova Z, Gruys E, Wilhelm J (2003) The role of free radicals in canine counterpart of senile dementia of the Alzheimer type. *Exp Gerontol* 38:711–9.

Su MY, Head E, Brooks WM, Wang Z, Muggenburg BA, Adam GE, Sutherland R, Cotman CW, Nalcioglu O (1998) Magnetic resonance imaging of anatomic and vascular characteristics in a canine model of human aging. *Neurobiol Aging* 19:479–85.

Su MY, Tapp PD, Vu L, Chen YF, Chu Y, Muggenburg B, Chiou JY, Chen C, Wang J, Bracco C, Head E (2005) A longitudinal study of brain morphometrics using serial magnetic resonance imaging analysis in a canine model of aging. *Prog Neuropsychopharmacol Biol Psychiatry* 29:389–97.

Tapp PD, Head K, Head E, Milgram NW, Muggenburg BA, Su MY (2006) Application of an automated voxel-based morphometry technique to assess regional gray and white matter brain atrophy in a canine model of aging. *Neuroimage* 29:234–44.

Tapp PD, Siwak CT, Gao FQ, Chiou JY, Black SE, Head E, Muggenburg BA, Cotman CW, Milgram NW, Su MY (2004) Frontal lobe volume, function, and β-amyloid pathology in a canine model of aging. *J Neurosci* 24:8205–13.

Thal DR, Rub U, Orantes M, Braak H (2002) Phases of A β-deposition in the human brain and its relevance for the development of AD. *Neurology* 58:1791–1800.

Tisserand DJ, Pruessner JC, Sanz Arigita EJ, van Boxtel MP, Evans AC, Jolles J, Uylings HB (2002) Regional frontal cortical volumes decrease differentially in aging: an MRI study to compare volumetric approaches and voxel-based morphometry. *Neuroimage* 17:657–69.

Torp R, Head E, Cotman CW (2000a) Ultrastructural analyses of β-amyloid in the aged dog brain: Neuronal β-amyloid is localized to the plasma membrane. *Prog Neuropsychopharmacol Biol Psychiatry* 24:801–10.

Torp R, Head E, Milgram NW, Hahn F, Ottersen OP, Cotman CW (2000b) Ultrastructural evidence of fibrillar β-amyloid associated with neuronal membranes in behaviorally characterized aged dog brains. *Neuroscience* 93:495–506.

Torp R, Ottersen OP, Cotman CW, Head E (2003) Identification of neuronal plasma membrane microdomains that colocalize β-amyloid and presenilin: implications for β-amyloid precursor protein processing. *Neuroscience* 120:291–300.

Uchida K, Kuroki K, Yoshino T, Yamaguchi R, Tateyama S (1997) Immunohistochemical study of constituents other than β-protein in canine senile plaques and cerebral amyloid angiopathy. *Acta Neuropathol* 93:277–84.

Uchida K, Miyauchi Y, Nakayama H, Goto N (1990) Amyloid angiopathy with cerebral hemorrhage and senile plaque in aged dogs. *Nippon Juigaku Zasshi* 52:605–11.

Uchida K, Nakayama H, Goto N (1991) Pathological studies on cerebral amyloid angiopathy, senile plaques and amyloid deposition in visceral organs in aged dogs. *J Vet Med Sci* 53:1037–42.

Uchida K, Nakayama H, Tateyama S, Goto N (1992a) Immunohistochemical analysis of constituents of senile plaques and cerebro-vascular amyloid in aged dogs. *J Vet Med Sci* 54:1023–9.

Uchida K, Okuda R, Yamaguchi R, Tateyama S, Nakayama H, Goto N (1993) Double-labeling immunohistochemical studies on canine senile plaques and cerebral amyloid angiopathy. *J Vet Med Sci* 55:637–42.

Uchida K, Tani Y, Uetsuka K, Nakayama H, Goto N (1992b) Immunohistochemical studies on canine cerebral amyloid angiopathy and senile plaques. *J Vet Med Sci* 54: 659–67.

Walker LC (1997) Animal models of cerebral β-amyloid angiopathy. *Brain Res Rev* 25:70–84.

Wegiel J, Wisniewski HM, Soltysiak Z (1998) Region- and cell-type-specific pattern of tau phosphorylation in dog brain. *Brain Res* 802:259–66.

West MJ (1993) Regionally specific loss of neurons in the aging human hippocampus. *Neurobiol Aging* 14:287–93.

West MJ, Coleman PD, Flood DG, Troncoso JC (1994) Differences in the pattern of hippocampal neuronal loss in normal ageing and Alzheimer's disease. *Lancet* 344: 769–72.

Wisniewski HM, Johnson AB, Raine CS, Kay WJ, Terry RD (1970) Senile plaques and cerebral amyloidosis in aged dogs. *Laboratory Investigations* 23:287–96.

Wisniewski HM, Wegiel J, Morys J, Bancher C, Soltysiak Z, Kim KS (1990) Aged dogs: an animal model to study β-protein amyloidogenesis. In: *Alzheimer's disease: Epidemiology, Neuropathology, Neurochemistry and Clinics* (K. Maurer PR, and H. Beckman, ed), pp 151–67. New York: Springer-Verlag.

Wisniewski T, Lalowski M, Bobik M, Russell M, Strosznajder J, Frangione B (1996) Amyloid Beta 1-42 deposits do not lead to Alzheimer's neuritic plaques in aged dogs. *Biochem J* 313:575–80.

Yoshino T, Uchida K, Tateyama S, Yamaguchi R, Nakayama H, Goto N (1996) A retrospective study of canine senile plaques and cerebral amyloid angiopathy. *Vet Pathol* 33:230–4.

Chapter Ten

_____

Alzheimer's Disease–Related Mechanisms of Neuronal Dysfunction and Degeneration: Studies in Human Cortical Neurons

Jorge Busciglio and Atul Deshpande

In this chapter we review recent work from our laboratory, which illustrates the utilization of human cortical neurons for the study of molecular mechanisms of β-amyloid (Aß) and tau-related neuronal degeneration relevant to Alzheimer's disease (AD). The results presented here have been previously published in Deshpande et al. (2006, 2008).

OLIGOMERIC AND FIBRILLAR Aß NEUROTOXICITY

The typical neuropathological features of Alzheimer's disease include the presence of senile plaques, neurofibrillary tangles, and neuronal loss in the cortex and hippocampal formation of affected individuals. Senile plaques are mainly composed of Aß peptide in its fibrillar form. Fibrillar Aß (Aßf) triggers a variety of pathological changes, including tau hyperphosphorylation, leading to neuronal dysfunction and degeneration (Pike et al. 1992; Busciglio et al. 1995; Scinto et al. 2001). In culture, chronic exposure of neurons to Aßf induces aberrant activation of adhesion signaling pathways, neuritic dystrophy, and synaptic loss (Grace et al. 2002). In vivo imaging in transgenic models shows neuritic dystrophy and distortion in direct apposition with Aßf deposits (Tsai et al. 2004; Spires et al. 2005), which cause alterations in neocortical synaptic responses (Stern et al.

2004). Fibrillization of Aß is preceded by multiple conformational changes, including trimer, pentamer, or higher molecular weight complex formation, also known as Aß-derived diffusible ligands (ADDLs) (Lambert et al. 1998), Aß oligomers composed of 15–20 monomers (AßO) (Kayed et al. 2003), protofibrils (string of oligomers) (Nguyen and Hall 2004), and dodecameric oligomers Aß*56 (Lesne et al. 2006). These intermediate Aß species are collectively designated as "soluble Aß" (Glabe 2004). Soluble Aß species are found in cerebrospinal fluid of AD patients (Kuo et al. 1996; Kayed et al. 2003; Georganopoulou et al. 2005), can be neurotoxic at low concentration, and induce inhibition of long-term potentiation and cognitive dysfunction in rodents (Lambert et al. 1998; Hartley et al. 1999; Dahlgren et al. 2002; Walsh et al. 2002). Most relevant, brain levels of soluble Aß species appear to correlate better than density of plaque deposition with severity of cognitive impairment (Lue et al. 1999; Naslund et al. 2000). In this regard, oligomers derived from different amyloidogenic proteins have been proposed as primary toxic species in several neurodegenerative diseases, including prion in spongiform encephalopathies, α-synuclein in Parkinson's disease, and polyglutamine in Huntington's disease (Lashuel et al. 2002a; Caughey and Lansbury 2003; Kayed et al. 2003; Sanchez et al. 2003). Oligomer toxicity appears to be related to a common conformational state, because various oligomers react with the conformation-dependent antibody A11 and oligomeric forms of non-disease-related proteins and peptides are equally toxic (Bucciantini et al. 2002; Kayed et al. 2003; Kayed et al. 2004; Demuro et al. 2005). These results raise the possibility that different conformations of Aß, including soluble and fibrillar Aß species, may contribute to AD pathology through different mechanisms.

To perform a side-by-side comparison of the effect of Aß species in human cortical neurons (HCN) we utilized homogeneous preparations of AßO, ADDLs, and Aßf, which have been well characterized by electron microscopy, high performance liquid chromatography (HPLC), and immunoreactivity to conformation-dependent antibodies (Lacor et al. 2004; Demuro et al. 2005). We found a very specific synaptic localization of AßO and ADDLs in HCN. The targeting of AßO and ADDLs to synaptic contacts was fast and accounted for approximately 45–50% of AßO total deposits present on HCN cultures after 1 hour of incubation (Figure 10.1). Similar results were obtained with ADDLs, which also show remarkable co-localization with synaptic sites in rat hippocampal neurons (Lacor et al. 2004).

The mechanism by which AßO and ADDLs are targeted to synaptic sites may be a crucial step in the pathological cascade. One possibility is that the high concentration of metal ions at synapses, particularly Cu^{+2} and Zn^{+2} (Frederickson and Bush 2001; Mocchegiani et al. 2005; Mathie et al. 2006), "attracts" Aß oligomers, given the high binding affinity of Aß for Cu^{+2} and Zn^{+2} (Bush et al. 1994; Atwood et al. 2000). Then, metal-Aß complexes in the synaptic area may initiate a toxic cascade (Cherny et al. 2001; Frederickson and Bush 2001), consistent with the synaptic alterations linked to soluble forms of Aß (Hartley et al. 1999; Walsh

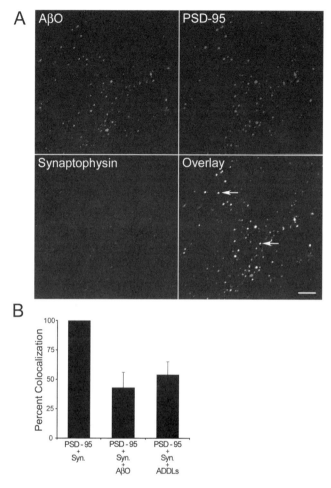

Figure 10.1. AßO colocalize with synaptic markers in HCN. (**A**) Triple immunofluores-cence of 18 DIV HCN with anti-Aß oligomers (AßO; A11, green, 1:2500), anti-PSD-95 (red, 1:1000), and anti-synaptophysin (blue, 1:500). Cultures were incubated with 5µm AßO for 1 hr before fixation. The overlay image shows the co-localization of the three an-tibodies. Triple co-localization is observed as light yellow fluorescent spots (arrows). Scale bar = 5µm. (**B**) Quantification of the frequency of co-localization of AßO and ADDLs (an-tibody A11) with the synaptic markers PSD-95 and synaptophysin (PSD-95+Syn.+AßO, PSD-95+Syn.+ADDLs). (See color Figure 10.1)

et al. 2002). Recent results suggest that ADDLs bind to and reduce the number of N-methyl-D-aspartic acid (NMDA) receptors, providing an alternative path-way by which soluble forms of Aß may cause synaptic failure (Lacor et al. 2007). Notably, most AßO and ADDLs not associated with synapses were found in close contact with cellular membranes, suggesting that soluble Aß may initiate toxicity not only at synapses, but also at multiple cellular locations.

The fast and highly toxic effect of Aßo (Figure 10.2) was correlated with a sequence of cellular alterations, which is consistent with the activation of a mito-chondrial death pathway, including early changes in mitochondrial membrane potential (MMP) and adenosine triphosphate (ATP) production; gradual decrease in mitochondrial oxidoreductase activity; cytoplasmic translocation of cytochrome C and apoptosis-inducing factor (AIF); caspase activation; and nuclear condensa-tion (Walker et al. 1988; Cai et al. 1998; Joza et al. 2001; van Loo et al. 2002). These toxic changes were concentration-dependent because lower Aßo concentra-tions induced chronic mitochondrial alterations but not cell death. In this regard, chronic and subtle impairment of mitochondrial function by low concentrations of Aß soluble species may underlie defective synaptic activity and cognitive impair-ment in AD patients. Furthermore, transport and localization of mitochondria into neuronal processes, an energy-dependent event, is necessary for the development and maintenance of both spines and synaptic plasticity (Li et al. 2004).

Despite inducing similar changes, the time course of ADDL toxicity was longer. ADDLs required approximately five times longer than Aßo to cause similar effects. Structural differences between Aßo and ADDLs influencing pore-forming or receptor-binding activities are likely to account for this disparity. An alternative possibility is that ADDLs' toxic effect could be receptor-mediated, leading to mitochondrial changes by downstream signals over a longer time course. We found that lowering extracellular calcium delayed significantly Aßo toxic process. How-ever, Aßo toxicity in low calcium approached that of Aßo in normal calcium after 24 hours. One interpretation is that the rapid toxic response induced by Aßo is accelerated by calcium influx (Mattson 1992; Mattson and Rydel 1992; Li et al. 1996; Berridge et al. 1998; LaFerla 2002; Pierrot et al. 2004), but in the absence of calcium, the pore-forming properties of Aß soluble species (Kagan et al. 2002; Lashuel et al. 2002b; Arispe 2004; Kayed et al. 2004; Quist et al. 2005; Thundimadathil et al. 2005) still trigger the apoptotic process. In this scenario, regardless of calcium influx, the progressive formation of Aß pores in the plasma membrane and internal endomembrane system leads to a general destabilization of ion homeostasis and activation of the apoptotic process.

Figure 10.3 summarizes the timeline of degenerative changes induced by Aßo, ADDLs, and Aßf. Aßo and ADDLs at μM concentrations result in similar mor-phological and biochemical changes. Aßo exert a faster effect, killing most neu-rons within 24 hours. Five to 7 days of incubation are required to generate a similar extent of cell death with ADDLs. Chronic incubation for 10 days and higher con-centrations of Aßf are required to produce generalized dystrophic changes but only modest cell death, whereas nM concentrations of Aßo and ADDLs result in chronic mitochondrial dysfunction and minor changes in cell viability.

Figure 10.4 illustrates a model of the toxic pathway(s) triggered by Aß soluble species. Aßo and ADDLs are recruited to synapses, possibly by metal ions enriched at synaptic sites and/or synaptic receptors. Another possibility is that Aß is

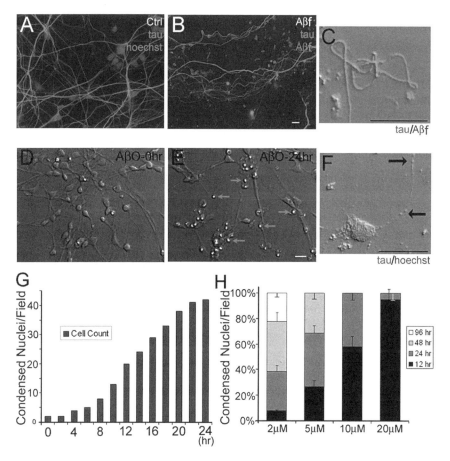

Figure 10.2. Aβo cause rapid and massive neuronal death. Double immunofluorescence
of 18 DIV HCN with anti-tau (red, 1:500) and anti-Aß (blue). (**A**) Neuronal processes in
vehicle-treated HCN exhibit considerable development and a normal, smooth appearance
(Ctrl). (**B**) After 10 days of treatment with 20μm Aßf, neuronal processes display aberrant morphologies, including tortuosity and irregular neuritic caliber. (**C**) Combined DIC/
fluorescence at higher magnification illustrates a neuronal process exhibiting loops and
sharp turns close to Aßf deposits (blue). (**D–F**) DIC images of living HCN cultures treated
with 5μm Aßo. Immediately after Aßo addition the culture exhibits normal appearance
(**D**); after 24 hr extensive cell death is indicated by retraction and disintegration of processes, and by nuclear condensation (arrows, **E**). At higher magnification, the beading and
disintegration of neuronal processes is clearly observed (arrows, **F**). Scale bars = 20μm.
(**G**) Quantification of condensed nuclei/field over the 24 hr period of Aßo treatment. The
graph illustrates one representative field. At least 20 different fields were analyzed with
similar results. (**H**) Bar graph illustrating the increase in condensed nuclei in HCN cultures treated with increasing concentrations of Aßo. The number of condensed nuclei was
scored at the indicated time points. Similar results were obtained in 5 independent experiments. (See color Figure 10.2)

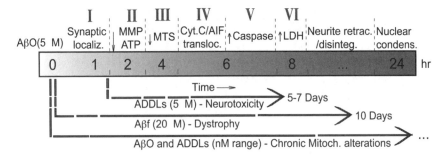

Figure 10.3. Timeline of neurodegenerative events induced by Aß toxic species. Progression of AßO- and ADDL-induced neurotoxicity: (**I**) synaptic localization of AßO and AD-DLs; (**II**) reduced mitochondrial membrane potential (MMP) and ATP levels; (**III**) reduced mitochondrial oxidoreductase activity (MTS); (**IV**) cyt C and AIF translocation from the mitochondrial matrix to the cytosol; (**V**) increase caspase activity; (**VI**) increased LDH levels in culture medium, massive neuritic retraction and disintegration, and nuclear condensation. The timeline for AßO is 24 hr. ADDLs are already detected at synaptic sites by 1 hr, but progression of similar alterations takes 96 hr. Aßf (20µm) requires 10 days to induce generalized neuronal dystrophy and modest cell death. Lower concentrations (nM range) of AßO and ADDLs lead to chronic mitochondrial dysfunction and minimal cell death over time. (See color Figure 10.3)

released at synapses, where it may undergo oligomerization (Gylys et al. 2004). Regardless, the pore-forming activity of Aß soluble species could channel a rapid influx of calcium inside cells at synaptic sites and other cellular locations. Mitochondria act as a major buffering system for calcium, but extreme calcium loads lead to the opening of the MTP (Korge et al. 2002; Scorrano et al. 2003; Miyamoto et al. 2005). This causes the collapse of the MMP and the release of cyt C and AIF from the mitochondrial matrix to the cytosol, where caspases are activated for the execution phase of the apoptotic process. The end stage is illustrated by the complete loss of cell membrane integrity and release of lactate dehydrogenase (LDH).

The emerging view of multiple Aß species capable of deleterious effects at multiple levels co-existing in AD will require a refined therapeutic strategy to address Aß-mediated neurotoxicity. Additional studies in AD brains will be necessary to: assess the synaptic localization of Aß soluble species, establish how the load of Aß soluble species changes during disease progression, determine whether there is a precursor–product relationship among oligomeric and/or fibrillar species, and understand how each of these factors contributes to neurodegeneration.

THE ROLE OF TAU IN AD PATHOLOGY

Neurofibrillary tangles are composed of bundles of highly phosphorylated tau protein paired into helical or coiled filaments (paired helical filaments [PHF])

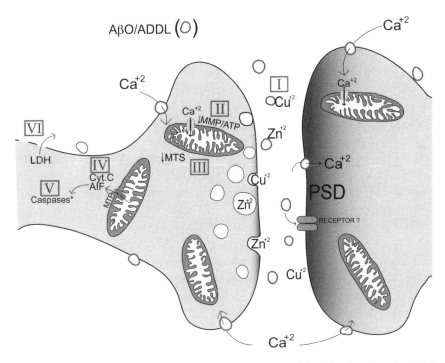

Figure 10.4. Proposed model of Aß soluble species neurotoxicity. The alterations included in the timeline in Fig. 10.3 (**I–VI**) are illustrated taking place at a synapse. AßO or ADDLs (red circles) are recruited to synaptic sites, where they associate with metal ions (Cu^{+2} and Zn^{+2}) or bind post-synaptic receptors (**I**). The pore-/channel-forming activity of Aß soluble species causes massive calcium influx, general destabilization of ion homeostasis, and mitochondrial alterations (**II**, reduced MMP and ATP; **III**, reduced MTS), leading to the opening of the mitochondrial transition pore (MTP) and cyt C and AIF translocation (**IV**), caspase activation (**V**), and cell death evidenced by LDH release (**VI**). PSD, post-synaptic density. (See color Figure 10.4)

(Grundke-Iqbal et al. 1986; Kosik et al. 1986; Goedert et al. 1998; Spillantini and Goedert 1998; Davies 2000; Lee et al. 2001; Iqbal and Grundke-Iqbal 2006). Hyperphosphorylated tau is also found in aberrant neuronal extensions called dystrophic neurites, which have been associated with synaptic loss and the cognitive decline observed in AD patients (McKee et al. 1991). Tau is a neuron-specific microtubule-associated protein preferentially localized in axons (Couchie et al. 1985; Peng et al. 1985; Kosik et al. 1986; Goedert et al. 1989a). Tau pathology involves the release of tau from microtubules, mislocalization in the somatodendritic compartment, and its hyperphosphorylation and self-association into PHF, which further aggregate into tangles. The molecular mechanism(s) and precise sequence of events leading to tangle formation remain poorly understood (Neve and Robakis 1998; Lee et al. 2001). Perturbations in tau are not only present in AD, but also in a number of other neurodegenerative diseases such as Down's syndrome, Parkinson's disease, prion diseases, fronto-temporal dementias, and Niemann-Pick disease type C, suggesting the existence of multiple genetic and epigenetic factors that induce and/or facilitate tau pathology (Spillantini and Goedert 1998; Buee et al. 2000; Lee et al. 2001).

Human tau is encoded by a single gene consisting of 16 exons present on chromosome 17q21. Alternate splicing of 11 of these exons results in 6 tau isoforms found in the central nervous system (CNS) (Neve et al. 1986; Goedert et al. 1988; Andreadis et al. 1992; Lee et al. 2001). These splice variants consist of either or all of the E2, E3, and E10 exons and range from 352 aa (fetal form) to 441 aa (full-length form) (Buee et al. 2000). They differ from each other by the presence of three (3R) or four (4R) C-terminal tandem repeats of 31–32 aa microtubule binding domains encoded by E9, E10, E11, and E12 (Goedert et al. 1989b; Goedert et al. 1989a; Andreadis et al. 1992). In addition, the triplets of 3R and 4R isoforms differ from one another by the presence or absence of E2 and E3 to generate tau isoforms with either 0 (form 0N), 29 (form 1N), or 58 (form 2N) amino acid inserts at the N-terminus (Fig. 10.1) (Goedert et al. 1989a). In the adult human brain, the 3R/4R ratio is approximately 1, but the ratio of 0N, 1N, and 2N isoforms is about 37:54:9 (Goedert and Jakes 1990; Hong et al. 1998).

The expression of tau isoforms is differentially and developmentally regulated. The fetal brain only expresses the shortest (3R-0N) isoform, whereas the adult brain expresses all six isoforms (Goedert et al. 1989b; Kosik et al. 1989). Structural differences among tau isoforms may underlie pathological significance. For instance, 4R isoforms have higher microtubule-binding affinity than 3R isoforms (Goode et al. 2000), and the ratio of 4R/3R expression and/or accumulation is altered in certain neurodegenerative diseases, such as progressive supranuclear palsy, in which 4R tau accumulates in the brain lesions (Lee et al. 2001; Johnson and Stoothoff 2004; Stoothoff and Johnson 2005). Current experimental models for the study of tau pathology include transgenic animals and cultured neurons or neuronal cell lines, which do not fully recapitulate tau pattern of expression in the adult human brain. Only three 4R tau isoforms are expressed in rat, four tau isoforms (three 3R plus one 4R) are found in mice (Kosik et al. 1989; Kampers et al. 1999; Hall et al. 2000), and isoforms expressed in immature neurons appear to predominate in human neuroblastoma cell lines (Smith et al. 1995).

The development and characterization of clinically relevant experimental models for the study of neurodegenerative conditions is critical to understand complex disease mechanisms at the molecular level. HCN develop a complex network of axons and dendrites and numerous synaptic contacts in culture (Deshpande et al. 2006). Synaptic loss is one of the earliest features associated with tau pathology (Yoshiyama et al. 2007), possibly as a consequence of alterations in microtubule-based transport of organelles and synaptic proteins due to increased tau solubilization (Alonso et al. 2006), expression (Thies and Mandelkow 2007), and/or filament formation (Hall et al. 2000). The establishment of numerous synapses by HCN (Deshpande et al. 2006) will allow us to perform a detailed examination of the time course of tau modifications and their effect on axonal transport and synaptic number and function (A.D. and J.B., studies in progress).

Immunofluorescence analysis using three different 4R isoform-specific antibodies resulted in a stippled pattern of staining along axonal processes, which differed from the smooth labeling obtained with antibodies that do not distinguish between tau isoforms (Figure 10.5) (Deshpande et al. 2008), or with a 3R tau-specific antibody (data not shown). This finding raises the possibility of tau isoform–specific subcellular localization and function in HCN, possibly related to distinct interactions of 3R and 4R, with different microtubular populations required to regulate dynamic instability in neuronal processes (Levy et al. 2005). In mature HCN, the 4R/3R expression ratio was approximately 1, similar to the 4R/3R ratio in the adult human brain, and in contrast with the elevated levels of 4R observed in the DS/AD brain. In fact, previous studies have reported an excess of 4R tau in several tauopathies and also in AD (Hong et al. 1998; Hutton et al. 1998; D'Souza et al. 1999; Grover et al. 1999; Yasojima et al. 1999). This is particularly relevant in light of recent experiments showing that 4R tau suppresses neuronal precursor proliferation and promotes neuronal differentiation and axonal growth in the hippocampus of tau knock-in/knock-out mice (Sennvik et al. 2007). Thus, alterations in tau isoform levels may lead to pathological changes ranging from unbalanced cytoskeletal modulation to perturbations in neuronal differentiation and process formation. These results underscore the importance of studying tau pathology in an experimental system that recapitulates as close as possible the expression pattern of tau in the human brain, and that can replicate the molecular changes present during the disease process. In this regard, HCN represent a valuable experimental model, which appears to recapitulate important molecular aspects of tau isoform expression in the human brain.

Protein phosphatases are the focus of intense research in the AD field because they are critical to counterbalance the effect of kinases on tau phosphorylation (Lee et al. 2001). Chronic treatment with specific phosphatase inhibitors demonstrated that inhibition of PP2A activity resulted in marked alterations in the band profile of tau isoforms, elevated levels of soluble tau, increased level of phosphorylated tau in the soluble fraction, and translocation of phosphorylated tau to the somatodendritic compartment (Figure 10.6). Consistent with these observations, PP2A is the major phosphatase activity toward phosphorylated tau in the brain (Goedert et al. 1992, 1995), it binds to tau, and it mediates its association with microtubules (Sontag et al. 1996; Liao et al. 1998), indicating an important role for PP2A in tau pathological changes. We have also detected dramatic

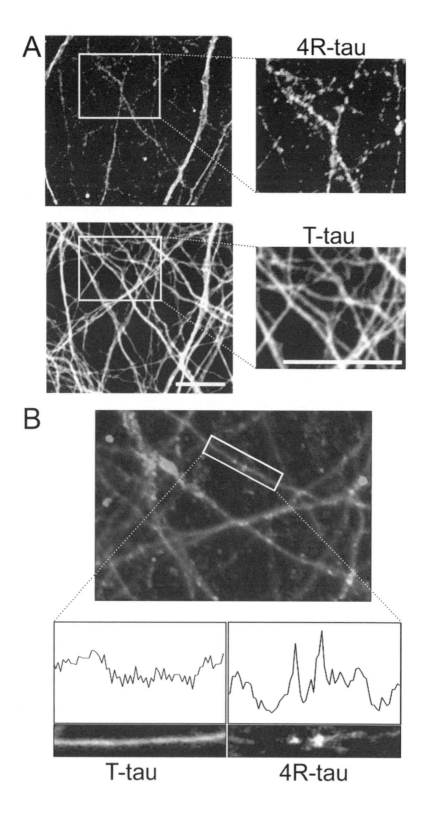

changes in tau phosphorylation and cystoskeletal association in HCN after treatment with a number of agents, including proteasomal inhibitors, lysosomal inhibitors, and kinase activators (data not shown), suggesting that tau phosphorylation is regulated at multiple levels and that alterations in a number of cellular pathways can lead to tau modifications, consistent with the conspicuous presence of tau pathology in neurological conditions with very different etiology.

Finally, we found tau oligomeric forms after phosphatase inhibition in HCN (Fig. 10.6). Berger and co-workers have recently identified tau multimers in the 140–170 kD range in tauopathy mouse models, as well as in FTDP-17 and AD brain homogenates (Berger et al. 2007). Furthermore, the appearance of tau multimers closely correlated with functional memory impairments in tau mutant mice, suggesting the involvement of tau multimeric species in the disease process. Tau multimers in HCN were clearly recognized by 4R tau-specific antibodies and by the conformation-dependent antibody A11, which recognizes oligomeric species regardless of the protein primary sequence (Kayed et al. 2003), indicating that 4R tau isoforms are principally involved in tau oligomerization. The intracellular accumulation of tau oligomeric forms appears to impair neuronal function independently of tau phosphorylation state, because tau multimers have been shown to derive from both nonhyperphosphorylated (~140 kD) and hyperphosphorylated tau (~170 kD) (Berger et al. 2007), and they are induced by multiple cellular insults (A.D. and J.B., unpublished observations). Ongoing studies in our laboratory are directed toward determining the functional consequences of tau oligomerization in neuronal function, including protein trafficking and synaptic activity.

In summary, these studies demonstrate a specific and complex pattern of tau isoform expression in HCN, which may play a critical role in the development of human tauopathies.

Figure 10.5. Differential distribution of 3R and 4R tau in HCN. (**A**) Double immunofluorescence analysis of HCN at 20 days in culture with anti-4R tau (clone 4RT) and polyclonal anti-total tau antibodies illustrate the stippled appearance of 4R immunoreactivity along axonal processes in sharp contrast with the smooth-textured appearance of total tau immunoreactivity. Insets in the left panels correspond to regions magnified in the right panels. (**B**) Densitometric analysis of immunofluorescence signal intensity along axonal processes revealed significantly larger peaks and valleys in the 4R tau densitometric profile compared to that of total tau. The images correspond to the same microscopic field. Scale bars = 20µm. (See color Figure 10.5)

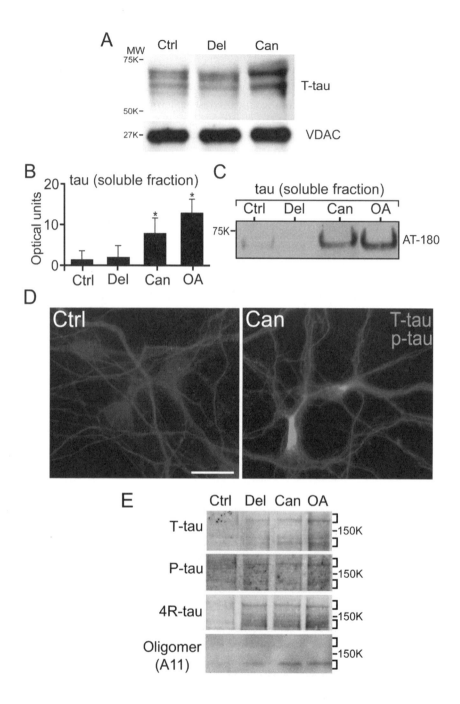

Figure 10.6. Phosphatase inhibitors enhance tau phosphorylation and oligomerization in HCN. (**A**) Western blot of HCN treated with 40 pM deltamethrin (Del) and 10 nM cantharidin (Can) for 10 days, homogenized, and probed with polyclonal anti-tau (T-tau) and anti-VDAC antibodies. All treatments were initiated at day 20 in culture. Note the change in the profile of tau isoforms after cantharidin treatment. (**B**) Dot blot quantification of total tau in the soluble fraction of cytoskeletal preparations after treatment with deltamethrin and cantharidin at the concentrations indicated above, and 5 nM okadaic acid (OA). (**C**) There is a significant increase in soluble tau after treatment with cantharidin and okadaic acid, which was accompanied by a marked elevation in phosphorylated tau in the soluble fraction, as shown after blotting with antibody AT-180, which recognizes tau phosphorylated at Thr231. (**D**) Double immunofluorescence analysis with polyclonal anti-tau (T-tau, blue channel) and PHF-1 (phosphorylated tau at Ser 396/404, red channel) illustrates both the increase in phosphorylated tau immunoreactivity and its translocation to the somatodendritic compartment after cantharidin (Can) treatment. PHF-1 immunoreactivity was negative in nontreated cells (Ctrl). (**E**) Western blot of HCN treated with cantharidin (Can) and okadaic acid (OA) showed induction of ~140–170 kD tau multimers, which labeled positive with an antibody that recognizes all tau isoforms (T-tau). Anti-phosphorylated tau antibody AT-180 preferentially labeled the ~170kD bands (P-tau). The multimers were also strongly labeled by anti-4R tau antibody (clone 4RT). Lower MW multimers (~140 kD) were detected by the conformation-dependent antibody A11, which recognizes oligomeric structures regardless of the protein sequence (A11). Scale bar = 20µm. (See color Figure 10.6)

ACKNOWLEDGMENTS

Supported by grants from the Alzheimer's Association, National Institutes of Health (HD38466), and the Institute for Brain Aging and Dementia at UCI.

REFERENCES

Alonso AD, Li B, Grundke I, Iqbal K (2006) O2-01-02. Treat abnormal hyperphosphorylation and not aggregation of tau. *Alzheimer's & Dementia: The Journal of the Alzheimer's Association* 2:S29–30.

Andreadis A, Brown WM, Kosik KS (1992) Structure and novel exons of the human tau gene. *Biochemistry* 31:10626–33.

Arispe N (2004) Architecture of the Alzheimer's A beta P ion channel pore. *J Membr Biol* 197:33–48.

Atwood CS, Scarpa RC, Huang X, Moir RD, Jones WD, Fairlie DP, Tanzi RE, Bush AI (2000) Characterization of copper interactions with alzheimer amyloid beta peptides: identification of an attomolar-affinity copper binding site on amyloid beta1-42. *J Neurochem* 75:1219–33.

Berger Z, Roder H, Hanna A, Carlson A, Rangachari V, Yue M, Wszolek Z, Ashe K, Knight J, Dickson D, Andorfer C, Rosenberry TL, Lewis J, Hutton M, Janus C (2007) Accumulation of pathological tau species and memory loss in a conditional model of tauopathy. *J Neurosci* 27:3650–62.

Berridge MJ, Bootman MD, Lipp P (1998) Calcium—a life and death signal. *Nature* 395:645–8.

Bucciantini M, Giannoni E, Chiti F, Baroni F, Formigli L, Zurdo J, Taddei N, Ramponi G, Dobson CM, Stefani M (2002) Inherent toxicity of aggregates implies a common mechanism for protein misfolding diseases. *Nature* 416:507–11.

Buee L, Bussiere T, Buee-Scherrer V, Delacourte A, Hof PR (2000) Tau protein isoforms, phosphorylation and role in neurodegenerative disorders. *Brain Res Brain Res Rev* 33:95–130.

Busciglio J, Lorenzo A, Yeh J, Yankner BA (1995) beta-amyloid fibrils induce tau phosphorylation and loss of microtubule binding. *Neuron* 14:879–88.

Bush AI, Pettingell WH Jr, Paradis MD, Tanzi RE (1994) Modulation of A beta adhesiveness and secretase site cleavage by zinc. *J Biol Chem* 269:12152–8.

Cai J, Yang J, Jones DP (1998) Mitochondrial control of apoptosis: the role of cytochrome c. *Biochim Biophys Acta* 1366:139–49.

Caughey B, Lansbury PT (2003) Protofibrils, pores, fibrils, and neurodegeneration: separating the responsible protein aggregates from the innocent bystanders. *Annu Rev Neurosci* 26:267–98.

Cherny RA, Atwood CS, Xilinas ME, Gray DN, Jones WD, McLean CA, Barnham KJ, Volitakis I, Fraser FW, Kim Y, Huang X, Goldstein LE, Moir RD, Lim JT, Beyreuther K, Zheng H, Tanzi RE, Masters CL, Bush AI (2001) Treatment with a copper-zinc chelator markedly and rapidly inhibits beta-amyloid accumulation in Alzheimer's disease transgenic mice. *Neuron* 30:665–76.

Couchie D, Fages C, Bridoux AM, Rolland B, Tardy M, Nunez J (1985) Microtubule-associated proteins and in vitro astrocyte differentiation. *J Cell Biol* 101:2095–103.

Dahlgren KN, Manelli AM, Stine WB Jr, Baker LK, Krafft GA, LaDu MJ (2002) Oligomeric and fibrillar species of amyloid-beta peptides differentially affect neuronal viability. *J Biol Chem* 277:32046–53.

Davies P (2000) A very incomplete comprehensive theory of Alzheimer's disease. *Ann N Y Acad Sci* 924:8–16.

Demuro A, Mina E, Kayed R, Milton SC, Parker I, Glabe CG (2005) Calcium dysregulation and membrane disruption as a ubiquitous neurotoxic mechanism of soluble amyloid oligomers. *J Biol Chem* 280:17294–300.

Deshpande A, Mina E, Glabe C, Busciglio J (2006) Different conformations of amyloid beta induce neurotoxicity by distinct mechanisms in human cortical neurons. *J Neurosci* 26:6011–8.

Deshpande A, Win KM, Busciglio J (2008) Tau isoform expression and regulation in human cortical neurons. *Faseb J*, published online February 8, 2008 as doi: 10.1096/ fj.07-096909

D'Souza I, Poorkaj P, Hong M, Nochlin D, Lee VM, Bird TD, Schellenberg GD (1999) Missense and silent tau gene mutations cause frontotemporal dementia with parkinsonism-chromosome 17 type, by affecting multiple alternative RNA splicing regulatory elements. *Proc Natl Acad Sci USA* 96:5598–603.

Frederickson CJ, Bush AI (2001) Synaptically released zinc: physiological functions and pathological effects. *Biometals* 14:353–66.

Georganopoulou DG, Chang L, Nam JM, Thaxton CS, Mufson EJ, Klein WL, Mirkin CA (2005) Nanoparticle-based detection in cerebral spinal fluid of a soluble pathogenic biomarker for Alzheimer's disease. *Proc Natl Acad Sci USA* 102:2273–6.

Glabe CG (2004) Conformation-dependent antibodies target diseases of protein misfolding. *Trends Biochem Sci* 29:542–7.

Goedert M, Cohen ES, Jakes R, Cohen P (1992) p42 MAP kinase phosphorylation sites in microtubule-associated protein tau are dephosphorylated by protein phosphatase 2A1. Implications for Alzheimer's disease [corrected]. *FEBS Lett* 312:95–9.

Goedert M, Jakes R (1990) Expression of separate isoforms of human tau protein: correlation with the tau pattern in brain and effects on tubulin polymerization. *Embo J* 9:4225–30.

Goedert M, Jakes R, Qi Z, Wang JH, Cohen P (1995) Protein phosphatase 2A is the major enzyme in brain that dephosphorylates tau protein phosphorylated by proline-directed protein kinases or cyclic AMP-dependent protein kinase. *J Neurochem* 65: 2804–7.

Goedert M, Spillantini MG, Davies SW (1998) Filamentous nerve cell inclusions in neurodegenerative diseases. *Curr Opin Neurobiol* 8:619–32.

Goedert M, Spillantini MG, Jakes R, Rutherford D, Crowther RA (1989b) Multiple isoforms of human microtubule-associated protein tau: sequences and localization in neurofibrillary tangles of Alzheimer's disease. *Neuron* 3:519–26.

Goedert M, Spillantini MG, Potier MC, Ulrich J, Crowther RA (1989a) Cloning and sequencing of the cDNA encoding an isoform of microtubule-associated protein tau containing four tandem repeats: differential expression of tau protein mRNAs in human brain. *Embo J* 8:393–9.

Goedert M, Wischik CM, Crowther RA, Walker JE, Klug A (1988) Cloning and sequencing of the cDNA encoding a core protein of the paired helical filament of Alzheimer disease: identification as the microtubule-associated protein tau. *Proc Natl Acad Sci USA* 85:4051–5.

Goode BL, Chau M, Denis PE, Feinstein SC (2000) Structural and functional differences between 3-repeat and 4-repeat tau isoforms. Implications for normal tau function and the onset of neurodegenetative disease. *J Biol Chem* 275:38182–9.

Grace EA, Rabiner CA, Busciglio J (2002) Characterization of neuronal dystrophy induced by fibrillar amyloid beta: implications for Alzheimer's disease. *Neuroscience* 114:265–73.

Grover A, Houlden H, Baker M, Adamson J, Lewis J, Prihar G, Pickering-Brown S, Duff K, Hutton M (1999) 5' splice site mutations in tau associated with the inherited dementia FTDP-17 affect a stem-loop structure that regulates alternative splicing of exon 10. *J Biol Chem* 274:15134–43.

Grundke-Iqbal I, Iqbal K, Tung YC, Quinlan M, Wisniewski HM, Binder LI (1986) Abnormal phosphorylation of the microtubule-associated protein tau (tau) in Alzheimer cytoskeletal pathology. *Proc Natl Acad Sci USA* 83:4913–7.

Gylys KH, Fein JA, Yang F, Wiley DJ, Miller CA, Cole GM (2004) Synaptic changes in Alzheimer's disease: increased amyloid-beta and gliosis in surviving terminals is accompanied by decreased PSD-95 fluorescence. *Am J Pathol* 165:1809–17.

Hall GF, Chu B, Lee G, Yao J (2000) Human tau filaments induce microtubule and synapse loss in an in vivo model of neurofibrillary degenerative disease. *J Cell Sci* 113(Pt 8):1373–87.

Hartley DM, Walsh DM, Ye CP, Diehl T, Vasquez S, Vassilev PM, Teplow DB, Selkoe DJ (1999) Protofibrillar intermediates of amyloid beta-protein induce acute electrophysiological changes and progressive neurotoxicity in cortical neurons. *J Neurosci* 19: 8876–84.

Hong M, Zhukareva V, Vogelsberg-Ragaglia V, Wszolek Z, Reed L, Miller BI, Geschwind DH, Bird TD, McKeel D, Goate A, Morris JC, Wilhelmsen KC, Schellenberg GD,

Trojanowski JQ, Lee VM (1998) Mutation-specific functional impairments in distinct tau isoforms of hereditary FTDP-17. *Science* 282:1914–7.

Hutton M, Lendon CL, Rizzu P, Baker M, Froelich S, Houlden H, Pickering-Brown S, Chakraverty S, Isaacs A, Grover A, Hackett J, Adamson J, Lincoln S, Dickson D, Davies P, Petersen RC, Stevens M, de Graaff E, Wauters E, van Baren J, Hillebrand M, Joosse M, Kwon JM, Nowotny P, Che LK, Norton J, Morris JC, Reed LA, Trojanowski J, Basun H, Lannfelt L, Neystat M, Fahn S, Dark F, Tannenberg T, Dodd PR, Hayward N, Kwok JB, Schofield PR, Andreadis A, Snowden J, Craufurd D, Neary D, Owen F, Oostra BA, Hardy J, Goate A, van Swieten J, Mann D, Lynch T, Heutink P (1998) Association of missense and 5'-splice-site mutations in tau with the inherited dementia FTDP-17. *Nature* 393:702–5.

Iqbal K, Grundke-Iqbal I (2006) Discoveries of tau, abnormally hyperphosphorylated tau and others of neurofibrillary degeneration: a personal historical perspective. *J Alzheimers Dis* 9:219–42.

Johnson GV, Stoothoff WH (2004) Tau phosphorylation in neuronal cell function and dysfunction. *J Cell Sci* 117:5721–9.

Joza N, Susin SA, Daugas E, Stanford WL, Cho SK, Li CY, Sasaki T, Elia AJ, Cheng HY, Ravagnan L, Ferri KF, Zamzami N, Wakeham A, Hakem R, Yoshida H, Kong YY, Mak TW, Zuniga-Pflucker JC, Kroemer G, Penninger JM (2001) Essential role of the mitochondrial apoptosis-inducing factor in programmed cell death. *Nature* 410: 549–54.

Kagan BL, Hirakura Y, Azimov R, Azimova R, Lin MC (2002) The channel hypothesis of Alzheimer's disease: current status. *Peptides* 23:1311–5.

Kampers T, Pangalos M, Geerts H, Wiech H, Mandelkow E (1999) Assembly of paired helical filaments from mouse tau: implications for the neurofibrillary pathology in transgenic mouse models for Alzheimer's disease. *FEBS Lett* 451:39–44.

Kayed R, Head E, Thompson JL, McIntire TM, Milton SC, Cotman CW, Glabe CG (2003) Common structure of soluble amyloid oligomers implies common mechanism of pathogenesis. *Science* 300:486–9.

Kayed R, Sokolov Y, Edmonds B, McIntire TM, Milton SC, Hall JE, Glabe CG (2004) Permeabilization of lipid bilayers is a common conformation-dependent activity of soluble amyloid oligomers in protein misfolding diseases. *J Biol Chem* 279:46363–6.

Korge P, Honda HM, Weiss JN (2002) Protection of cardiac mitochondria by diazoxide and protein kinase C: implications for ischemic preconditioning. *Proc Natl Acad Sci USA* 99:3312–7.

Kosik KS, Joachim CL, Selkoe DJ (1986) Microtubule-associated protein tau (tau) is a major antigenic component of paired helical filaments in Alzheimer disease. *Proc Natl Acad Sci USA* 83:4044–8.

Kosik KS, Orecchio LD, Bakalis S, Neve RL (1989) Developmentally regulated expression of specific tau sequences. *Neuron* 2:1389–97.

Kuo YM, Emmerling MR, Vigo-Pelfrey C, Kasunic TC, Kirkpatrick JB, Murdoch GH, Ball MJ, Roher AE (1996) Water-soluble Abeta (N-40, N-42) oligomers in normal and Alzheimer disease brains. *J Biol Chem* 271:4077–81.

Lacor PN, Buniel MC, Chang L, Fernandez SJ, Gong Y, Viola KL, Lambert MP, Velasco PT, Bigio EH, Finch CE, Krafft GA, Klein WL (2004) Synaptic targeting by Alzheimer's-related amyloid beta oligomers. *J Neurosci* 24:10191–200.

Lacor PN, Buniel MC, Furlow PW, Clemente AS, Velasco PT, Wood M, Viola KL, Klein WL (2007) Abeta oligomer-induced aberrations in synapse composition, shape, and density provide a molecular basis for loss of connectivity in Alzheimer's disease. *J Neurosci* 27:796–807.

LaFerla FM (2002) Calcium dyshomeostasis and intracellular signalling in Alzheimer's disease. *Nat Rev Neurosci* 3:862–72.

Lambert MP, Barlow AK, Chromy BA, Edwards C, Freed R, Liosatos M, Morgan TE, Rozovsky I, Trommer B, Viola KL, Wals P, Zhang C, Finch CE, Krafft GA, Klein WL (1998) Diffusible, nonfibrillar ligands derived from Abeta1-42 are potent central nervous system neurotoxins. *Proc Natl Acad Sci USA* 95:6448–53.

Lashuel HA, Hartley DM, Balakhaneh D, Aggarwal A, Teichberg S, Callaway DJ (2002a) New class of inhibitors of amyloid-beta fibril formation. Implications for the mechanism of pathogenesis in Alzheimer's disease. *J Biol Chem* 277:42881–90.

Lashuel HA, Petre BM, Wall J, Simon M, Nowak RJ, Walz T, Lansbury PT Jr (2002b) Alpha-synuclein, especially the Parkinson's disease-associated mutants, forms pore-like annular and tubular protofibrils. *J Mol Biol* 322:1089–102.

Lee VM, Goedert M, Trojanowski JQ (2001) Neurodegenerative tauopathies. *Annu Rev Neurosci* 24:1121–59.

Lesne S, Koh MT, Kotilinek L, Kayed R, Glabe CG, Yang A, Gallagher M, Ashe KH (2006) A specific amyloid-beta protein assembly in the brain impairs memory. *Nature* 440:352–7.

Levy SF, Leboeuf AC, Massie MR, Jordan MA, Wilson L, Feinstein SC (2005) Three- and four-repeat tau regulate the dynamic instability of two distinct microtubule subpopulations in qualitatively different manners. Implications for neurodegeneration. *J Biol Chem* 280:13520–8.

Li YP, Bushnell AF, Lee CM, Perlmutter LS, Wong SK (1996) Beta-amyloid induces apoptosis in human-derived neurotypic SH-SY5Y cells. *Brain Res* 738:196–204.

Li Z, Okamoto K, Hayashi Y, Sheng M (2004) The importance of dendritic mitochondria in the morphogenesis and plasticity of spines and synapses. *Cell* 119:873–87.

Liao H, Li Y, Brautigan DL, Gundersen GG (1998) Protein phosphatase 1 is targeted to microtubules by the microtubule-associated protein Tau. *J Biol Chem* 273: 21901–8.

Lue LF, Kuo YM, Roher AE, Brachova L, Shen Y, Sue L, Beach T, Kurth JH, Rydel RE, Rogers J (1999) Soluble amyloid beta peptide concentration as a predictor of synaptic change in Alzheimer's disease. *Am J Pathol* 155:853–62.

Mathie A, Sutton GL, Clarke CE, Veale EL (2006) Zinc and copper: Pharmacological probes and endogenous modulators of neuronal excitability. *Pharmacol Ther* 111: 567–83.

Mattson MP (1992) Calcium as sculptor and destroyer of neural circuitry. *Exp Gerontol* 27:29–49.

Mattson MP, Rydel RE (1992) beta-Amyloid precursor protein and Alzheimer's disease: the peptide plot thickens. *Neurobiol Aging* 13:617–21.

McKee AC, Kosik KS, Kowall NW (1991) Neuritic pathology and dementia in Alzheimer's disease. *Ann Neurol* 30:156–65.

Miyamoto S, Howes AL, Adams JW, Dorn GW 2nd, Brown JH (2005) Ca2+ dysregulation induces mitochondrial depolarization and apoptosis: role of Na+/Ca2+ exchanger and AKT. *J Biol Chem* 280:38505–12.

Mocchegiani E, Bertoni-Freddari C, Marcellini F, Malavolta M (2005) Brain, aging and neurodegeneration: role of zinc ion availability. *Prog Neurobiol* 75:367–90.

Naslund J, Haroutunian V, Mohs R, Davis KL, Davies P, Greengard P, Buxbaum JD (2000) Correlation between elevated levels of amyloid beta-peptide in the brain and cognitive decline. *JAMA* 283:1571–7.

Neve RL, Harris P, Kosik KS, Kurnit DM, Donlon TA (1986) Identification of cDNA clones for the human microtubule-associated protein tau and chromosomal localization of the genes for tau and microtubule-associated protein 2. *Brain Res* 387: 271–80.

Neve RL, Robakis NK (1998) Alzheimer's disease: a re-examination of the amyloid hypothesis. *Trends Neurosci* 21:15–9.

Nguyen HD, Hall CK (2004) Molecular dynamics simulations of spontaneous fibril formation by random-coil peptides. *Proc Natl Acad Sci USA* 101:16180–5.

Peng I, Binder LI, Black MM (1985) Cultured neurons contain a variety of microtubule-associated proteins. *Brain Res* 361:200–11.

Pierrot N, Ghisdal P, Caumont AS, Octave JN (2004) Intraneuronal amyloid-beta1-42 production triggered by sustained increase of cytosolic calcium concentration induces neuronal death. *J Neurochem* 88:1140–50.

Pike CJ, Cummings BJ, Cotman CW (1992) beta-Amyloid induces neuritic dystrophy in vitro: similarities with Alzheimer pathology. *NeuroReport* 3:769–72.

Quist A, Doudevski I, Lin H, Azimova R, Ng D, Frangione B, Kagan B, Ghiso J, Lal R (2005) Amyloid ion channels: a common structural link for protein-misfolding disease. *Proc Natl Acad Sci USA* 102:10427–32.

Sanchez I, Mahlke C, Yuan J (2003) Pivotal role of oligomerization in expanded polyglutamine neurodegenerative disorders. *Nature* 421:373–9.

Scinto LF, Frosch M, Wu CK, Daffner KR, Gedi N, Geula C (2001) Selective cell loss in Edinger-Westphal in asymptomatic elders and Alzheimer's patients. *Neurobiol Aging* 22:729–36.

Scorrano L, Oakes SA, Opferman JT, Cheng EH, Sorcinelli MD, Pozzan T, Korsmeyer SJ (2003) BAX and BAK regulation of endoplasmic reticulum Ca2+: a control point for apoptosis. *Science* 300:135–9.

Sennvik K, Boekhoorn K, Lasrado R, Terwel D, Verhaeghe S, Korr H, Schmitz C, Tomiyama T, Mori H, Krugers H, Joels M, Ramakers GJ, Lucassen PJ, Van Leuven F (2007) Tau-4R suppresses proliferation and promotes neuronal differentiation in the hippocampus of tau knockin/knockout mice. *FASEB J*.

Smith CJ, Anderton BH, Davis DR, Gallo JM (1995) Tau isoform expression and phosphorylation state during differentiation of cultured neuronal cells. *FEBS Lett* 375:243–8.

Sontag E, Nunbhakdi-Craig V, Lee G, Bloom GS, Mumby MC (1996) Regulation of the phosphorylation state and microtubule-binding activity of Tau by protein phosphatase 2A. *Neuron* 17:1201–7.

Spillantini MG, Goedert M (1998) Tau protein pathology in neurodegenerative diseases. *Trends Neurosci* 21:428–33.

Spires TL, Meyer-Luehmann M, Stern EA, McLean PJ, Skoch J, Nguyen PT, Bacskai BJ, Hyman BT (2005) Dendritic spine abnormalities in amyloid precursor protein transgenic mice demonstrated by gene transfer and intravital multiphoton microscopy. *J Neurosci* 25:7278–87.

Stern EA, Bacskai BJ, Hickey GA, Attenello FJ, Lombardo JA, Hyman BT (2004) Cortical synaptic integration in vivo is disrupted by amyloid-beta plaques. *J Neurosci* 24:4535–40.

Stoothoff WH, Johnson GV (2005) Tau phosphorylation: physiological and pathological consequences. *Biochim Biophys Acta* 1739:280–97.

Thies E, Mandelkow EM (2007) Missorting of tau in neurons causes degeneration of synapses that can be rescued by the kinase MARK2/Par-1. *J Neurosci* 27:2896–907.

Thundimadathil J, Roeske RW, Jiang HY, Guo L (2005) Aggregation and porin-like channel activity of a beta sheet peptide. *Biochemistry* 44:10259–70.

Tsai J, Grutzendler J, Duff K, Gan WB (2004) Fibrillar amyloid deposition leads to local synaptic abnormalities and breakage of neuronal branches. *Nat Neurosci* 7:1181–3.

van Loo G, Saelens X, van Gurp M, MacFarlane M, Martin SJ, Vandenabeele P (2002) The role of mitochondrial factors in apoptosis: a Russian roulette with more than one bullet. *Cell Death Differ* 9:1031–42.

Walker NI, Harmon BV, Gobe GC, Kerr JF (1988) Patterns of cell death. *Methods Achiev Exp Pathol* 13:18–54.

Walsh DM, Klyubin I, Fadeeva JV, Rowan MJ, Selkoe DJ (2002) Amyloid-beta oligomers: their production, toxicity and therapeutic inhibition. *Biochem Soc Trans* 30: 552–7.

Yasojima K, McGeer EG, McGeer PL (1999) Tangled areas of Alzheimer brain have upregulated levels of exon 10 containing tau mRNA. *Brain Res* 831:301–5.

Yoshiyama Y, Higuchi M, Zhang B, Huang SM, Iwata N, Saido TC, Maeda J, Suhara T, Trojanowski JQ, Lee VM (2007) Synapse loss and microglial activation precede tangles in a P301S tauopathy mouse model. *Neuron* 53:337–51.

Chapter Eleven

Aberrant Cells and Synaptic Circuits in Pediatric Epilepsy Surgery Patients

Carlos Cepeda, Véronique M. André, Irene Yamazaki,
Max Kleiman-Weiner, Robin S. Fisher, Harry V. Vinters,
Michael S. Levine, and Gary W. Mathern

INTRODUCTION

One of the key elements for the success of Cajal and his neuron theory was the use of ontogenetic analyses. The application of a modified Golgi technique to embryonic and early postnatal brain tissue allowed Cajal to trace developing neurons while their processes were still growing (De Castro et al. 2007). This permitted better visualization of the rudimentary patterns of early neuronal connectivity, which contrasts to the intricate mesh of dendrites and axons observed in adults.

Although much simpler, it would be naïve to think that a developing brain is just a small version of an adult brain. In fact, throughout development transient cellular elements and connections emerge and disappear, leaving their place to the neurons and synapses that will eventually constitute the mature cerebral cortex. Also, from a functional perspective, the mechanisms that govern neuronal communication in adult brains are often different from those in developing brains (Ben-Ari 2006).

The progressive refinement of neuronal architecture and connectivity during brain development is well exemplified by the cerebral cortex, a laminar structure in which neurogenesis and final positioning of neurons in the cortical plate follow a series of precisely regulated steps in both space and time (Rakic 2006). In some pathological conditions the sequence of events leading to cortical formation is perturbed, causing neuronal disarray and/or the presence of aberrant cells. This is best represented by cortical dysplasia (CD), a neuronal migration and differentiation disorder (Gleeson 2001) that constitutes the leading cause of seizures in pediatric epilepsy surgery cases (Mathern et al. 1999; Harvey et al. 2008).

Focal CD was first described by David Taylor and associates as a histopathological abnormality in a subset of surgical specimens from epileptic patients. CD is characterized by cortical dyslamination, misoriented pyramidal cells, and the presence of dysmorphic cells, in particular cytomegalic neurons and balloon cells (Taylor et al. 1971). The potential role of these cells in epileptogenesis has long been hypothesized (Spreafico et al. 1998; Kerfoot et al. 1999; Schwartzkroin and Walsh 2000), and a number of studies demonstrated that human CD tissue is exquisitely sensitive to epileptogenic agents such as 4-aminopyridine (Mattia et al. 1995). However, technical limitations prevented the visualization and electrophysiological characterization of these abnormal cells (Dudek et al. 1995).

The introduction of new optical methods to visualize individual cells in live tissue specimens permitted the correlation of electrophysiology with morphology of neurons. This chapter will summarize studies in our laboratory—at the University of California Los Angeles (UCLA)—describing the properties of abnormal cells and synaptic circuits in pediatric CD tissue, as well as provide a working hypothesis concerning how CD tissue may be able to generate epileptic discharges. Before describing our observations in pediatric CD tissue, a succinct overview of normal cortical development is required.

NORMAL DEVELOPMENT OF THE CEREBRAL CORTEX

In humans, telencephalic development begins with progenitor cell proliferation in the germinal zone and migration toward the cortical surface. Neurogenesis takes place in the ventricular and subventricular zones predominantly during the first and early second trimesters. Recent studies in rodents have shown that the traditional belief that glial and neuronal cells have different lineages is not entirely true. In fact, there is evidence that a substantial number of radial glial cells are self-renewing neural stem cells that can generate neurons during neurogenesis and then produce astrocytes (Chanas-Sacré et al. 2000; Malatesta et al. 2000; Kriegstein 2005). Thus, radial glial cells can no longer be viewed just as a scaffolding for migration of newly generated neurons, but as producers of neurons in the developing neocortex (Noctor et al. 2002). In addition to radial glial cells, another source of cortical neurons is the intermediate progenitor cells, themselves derived from radial glia, located in the subventricular zone (Noctor et al. 2007). Radial glia express—among other protein and transcription factors—vimentin, nestin, and Pax6, whereas intermediate progenitors express growth-associated protein-43 (GAP-43), Svet1[6], and Tbr2[7], as well as a number of markers also found in radial glia such as phosphorylated vimentin (Noctor et al. 2007).

Many of these observations in rodents also apply to human brains. However, species-specific differences also have been described (Rakic 2003; Bystron et al. 2008). For example, in humans at early embryonic stages (5.5–6 gestational weeks [g.w.]) three different classes of progenitor cells were found. A vast majority of dividing cells in the ventricular zone expressed radial glia markers, a minority expressed restricted neuronal markers, and a third population of cells co-expressed glial and neuronal markers (Zecevic 2004). In mid-gestation the subventricular zone is the main proliferative zone and about 10% of cells around 18–24 g.w. are still proliferating. However, the main events during the second trimester post-gestation are neuronal migration and differentiation.

The earliest migrating cells form the preplate, which is split by subsequent generations of cortical plate neurons into a primordial plexiform layer (the marginal zone that becomes the molecular layer or layer I) and a subplate zone. In primates and humans the subplate zone is the most prominent structure during mid-gestation, and it progressively dissolves during late gestation and the early postnatal period along with most of the preplate elements of the molecular layer (often termed Cajal–Retzius neurons). Vestiges of the subplate deepest elements persist in adult layer VI and the white matter. Differentiated neurons and abundant terminals intercalate with and pass through the subplate until many of its constituent neurons undergo apoptotic cell death and the axons relocate in the cortical plate. It has been hypothesized that the subplate zone may serve as a waiting compartment for transient cellular interactions and a substrate for guidance, competition, segregation, and growth of afferents (Kostovic and Rakic 1990).

Diverse cell types exist in the subplate and include five well-differentiated classes: (1) giant multipolar neurons, (2) pyramidal neurons with the main apical dendrite directed toward the piamater, (3) large fusiform neurons with a long main dendrite and few side branches, (4) pyramidal neurons with their apical dendrites oriented away from the piamater, and (5) polymorphous neurons (Mrzljak et al. 1988). The subplate neurons, along with the Cajal–Retzius neurons that populate the marginal zone, are the more mature neurons before birth and animal studies have shown they display spontaneous electrophysiological activity (Friauf et al. 1990; Allendoerfer and Shatz 1994; Hanganu et al. 2002) and receive functional glutamatergic and GABAergic inputs (Hanganu et al. 2001). Low calcium influx appears to play an important role in programmed cell death of both Cajal–Retzius and subplate neurons (Luhmann et al. 2000).

The last period of normal cortical development consists of neuronal and glial differentiation, alignment and orientation of pyramidal neurons in the proper cortical layers, synaptic remodeling, and cell death. Interference with normal development of cortical formation either during proliferation, migration, differentiation, or programmed cell death can lead to numerous pathologies in human brains (Volpe 2000). Focal CD is primarily a disorder of cell migration and differentiation, but other processes may be involved, as discussed later.

In the past 10 years we have examined, using correlative morphological and electrophysiological methods, more than 150 cases of pediatric epilepsy undergoing surgical treatment for therapy-resistant epilepsy. About two-thirds of those cases presented with CD, from mild to severe forms. The remainder comprised non-CD pathologies, including Rasmussen's encephalitis, tumor, stroke, and hippocampal sclerosis. The ages of tissue examined ranged from 2 months to about 14 years.

METHODOLOGICAL ASPECTS

Tissue Selection

CD is not a homogeneous pathological entity, as several types have been described. In our initial studies the pathology group at UCLA divided CD into mild and severe (Mischel et al. 1995). More recently CD tissue has been classified using the Palmini nomenclature (Palmini et al. 2004). These include CD Type I, in which only architectural abnormalities of the cerebral cortex are found, and more severe cases in which, in addition to cortical dyslamination, the sample contains abnormal cells; CD Type IIA (with dysmorphic neurons); and CD Type IIB (with balloon cells). Even within the same patient, areas removed at surgery have different degrees of abnormality. Accordingly, we separate the tissue samples into most abnormal and least abnormal areas based on degree of electrocorticography (ECoG), magnetic resonance imaging (MRI), and positron emission tomography abnormalities. Areas with the greatest degree of ECoG abnormalities consisting of rhythmic high amplitude slow waves correlate with severest MRI and pathological findings (Cepeda et al. 2005b). It is in these samples with the worse ECoG and neuroimaging findings in which the likelihood of finding abnormal cells is greatest. Tuberous sclerosis complex (TSC), an autosomal dominant disease caused by mutations in TSC genes encoding for hamartin and tuberin that shares histopathological similarities with severe CD, also presents with abnormal cells, particularly in the vicinity of the cortical tuber.

Cell Identification

Infrared videomicroscopy in combination with differential interference contrast optics (IR-DIC) permitted, for the first time, visualization of individual cells in living slices (Dodt and Zieglgänsberger 1994). IR-DIC and whole-cell patch clamp recordings have become a powerful tool for the characterization of different cellular types in specific brain regions. In CD, this technology played a critical role in the identification and systematic characterization of abnormal cells (Cepeda et al. 1999, 2003; Mathern et al. 2000). However, similar to the drawbacks noted by Cajal using the Golgi method, heavy myelination precludes adequate visualization of individual cells in older nervous tissue. Younger tissue, with less myelination, is more amenable to adequate visualization using IR-DIC. In our experience, the best tissue samples are from patients younger than 5 years of age. Also the health of the cells and the possibility of maintaining the slices for long periods of time are best in the younger tissue samples. In our cohort, most cases are less than 2 years of age at the time of surgery—particularly in severe CD cases—which permits electrophysiological recordings in optimal conditions.

In CD there are the two main types of morphologically abnormal cells described in the literature: cytomegalic pyramidal neurons and balloon cells. Cytomegalic pyramidal neurons and balloon cells occur in severe CD cases (CD Type IIA and B). Under IR-DIC cytomegalic pyramidal neurons are easy to recognize by their large size, a typical triangular somatic shape, and a prominent apical dendrite. In contrast, balloon cells are usually large and round and have a pale appearance. Numerous small processes can be seen protruding from their cell somata.

Cell Recordings

In our electrophysiological studies we use standard whole-cell patch recording techniques in current and voltage clamp modes. Cells are recorded in slices or after enzymatic treatment and mechanical dissociation. There are some limitations and caveats associated with these techniques. Selecting the cells for electrophysiological recording in slices or after dissociation requires careful and systematic examination of the entire preparation in order to distinguish the normal-appearing from the putative abnormal cells. In addition, a limitation of in vitro preparations is that the normal connectivity patterns are altered by the slicing technique. As a consequence, the epileptogenicity of CD tissue in situ is not maintained in the slice. Finally, sampling in the gray matter is easier than sampling in the white matter due to dense myelination that precludes systematic examination of interstitial cells. In spite of those limitations, we have been able to record and characterize all the abnormal cell types described by morphological studies.

ABNORMAL CELL TYPES IN PEDIATRIC CD

Normal-Sized Misoriented Pyramidal Neurons

Besides cortical dyslamination, a hallmark of CD is the presence of misoriented pyramidal neurons. Misorientation is manifested by a rotation of the cell body and deviation of the apical dendrite from the normal perpendicular orientation with respect to the pial surface. In some pyramidal cells misorientation is very subtle (approximately 15–30° rotation), but in other cases it is more noticeable and complete inversion of the soma is not uncommon. In nearly all of our CD tissue samples we encountered misoriented pyramidal neurons. Despite their abnormal orientation, membrane cell capacitance, input resistance, and time constant were very similar to those of normal-appearing pyramidal neurons (Cepeda et al. 2003). Also, action potential firing induced by membrane depolarization did not reveal signs of hyperexcitability. This indicates that misoriented neurons probably do not contribute significantly to the intrinsic epileptogenicity of CD tissue. This is in line with the finding that a mouse model of cortical migration disorder, the *Reeler* mouse, does not display spontaneous seizures (Caviness 1976; Schwartzkroin and Walsh 2000), although *Reeler* mice have lowered thresholds for epileptic activity (Patrylo et al. 2006).

The underlying mechanisms that induce dyslamination and cell misorientation are unknown. However, important clues have been provided by the isolation of genes related to neuronal guidance and final positioning in the cortical plate, such as *Reelin* (D'Arcangelo et al. 1995). The glycoprotein *Reelin* appears early during embryogenesis (by 11 g.w. in humans) and is expressed prominently in the marginal zone by the Cajal–Retzius neurons, as well as by subpial granular cells (Meyer and Goffinet 1998). *Reelin* promotes neuronal migration toward the cortical surface and this has been proposed to occur via a differential gradient of extracellular *Reelin* so that a low level promotes upward migration, whereas a high level induces cell detachment from the radial glia and migration arrest (D'Arcangelo 2006). Interestingly, the number of Cajal–Retzius neurons appears increased in some types of CD, suggesting a role in migration abnormalities (Mischel et al. 1995; Garbelli et al. 2001; Thom et al. 2003).

Pyramidal Neurons with Dysmorphic Neurites

Another morphological finding in CD tissue is the presence of normal-sized pyramidal neurons with dysmorphic or dystrophic neurites. These neurons have normal somata, but the apical or basilar dendrites and sometimes the axon display segments that are tortuous (Figure 11.1). Many cells with dysmorphic dendrites also show misorientation. Dystrophic neurites can be seen in many neurological pathologies, including temporal lobe epilepsy (Porter et al. 2003). However, the occurrence of dystrophic neurites appears to be relatively specific to CD (Judkins et al. 2006). The role of dystrophic neurites in epileptogenesis is presently unknown. Our single-cell electrophysiological recordings revealed neither clear differences in basic membrane properties nor clear signs of hyperexcitability compared with normal pyramidal neurons (Cepeda et al. 2003).

What causes dystrophic dendritic and axonal growth? The observation that many misoriented neurons also showed dystrophic neurites suggests common mechanisms.

Pyramidal Cells

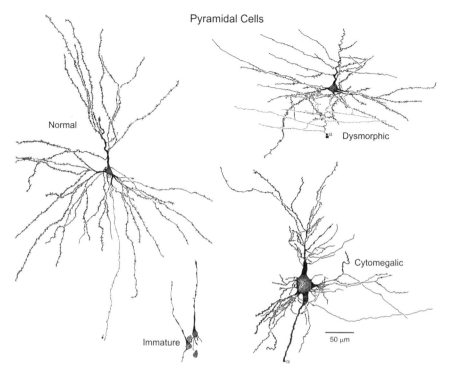

Figure 11.1. Camera lucida drawings of pyramidal neurons recorded electrophysiologically and filled with biocytin. **Top left:** normal pyramidal neuron; **top right:** pyramidal neuron with dysmorphic neurites; **bottom left:** immature pyramidal neuron; **bottom right:** cytomegalic pyramidal neuron.

In fact, some of the mechanisms involved in axonal growth are also implicated in cell migration (Ridley et al. 2003). Intrinsic and extrinsic signals aid pathfinding by neurites. Among the most important signals, calcium (Gomez and Zhen 2006), the surface receptor Notch1 (Šestan et al. 1999; Redmond et al. 2000), semaphorins (Polleux et al. 1998), netrins (Round and Stein 2007), and integrins (Clegg et al. 2003) are intimately involved in this process. For example, the growth of apical dendrites toward the pial surface is regulated by chemoattractant molecules located in the marginal zone and semaphorin 3A, a chemorepellant for cortical axons, is also a chemoattractant for apical dendrites (Polleux et al. 2000). Alterations in radial glia and adhesive surface molecules may also contribute to abnormal neurite pathfinding.

Balloon Cells

These cells are some of the most bizarre and unusual cells present in severe CD tissue and, from an electrophysiological perspective regarding epileptogenesis, they are a paradox. Balloon cells are found in severe CD tissue from approximately

40% of pediatric surgery cases and are also very abundant in children with TSC. Morphologically, they are reminiscent of fibrillary astrocytes (Figure 11.2). They lack dendritic spines and an axon is not visible. They usually display very abundant, tortuous processes that extend for several hundred microns and become progressively thinner with greater distances. Immunocytochemical studies revealed that balloon cells may display neuronal and glial markers alone or in combination (Farrell et al. 1992; Mathern et al. 2000). This suggests that balloon cells do not commit to a neuronal or glial phenotype and remain undifferentiated.

For some time it was believed that balloon cells could be the culprits of epileptogenicity in CD. However, our electrophysiological recordings demonstrated that these cells are unable to generate sodium- or calcium-inward currents and do not depolarize when excitatory amino acids are applied (Cepeda et al. 2003, 2005a). In more recent studies balloon cells were found not to be completely inert, as they produced minor membrane oscillations in the presence of the K^+ channel blocker 4-aminopyridine, similar to those generated by glial cells. The role of balloon cells in the generation of epileptic activity in severe CD is still an open question, but based on the fact that these cells are unable to generate action potentials, their role in epileptogenesis is probably only minor.

The origin of balloon cells in severe CD and in TSC is still an enigma. However, understanding their origin can provide important clues about timing of the cortical lesion that produces CD. From the outset these cells have been difficult

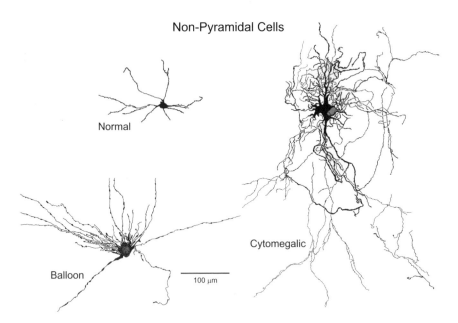

Figure 11.2. Camera lucida drawings of non-pyramidal cells. **Top left:** normal interneuron; **top right:** cytomegalic interneuron; and **bottom:** balloon cell.

to classify due to their similarities to both neurons and glia. Although they may express neuronal markers, the absence of an axon casts doubts about their neuronal phenotype. The first clues about the origin of these atypical cells came from anatomical studies suggesting they were undifferentiated cells (Probst and Ohnacker 1977; Huttenlocher and Heydemann 1984) that, in a sense, mimicked features of neuroembryonic development (Trombley and Mirra 1981). Stronger evidence came from immunocytochemical and molecular biological studies demonstrating that balloon cells express both neuronal and glial markers (Farrell et al. 1992; Mathern et al. 2000; Englund et al. 2005), as well as a wide variety of embryological markers characteristic of undifferentiated progenitors (Fukutani et al. 1992; Hirose et al. 1995; Crino et al. 1996, 1997; Thom et al. 2005, 2007; Ying et al. 2005). More specifically, we and others have proposed that balloon cells may be remnants of radial glial progenitor cells (Cepeda et al. 2006; Lamparello et al. 2007) and/or from the minority of embryonic progenitors that co-express neuronal and glial markers described by Zecevic et al. (2004). Why balloon cells do not differentiate remains unknown. However, a recent study found that many balloon cells fail to complete the cell cycle, suggesting that cell arrest occurs at an early point of the G_1 phase (Thom et al. 2007).

Cytomegalic Pyramidal Neurons

The presence of cytomegalic pyramidal neurons is another hallmark of severe CD and occurs in approximately 60% of pediatric CD cases. These cells are 2–3 times larger than normal pyramidal neurons and also display very thick processes including the axon hillock (Fig. 11.1). Spines are present and can be abundant in some dendritic segments, whereas in others they are scarce. Cytomegalic pyramidal neurons have abnormal membrane properties. Due to their large size, the membrane capacitance and time constants are significantly larger compared to normal pyramidal neurons. In contrast, their input resistance is very low. The resting membrane potential of cytomegalic pyramidal neurons is relatively hyperpolarized (Cepeda et al. 2005a). One of the most distinct features of cytomegalic pyramidal neurons is their capacity to generate repetitive calcium oscillations once depolarized, suggesting upregulation of calcium channels (Cepeda et al. 2003). Cytomegalic pyramidal neurons also display reduced Mg^{2+} sensitivity (André et al. 2004). This implies that N-methyl-D-aspartate (NMDA) receptors can be activated at more hyperpolarized membrane potentials, which can also lead to cellular hyperexcitability.

Cytomegalic GABAergic Interneurons

In some severe CD cases, particularly in children with hemimegalencephaly, we recently described another type of abnormal neuron, the cytomegalic interneuron (André et al. 2007). Cytomegalic interneurons are found in the areas of greatest

CD abnormality, and in close proximity to cytomegalic pyramidal neurons. Cyto-megalic interneurons are 2–3 times larger than normal interneurons and can be labeled with GABAergic markers such as GAD, calbindin, and parvalbumin. They are generally basket-like cells and display increased numbers of dendrites (Fig. 11.2). These cells display signs of cellular hyperexcitability such as non-inactivating sodium spikes when a depolarizing ramp voltage command is applied. An important feature of a subpopulation of cytomegalic interneurons is that these are the only cells in which we have observed spontaneous paroxysmal depolarizing shifts in the in vitro slice preparation. It is thus likely that cytome-galic interneurons play an important role in the generation of epileptic activity in those CD patients who display these cells.

The origin of cytomegalic pyramidal neurons and interneurons is another riveting question in the CD puzzle. One possibility is that these cells are a normal constitu-ent of cortical development but do not undergo programmed cell death, a normal process common in mid- and late-gestational periods (Rakic and Zecevic 2000). The fact that cytomegalic neurons resemble cells previously described in the human subplate (Mrzljiak et al. 1988) supports this hypothesis (Cepeda et al. 2003, 2006; Andres et al. 2005). Alterations in the mTOR pathway, which controls cell growth, could also explain the presence of cytomegalic neurons. For example, using micro-array analysis of gene expression and immunohistochemistry, it has been shown that some proteins in this pathway such as the ribosomal protein S6, eIF4G, and Akt are hyperphosphorylated in cytomegalic neurons from human CD tissue (Ljungberg et al. 2006). If this is correct, these findings open avenues for novel treatments by targeting the mTOR pathway (Franz et al. 2006; Rüegg et al. 2007).

The presence of cytomegalic interneurons in severe CD cases is particularly intriguing. These cells are unique in that they can generate spontaneous depolar-izing shifts, making them suitable as generators of synchronous activity. It is interesting that, in cell cultures from the embryonic cerebral rat cortex, a distinct subpopulation of large GABAergic neurons, which constitute only a small minor-ity, are a key element in the generation of synchronous oscillatory network activity (Voigt et al. 2001). In addition, these basket-like neurons are derived from the primordial plexiform layer and reside in the subplate at the time of birth, placing them in an ideal position to distribute activity in the local networks (Voigt et al. 2001). Finally, in the case of cytomegalic interneurons observed in severe CD, another possibility is that a subset of normal interneurons became hyperplastic due to the epileptic activity and to keep in check the hyperexcitability of cytome-galic pyramidal neurons. However, this does not explain why in cases of mild CD that also sustain epileptic activity cytomegalic neurons are not observed.

Immature Pyramidal Neurons

Immature-looking pyramidal neurons can be observed in mild and severe CD tissue from patients generally younger than 2 years of age. They tend to occur in clusters, similar to the clones occurring during early neuroblast migration (Fig. 11.1). Their morphological and electrophysiological properties are typical of immature pyramidal neurons, i.e., incipient dendrites and spines, very high membrane input resistance, low capacitance, fast time constants, and small inward currents. Although rigorously speaking these cells are not abnormal, their presence in postnatal tissue was unexpected, as we have not observed similar cells in patients with non-CD pathologies. What could be the significance of islands of immature pyramidal neurons surrounded by otherwise normal-appearing, mature neurons? Are these immature neurons still in the process of migration and differentiation? Are they the product of late proliferation? These remain open questions.

SYNAPTIC CIRCUITS IN PEDIATRIC CD

Spontaneous synaptic activity, mostly due to activation of glutamatergic and GABAergic receptors, is an accurate index of synaptic inputs onto the cell. In our studies we routinely record spontaneous synaptic currents at two holding potentials (−70 and +10 mV) to isolate glutamatergic and GABAergic inputs, respectively. In addition, selective blockers of these receptors allow pharmacological isolation. Using these methods we found that some abnormal cells also display abnormal synaptic activity. Although misoriented pyramidal neurons with dysmorphic neurites do not show obvious changes in spontaneous synaptic activity, balloon cells are unique in that no synaptic activity is observed (Cepeda et al. 2003, 2005a), supporting observations that these cells do not form synapses with neighboring neurons (Lippa et al. 1993; Hirose et al. 1995; Alonso-Nanclares et al. 2005). Cytomegalic pyramidal neurons are very diverse in terms of the nature and abundance of synaptic inputs. Whereas some cells display abundant synaptic activity, others display very little activity. Further, in some cytomegalic neurons the main inputs are GABAergic. In the case of immature neurons the most remarkable feature is the presence of abundant, rhythmic spontaneous GABAergic synaptic activity (Cepeda et al. 2003, 2006). In current clamp recordings GABAergic synaptic events are depolarizing and may induce action potentials that can be blocked with bicuculline, a $GABA_A$ receptor antagonist, suggesting that some local circuits in CD are immature (Cepeda et al. 2007) and supporting the belief that GABA can be excitatory in early development (Cherubini et al. 1991).

These observations led us to ask what types of inputs are present in normal-appearing pyramidal neurons in CD tissue. Recordings of spontaneous synaptic activity in these neurons indicated that in CD tissue GABAergic activity is not reduced compared to relatively normal tissue, even in the most abnormal areas. In fact, in severe CD it is the glutamatergic activity that is reduced (Cepeda et al. 2005b). Paradoxically, immunohistological studies using calcium-binding proteins, an indirect marker of inhibitory cells, have consistently found that the number of GABAergic interneurons is decreased in CD tissue. How can this be reconciled with the observation of relatively high spontaneous synaptic activity in pediatric CD tissue? One possibility is that compensatory changes and/or synaptic reorganization from the remaining GABA interneurons occur. In human temporal lobe epilepsy, calbindin-positive cells in the hilus become hypertrophic to compensate for the loss of interneurons (Magloczky et al. 2000). Similarly, in focal CD and microdysgenesis hypertrophic calbindin- and pavalbumin-positive neurons have been reported (Ferrer et al. 1992; Thom et al. 2003). The demonstration of extensive GABA synaptic reorganization in CD—for example, the hypertrophic parvalbumin-positive basket formations surrounding cytomegalic pyramidal neurons (Ferrer et al. 1992; Spreafico et al. 1998; Garbelli et al. 1999; Alonso-Nanclares et al. 2005)—reinforces the idea of compensatory mechanisms in CD. Another possibility is that, in severe CD cases, cytomegalic interneurons provide rich innervation onto cytomegalic, normal, and immature pyramidal neurons.

What Makes CD Tissue Epileptogenic?

Hypotheses attempting to explain the intrinsic epileptogenicity of CD tissue range from those proposing that abnormal neurons can generate epileptic activity (Kerfoot et al. 1999; Schwartzkroin and Walsh 2000) to those suggesting a more prominent involvement of aberrant circuits, including abnormal NMDA receptor function (Ying et al. 1999; André et al. 2004) or reduced $GABA_A$ receptor-mediated synaptic activity (Spreafico et al. 1998; Calcagnotto et al. 2005). A combination of those factors is a more parsimonious explanation. Among the diverse classes of abnormal cells described above, we believe that cytomegalic and immature neurons have membrane properties that could contribute to the mechanisms involved in epileptogenesis. In contrast, the balloon cells, which are unable to generate action potentials and lack synaptic connections and axonal processes, are unlikely candidates to play a direct role in epileptogenesis. Cytomegalic interneurons have the potential to generate spontaneous depolarizing shifts, making them good candidates as generators of synchronous activity. If GABAergic basket formations surrounding cytomegalic pyramidal neurons are depolarizing in these neurons, upregulated calcium channels could indeed generate synchronous oscillations. This could serve as an amplifier for the synchronization of cortical networks and the propagation of epileptic activity. Immature pyramidal neurons are also candidate hyperexcitable elements in younger, severe forms of CD. High membrane-input resistances can amplify incoming signals. Immature properties also include depolarizing GABA actions (Cepeda et al. 2007), an observation supported by immunocytochemical studies showing altered expression of chloride transporters NKCC1 and reduced KCC2 in CD tissue (Aronica et al. 2007; Munakata et al. 2007). However, it is important to note that there are many CD patients with intractable epilepsy in which the tissue specimen does not contain cytomegalic neurons. Thus, mechanisms of epileptogenesis are probably multifactorial and understanding how cells interact with each other in CD will require additional studies.

CONCLUSIONS AND IMPLICATIONS

Based on our initial studies, we proposed that CD pathogenesis probably involves partial failure of events occurring during later phases of corticogenesis resulting in incomplete cortical development (Andres et al. 2005; Cepeda et al. 2006). The timing of these events during cortical development would explain the different forms of CD. Developmental alterations during the late second or early third trimester would account for severe CD with numerous dysmorphic and cytomegalic cells (CDII Type A and B), whereas events occurring closer to birth after the subplate has nearly degenerated would explain mild CD (CD Type I). As a consequence, subplate and radial glial degeneration and transformation would be prevented, giving the appearance of abnormal dysmorphic cells in the postnatal human brain. In addition, failure of late cortical maturation could explain the presence of thickened, abnormally placed gyri with indistinct cortical gray–white matter junctions in postnatal CD tissue. However, it is important to acknowledge that these observations do not exclude that elements of severe CD pathogenesis might begin much earlier during neurogenesis and involve the generation of the preplate itself. Such early defects may be of particular importance in large-scale congenital dysplasias associated with severe epileptogenesis such as hemimegalencephaly.

The presence of undifferentiated cells, retained embryonic neurons, and immature pyramidal neurons; the predominance of GABAergic synaptic activity; and the depolarizing actions of GABA, all point to the idea that in CD we are probably dealing with a problem of tissue and cellular dysmaturity (Cepeda et al. 2006). Interestingly, the ECoG in severe CD is characterized by high-amplitude slow waves that resemble the EEG patterns of preterm infants including the "tracé alternant" (Khazipov and Luhmann 2006). Slow EEG transients decrease toward full term in association with an increase in the expression of KCC2 (Vanhatalo et al. 2005). Because GABAergic markers, including the vesicular GABA transporter, have been observed in the subplate of human embryos as early as 11.5 g.w., it has been proposed that GABA receptor–mediated synaptic activity occurs at this stage of brain development (Bayatti et al. 2007) and could play an important role in brain development (Owens and Kriegstein 2002). Thus, many of the observations reported here are congruent with the idea that, in severe CD, the pre- and subplate or some of their elements do not dissolve before birth and retain immature features.

The differences between mild and severe CD in terms of the timing and severity of the cortical lesion indicate that different therapeutic approaches may be necessary to control seizures. For example, if GABA activity is not significantly affected in CD, medications used to upregulate GABA receptor function may not be useful and could be detrimental if GABA is excitatory. Interestingly, in a rodent model of neonatal seizures it was shown recently that whereas Phenobarbital alone fails to abolish seizure activity, when combined with bumetanide, which blocks the NKCC1 transporter, it becomes a very effective seizure suppressor (Dzhala et al. 2007). It is clear that a better understanding of the basic mechanisms of epileptogenesis in pediatric CD will further our therapeutic perspective.

ACKNOWLEDGMENTS

We would like to thank the young patients and their parents for allowing use of resected tissue samples for research purposes. We also thank Drs. Raymond S. Hurst, Jorge Flores-Hernández, Elizabeth Hernández-Echeagaray, Nanping Wu, Marea K. Boylan, as well as a multitude of undergraduate students for their assistance in electrophysiological data collection and cellular morphological analyses. Julia Chang, Snow Nguyen, My Huynh, and others assisted in the anatomical studies. The expertise and dedication of the UCLA Hospital Pediatric Neurology Staff are also greatly appreciated. This work was supported by NIH grant NS 38992 from the NINDS.

REFERENCES

Allendoerfer KL, Shatz CJ (1994) The subplate, a transient neocortical structure: its role in the development of connections between thalamus and cortex. *Annu Rev Neurosci* 17:185–218.

Alonso-Nanclares L, Garbelli R, Sola RG, Pastor J, Tassi L, Spreafico R, DeFelipe J (2005) Microanatomy of the dysplastic neocortex from epileptic patients. *Brain* 128: 158–73.

André VM, Flores-Hernández J, Cepeda C, Starling AJ, Nguyen S, Lobo MK, Vinters HV, Levine MS, Mathern GW (2004) NMDA receptor alterations in neurons from pediatric cortical dysplasia tissue. *Cereb Cortex* 14:634–46.

André VM, Wu N, Yamazaki I, Nguyen ST, Fisher RS, Vinters HV, Mathern GW, Levine MS, Cepeda C (2007) Cytomegalic interneurons: a new abnormal cell type in severe pediatric cortical dysplasia. *J Neuropathol Exp Neurol* 66:491–504.

Andres M, André VM, Nguyen S, Salamon N, Cepeda C, Levine MS, Leite JP, Neder L, Vinters HV, Mathern GW (2005) Human cortical dysplasia and epilepsy: an ontogenetic hypothesis based on volumetric MRI and NeuN neuronal density and size measurements. *Cereb Cortex* 15:194–210.

Aronica E, Boer K, Redeker S, Spliet WG, van Rijen PC, Troost D, Gorter JA (2007) Differential expression patterns of chloride transporters, Na$^+$-K$^+$-2Cl$^-$-cotransporter and K$^+$-Cl$^-$-cotransporter, in epilepsy-associated malformations of cortical development. *Neuroscience* 145:185–96.

Bayatti N, Moss JA, Sun L, Ambrose P, Ward JF, Lindsay S, Clowry GJ (2007) A molecular neuroanatomical study of the developing human neocortex from 8 to 17 postconceptional weeks revealing the early differentiation of the subplate and subventricular zone. *Cereb Cortex* [Epub ahead of print, doi: 10.1093/cercor/bhm184].

Ben-Ari Y (2006) Basic developmental rules and their implications for epilepsy in the immature brain. *Epileptic Disord* 8:91–102.

Bystron I, Blakemore C, Rakic P (2008) Development of the human cerebral cortex: Boulder Committee revisited. *Nat Rev Neurosci* 9:110–22.

Calcagnotto ME, Paredes MF, Tihan T, Barbaro NM, Baraban SC (2005) Dysfunction of synaptic inhibition in epilepsy associated with focal cortical dysplasia. *J Neurosci* 25:9649–57.

Caviness VS Jr (1976) Patterns of cell and fiber distribution in the neocortex of the reeler mutant mouse. *J Comp Neurol* 170:435–47.

Cepeda C, André VM, Flores-Hernández J, Nguyen OK, Wu N, Klapstein GJ, Nguyen S, Koh S, Vinters HV, Levine MS, Mathern GW (2005b) Pediatric cortical dysplasia: correlations between neuroimaging, electrophysiology and location of cytomegalic neurons and balloon cells and glutamate/GABA synaptic circuits. *Dev Neurosci* 27:59–76.

Cepeda C, André VM, Levine MS, Salamon N, Miyata H, Vinters HV, Mathern GW (2006) Epileptogenesis in pediatric cortical dysplasia: the dysmature cerebral developmental hypothesis. *Epilepsy Behav* 9:219–35.

Cepeda C, André VM, Vinters HV, Levine MS, Mathern GW (2005a) Are cytomegalic neurons and balloon cells generators of epileptic activity in pediatric cortical dysplasia? *Epilepsia* 46(Suppl 5):82–8.

Cepeda C, André VM, Wu N, Yamazaki I, Uzgil B, Vinters HV, Levine MS, Mathern GW (2007) Immature neurons and GABA networks may contribute to epileptogenesis in pediatric cortical dysplasia. *Epilepsia* 48(Suppl 5):79–85.

Cepeda C, Hurst RS, Flores-Hernández J, Hernández-Echeagaray E, Klapstein GJ, Boylan MK, Calvert CR, Jocoy EL, Nguyen OK, André VM, Vinters HV, Ariano MA, Levine MS, Mathern GW (2003) Morphological and electrophysiological characterization of abnormal cell types in pediatric cortical dysplasia. *J Neurosci Res* 72:472–86.

Cepeda C, Li Z, Cromwell HC, Altemus KL, Crawford CA, Nansen EA, Ariano MA, Sibley DR, Peacock WJ, Mathern GW, Levine MS (1999) Electrophysiological and morphological analyses of cortical neurons obtained from children with catastrophic epilepsy: dopamine receptor modulation of glutamatergic responses. *Dev Neurosci* 21:223–35.

Chanas-Sacré G, Rogister B, Moonen G, Leprince P (2000) Radial glia phenotype: origin, regulation, and transdifferentiation. *J Neurosci Res* 61:357–63.

Cherubini E, Gaiarsa JL, Ben-Ari Y (1991) GABA: an excitatory transmitter in early postnatal life. *Trends Neurosci* 14:515–9.

Clegg DO, Wingerd KL, Hikita ST, Tolhurst EC (2003) Integrins in the development, function and dysfunction of the nervous system. *Front Biosci* 8:d723–50.

Crino PB, Trojanowski JQ, Dichter MA, Eberwine J (1996) Embryonic neuronal markers in tuberous sclerosis: single-cell molecular pathology. *Proc Natl Acad Sci USA* 93:14152–7.

Crino PB, Trojanowski JQ, Eberwine J (1997) Internexin, MAP1B, and nestin in cortical dysplasia as markers of developmental maturity. *Acta Neuropathol* 93:619–27.

D'Arcangelo G (2006) Reelin mouse mutants as models of cortical development disorders. *Epilepsy Behav* 8:81–90.

D'Arcangelo G, Miao GG, Chen SC, Soares HD, Morgan JI, Curran T (1995) A protein related to extracellular matrix proteins deleted in the mouse mutant reeler. *Nature* 374:719–23.

De Castro F, López-Mascaraque L, De Carlos JA (2007) Cajal: lessons on brain development. *Brain Res Rev* 55:481–9.

Dodt HU, Zieglgänsberger W (1994) Infrared videomicroscopy: a new look at neuronal structure and function. *Trends Neurosci* 17:453–8.

Dudek FE, Wuarin JP, Tasker JG, Kim YI, Peacock WJ (1995) Neurophysiology of neocortical slices resected from children undergoing surgical treatment for epilepsy. *J Neurosci Methods* 59:49–58.

Dzhala VI, Brumback AC, Staley KJ (2007) Bumetanide enhances phenobarbital efficacy in a neonatal seizure model. *Ann Neurol.* [Epub ahead of print].

Englund C, Folkerth RD, Born D, Lacy JM, Hevner RF (2005) Aberrant neuronal-glial differentiation in Taylor-type focal cortical dysplasia (type IIA/B). *Acta Neuropathol* 109:519–33.

Farrell MA, DeRosa MJ, Curran JG, Secor DL, Cornford ME, Comair YG, Peacock WJ, Shields WD, Vinters HV (1992) Neuropathologic findings in cortical resections (including hemispherectomies) performed for the treatment of intractable childhood epilepsy. *Acta Neuropathol* 83:246–59.

Ferrer I, Pineda M, Tallada M, Oliver B, Russi A, Oller L, Noboa R, Zujar MJ, Alcantara S (1992) Abnormal local-circuit neurons in epilepsia partialis continua associated with focal cortical dysplasia. *Acta Neuropathol* (Berl) 83:647–52.

Franz DN, Leonard J, Tudor C, Chuck G, Care M, Sethuraman G, Dinopoulos A, Thomas G, Crone KR (2006) Rapamycin causes regression of astrocytomas in tuberous sclerosis complex. *Ann Neurol* 59:490–8.

Friauf E, McConnell SK, Shatz CJ (1990) Functional synaptic circuits in the subplate during fetal and early postnatal development of cat visual cortex. *J Neurosci* 10: 2601–13.

Fukutani Y, Yasuda M, Saitoh C, Kyoya S, Kobayashi K, Miyazu K, Nakamura I (1992) An autopsy case of tuberous sclerosis. Histological and immunohistochemical study. *Histol Histopathol* 7:709–14.

Garbelli R, Frassoni C, Ferrario A, Tassi L, Bramerio M, Spreafico R (2001) Cajal–Retzius cell density as marker of type of focal cortical dysplasia. *NeuroReport* 12: 2767–71.

Garbelli R, Munari C, De Biasi S, Vitellaro-Zuccarello L, Galli C, Bramerio M, Mai R, Battaglia G, Spreafico R (1999) Taylor's cortical dysplasia: a confocal and ultrastructural immunohistochemical study. *Brain Pathol* 9:445–61.

Gleeson JG (2001) Neuronal migration disorders. *Ment Retard Dev Disabil Res Rev* 7:167–71.

Gomez TM, Zheng JQ (2006) The molecular basis for calcium-dependent axon pathfinding. *Nat Rev Neurosci* 7:115–25.

Hanganu IL, Kilb W, Luhmann HJ (2001) Spontaneous synaptic activity of subplate neurons in neonatal rat somatosensory cortex. *Cereb Cortex* 11:400–10.

Hanganu IL, Kilb W, Luhmann HJ (2002) Functional synaptic projections onto subplate neurons in neonatal rat somatosensory cortex. *J Neurosci* 22:7165–76.

Harvey AS, Cross JH, Shinnar S, Mathern GW; the Pediatric Epilepsy Surgery Survey Taskforce (2008) Defining the spectrum of international practice in pediatric epilepsy surgery patients. *Epilepsia* 49:146–55.

Hirose T, Scheithauer BW, Lopes MB, Gerber HA, Altermatt HJ, Hukee MJ, VandenBerg SR, Charlesworth JC (1995) Tuber and subependymal giant cell astrocytoma associated with tuberous sclerosis: an immunohistochemical, ultrastructural, and immunoelectron and microscopic study. *Acta Neuropathol* 90:387–99.

Huttenlocher PR, Heydemann PT (1984) Fine structure of cortical tubers in tuberous sclerosis: a Golgi study. *Ann Neurol* 16:595–602.

Judkins AR, Porter BE, Cook N, Clancy RR, Duhaime AC, Golden JA (2006) Dystrophic neuritic processes in epileptic cortex. *Epilepsy Res* 70:49–58.

Kerfoot C, Vinters HV, Mathern GW (1999) Cerebral cortical dysplasia: giant neurons show potential for increased excitation and axonal plasticity. *Dev Neurosci* 21: 260–70.

Khazipov R, Luhmann HJ (2006) Early patterns of electrical activity in the developing cerebral cortex of humans and rodents. *Trends Neurosci* 29:414–8.

Kostovic I, Rakic P (1990) Developmental history of the transient subplate zone in the visual and somatosensory cortex of the macaque monkey and human brain. *J Comp Neurol* 297:441–70.

Kriegstein AR (2005) Constructing circuits: neurogenesis and migration in the developing neocortex. *Epilepsia* 46(Suppl 7):15–21.

Lamparello P, Baybis M, Pollard J, Hol EM, Eisenstat DD, Aronica E, Crino PB (2007) Developmental lineage of cell types in cortical dysplasia with balloon cells. *Brain* 130:2267–76.

Lippa CF, Pearson D, Smith TW (1993) Cortical tubers demonstrate reduced immunoreactivity for synapsin I. *Acta Neuropathol* 85:449–51.

Ljungberg MC, Bhattacharjee MB, Lu Y, Armstrong DL, Yoshor D, Swann JW, Sheldon M, D'Arcangelo G (2006) Activation of mammalian target of rapamycin in cytomegalic neurons of human cortical dysplasia. *Ann Neurol* 60:420–9.

Luhmann HJ, Reiprich RA, Hanganu I, Kilb W (2000) Cellular physiology of the neonatal rat cerebral cortex: intrinsic membrane properties, sodium and calcium currents. *J Neurosci Res* 62:574–84.

Magloczky Z, Wittner L, Borhegyi Z, Halasz P, Vajda J, Czirjak S, Freund TF (2000) Changes in the distribution and connectivity of interneurons in the epileptic human dentate gyrus. *Neuroscience* 96:7–25.

Malatesta P, Hartfuss E, Götz M (2000) Isolation of radial glial cells by fluorescent-activated cell sorting reveals a neuronal lineage. *Development* 127:5253–63.

Mathern GW, Cepeda C, Hurst RS, Flores-Hernandez J, Mendoza D, Levine MS (2000) Neurons recorded from pediatric epilepsy surgery patients with cortical dysplasia. *Epilepsia* 41(Suppl. 6):S162–7.

Mathern GW, Giza CC, Yudovin S, Vinters HV, Peacock WJ, Shewmon DA, Shields WD (1999) Postoperative seizure control and antiepileptic drug use in pediatric epilepsy surgery patients: the UCLA experience, 1986–1997. *Epilepsia* 40:1740–9.

Mattia D, Olivier A, Avoli M (1995) Seizure-like discharges recorded in human dysplastic neocortex maintained in vitro. *Neurology* 45:1391–5.

Meyer G, Goffinet AM (1998) Prenatal development of reelin-immunoreactive neurons in the human neocortex. *J Comp Neurol* 397:29–40.

Mischel PS, Nguyen LP, Vinters HV (1995) Cerebral cortical dysplasia associated with pediatric epilepsy. Review of neuropathologic features and proposal for a grading system. *J Neuropathol Exp Neurol* 54:137–53.

Mrzljak L, Uylings HB, Kostovic I, Van Eden CG (1988) Prenatal development of neurons in the human prefrontal cortex: I. A qualitative Golgi study. *J Comp Neurol* 271:355–86.

Munakata M, Watanabe M, Otsuki T, Nakama H, Arima K, Itoh M, Nabekura J, Iinuma K, Tsuchiya S (2007) Altered distribution of KCC2 in cortical dysplasia in patients with intractable epilepsy. *Epilepsia* 48:837–44.

Noctor SC, Flint AC, Weissman TA, Wong WS, Clinton BK, Kriegstein AR (2002) Dividing precursor cells of the embryonic cortical ventricular zone have morphological and molecular characteristics of radial glia. *J Neurosci* 22:3161–73.

Noctor SC, Martínez-Cerdeño V, Kriegstein AR (2007) Contribution of intermediate progenitor cells to cortical histogenesis. *Arch Neurol* 64:639–42.

Owens DF, Kriegstein AR (2002) Is there more to GABA than synaptic inhibition? *Nat Rev Neurosci.* 3:715–27.

Palmini A, Najm I, Avanzini G, Babb T, Guerrini R, Foldvary-Schaefer N, Jackson G, Lüders HO, Prayson R, Spreafico R, Vinters HV (2004) Terminology and classification of the cortical dysplasias. *Neurology* 62(6 Suppl 3):S2–8.

Patrylo PR, Browning RA, Cranick S (2006) Reeler homozygous mice exhibit enhanced susceptibility to epileptiform activity. *Epilepsia* 47:257–66.

Polleux F, Giger RJ, Ginty DD, Kolodkin AL, Ghosh A (1998) Patterning of cortical efferent projections by semaphorin-neuropilin interactions. *Science* 282:1904–6.

Polleux F, Morrow T, Ghosh A (2000) Semaphorin 3A is a chemoattractant for cortical apical dendrites. *Nature* 404:567–73.

Porter BE, Judkins AR, Clancy RR, Duhaime A, Dlugos DJ, Golden JA (2003) Dysplasia: a common finding in intractable pediatric temporal lobe epilepsy. *Neurology* 61:365–8.

Probst A, Ohnacker H (1977) Sclérose tubereuse de Bourneville chez un prématuré. Ultrastructure des cellules atypiques: Présence de microvillosités. *Acta Neuropathol* 40:157–61.

Rakic P (2003) Developmental and evolutionary adaptations of cortical radial glia. *Cereb Cortex* 13:541–9.

Rakic P (2006) A century of progress in corticoneurogenesis: from silver impregnation to genetic engineering. *Cereb Cortex* 16(Suppl 1):i3–17.

Rakic S, Zecevic N (2000) Programmed cell death in the developing human telencephalon. *Eur J Neurosci* 12:2721–34.

Redmond L, Oh SR, Hicks C, Weinmaster G, Ghosh A (2000) Nuclear Notch1 signaling and the regulation of dendritic development. *Nat Neurosci* 3:30–40.

Ridley AJ, Schwartz MA, Burridge K, Firtel RA, Ginsberg MH, Borisy G, Parsons JT, Horwitz AR (2003) Cell migration: integrating signals from front to back. *Science* 302:1704–9.

Round J, Stein E (2007) Netrin signaling leading to directed growth cone steering. *Curr Opin Neurobiol* 17:15–21.

Rüegg S, Baybis M, Juul H, Dichter M, Crino PB (2007) Effects of rapamycin on gene expression, morphology, and electrophysiological properties of rat hippocampal neurons. *Epilepsy Res* 77:85–92.

Schwartzkroin PA, Walsh CA (2000) Cortical malformations and epilepsy. *Ment Retard Dev Disabil Res Rev* 6:268–80.

Šestan N, Artavanis-Tsakonas S, Rakic P (1999) Contact-dependent inhibition of cortical neurite growth mediated by notch signaling. *Science* 286:741–6.

Spreafico R, Battaglia G, Arcelli P, Andermann F, Dubeau F, Palmini A, Olivier A, Villemure JG, Tampieri D, Avanzini G, Avoli M (1998) Cortical dysplasia: an immunocytochemical study of three patients. *Neurology* 50:27–36.

Taylor DC, Falconer MA, Bruton CJ, Corsellis JA (1971) Focal dysplasia of the cerebral cortex in epilepsy. *J Neurol Neurosurg Psychiatry* 34:369–87.

Thom M, Harding BN, Lin WR, Martinian L, Cross H, Sisodiya SM (2003) Cajal–Retzius cells, inhibitory interneuronal populations and neuropeptide Y expression in focal cortical dysplasia and microdysgenesis. *Acta Neuropathol* 105:561–9.

Thom M, Martinian L, Sen A, Squier W, Harding BN, Cross JH, Harkness W, McEvoy A, Sisodiya SM (2007) An investigation of the expression of G1-phase cell cycle proteins in focal cortical dysplasia type IIB. *J Neuropathol Exp Neurol* 66:1045–55.

Thom M, Martinian L, Sisodiya SM, Cross JH, Williams G, Stoeber K, Harkness W, Harding BN (2005) Mcm2 labelling of balloon cells in focal cortical dysplasia. *Neuropathol Appl Neurobiol* 31:580–8.

Trombley IK, Mirra SS (1981) Ultrastructure of tuberous sclerosis: cortical tuber and subependymal tumor. *Ann Neurol* 9:174–81.

Vanhatalo S, Palva JM, Andersson S, Rivera C, Voipio J, Kaila K (2005) Slow endogenous activity transients and developmental expression of K⁺-Cl⁻ cotransporter 2 in the immature human cortex. *Eur J Neurosci* 22:2799–804.

Voigt T, Opitz T, de Lima AD (2001) Synchronous oscillatory activity in immature cortical network is driven by GABAergic preplate neurons. *J Neurosci* 21:8895–905.

Volpe JJ (2000) Overview: normal and abnormal human brain development. *Ment Retard Dev Disabil Res Rev* 6:1–5.

Ying Z, Babb TL, Mikuni N, Najm I, Drazba J, Bingaman W (1999) Selective coexpression of NMDAR2A/B and NMDAR1 subunit proteins in dysplastic neurons of human epileptic cortex. *Exp Neurol* 159:409–18.

Ying Z, Gonzalez-Martinez J, Tilelli C, Bingaman W, Najm I (2005) Expression of neural stem cell surface marker CD133 in balloon cells of human focal cortical dysplasia. *Epilepsia* 46:1716–23.

Zecevic N (2004) Specific characteristic of radial glia in the human fetal telencephalon. *Glia* 48:27–35.

Part 4

Neural Plasticity and Regeneration

Chapter Twelve

Developmental Profile of Newly Generated Granule Cells in the Adult Rodent Dentate Gyrus

Charles E. Ribak, Zachary D. Perez, and Lee A. Shapiro

INTRODUCTION

The phenomenon of neurogenesis in the adult hippocampus has recently received a great deal of public attention. This is because of the therapeutic potential that newborn neurons and their progenitor cells have in the adult brain. However, long before the "modern" popularity of this concept, there was earlier evidence in the 1960s for neurogenesis in the adult rat brain using autoradiography for tritiated thymidine (Altman and Das 1965). The pioneering work of Altman and Das was not expanded on until about a decade later, when Kaplan and Hinds (1977) used higher resolution methods to provide more compelling evidence of the neurogenic potential of the rodent dentate gyrus. Later studies from Gage and colleagues (Kempermann et al. 1997; van Praag et al. 1999) demonstrated a greater magnitude of adult hippocampal neurogenesis than previously observed in these earlier studies, and this work subsequently paved the way for the burgeoning field of adult neurogenesis in twenty-first century neuroscience. In addition, this phenomenon has now encompassed several brain regions in the adult mammalian brain, including the olfactory bulb, striatum, and piriform cortex (Lois and Alvarez-Buylla 1994; De Marchis et al. 2004; Dayer et al. 2005; Shapiro et al. 2007a). Although there is evidence for neurogenesis throughout several regions of the adult rodent brain, this chapter will focus specifically on the newly generated dentate granule cells in the adult rodent and will describe the developmental profile of their dendrites and axons.

PROGENITOR CELL TYPES IN THE ADULT DENTATE GYRUS

There are several types of progenitor cells found in the adult dentate gyrus, and it remains unknown whether these same progenitors are present in the developing brain. The progenitor cells of the adult dentate gyrus are primarily found within the subgranular zone. However, a subset of doublecortin (DCX) expressing cells found at the base of, or within, the granule cell layer, have also been shown to display a proliferative capacity. Although the nomenclature for these cells is not completely agreed on, these progenitor cells have been identified by double-labeling for bromodeoxyuridine (BrdU) combined with several different markers, such as DCX, ß-III-tubulin, GFAP, nestin, TUC-4, and Prox-1 (Parent et al. 1997; Filippov 2003; Seri et al. 2004). In addition, molecular methods incorporating fluorescent labeling using viral or retroviral vectors have been used to identify progenitor cells in the adult dentate gyrus (van Praag et al. 2002; Zhao 2007).

One of the most prominent types of dentate gyrus progenitor cells is the radial glial-like cell that has the following features: short tangential or horizontal processes extending within the subgranular zone of the dentate gyrus, a radial process that extends through the granule cell layer, and intermediate filaments rich in glial fibrillary acidic protein (GFAP) (Alvarez-Buylla et al. 2002; Kempermann et al. 2004; Seri et al. 2004; Shapiro et al. 2005). This progenitor cell type is referred to as type 1 by Kempermann et al. (2004) and as a radial astrocyte by Seri et al. (2004). It also should be noted that this cell has a vascular end-foot that contacts blood vessels in the subgranular zone (Filippov et al. 2003), and this neurogenesis in the hippocampus is said to occur within an angiogenic niche (Palmer et al. 2000). This cell type does not express another astrocyte marker, S100B, but it does express the radial glial marker brain lipid-binding protein (BLBP) and a stem cell protein, Sox2 (Steiner et al. 2006). Together, these light and electron microscopic features have provided a clear-cut identification for this radial glial-like progenitor cell type.

A second progenitor cell type in the dentate gyrus consists of two subtypes, type 2a and type 2b, distinguished from type 1 cells by their immunoreactivity for DCX and PSA-NCAM, two proteins expressed by immature neurons (Horesh et al. 1999; Seki and Arai 1993). Both type 2 subtypes express BLBP and nestin. Type 2a is considered to be less mature than type 2b because the latter subtype expresses NeuroD and Prox1 (Kempermann et al. 2004). Both of these subtypes have round or ovoid-shaped nuclei and the somata of these cells are smaller than those of the type 1 cells. In contrast to type 1 radial glial-like progenitor cells, the type 2 progenitor cells lack the long radial processes of radial glial cells, and instead have short cytoplasmic extensions oriented tangentially to the granule cell layer (Filippov et al. 2003). It appears that the type 2 cells proliferate following exercise in rodents (Kempermann et al. 2003), and possibly in response to other nonspecific stimuli, such as seizures (Ehninger and Kempermann 2008).

The third dentate gyrus progenitor cell type is the type 3 cells, and they are considered the final stage of transiently amplifying progenitor cells. These cells are similar to the type 2 cells in that they also display labeling for nestin and DCX. They are also similar in that glial markers are not expressed by these cells, whereas neuronal lineage markers are invariably seen (Ehninger and Kempermann 2008). This indicates that type 2 and type 3 cells have become committed solely to neuronal development. Although the type 3 cells are less proliferative than type 2 cells and have round nuclei, their similar features have led to the hypothesis that type 2 and type 3 cells may actually represent a continuum of progenitor cell development during adult hippocampal neurogenesis (Kempermann et al. 2004).

DENDRITIC GROWTH OF NEWLY GENERATED GRANULE CELLS IN ADULT RATS

The newly generated granule cells in adult rats that will be described were either labeled with DCX, BrdU, PSA-NCAM, or a retrovirus. The DCX- and PSA-NCAM-labeled cells are often observed adjacent to the type 1 progenitor cell or radial glial cell in the normal animal (Seki and Arai 1999; Shapiro et al. 2005). This close relationship between the cell body and proximal apical dendrite of newly generated granule cells and type 1 progenitor cells suggests that the DCX-labeled cell is derived from the type 1 cell. In the following paragraphs, data will be provided that show the importance of this relationship for dendritic outgrowth from newborn neurons in the adult brain. It should be noted that the dendrites of these newly generated granule cells face a difficult challenge. They must grow through the granule cell layer, where somata of mature granule cells are closely apposed, resulting in a situation in which little room is available for a young neuron to squeeze its process through. Furthermore, once this growing dendrite enters the molecular layer of the dentate gyrus, it encounters a more elaborate, mature, and denser neuropil in the adult brain than that found in the developing brain. Thus, a newborn neuron in the adult brain faces unique challenges for it to successfully establish its dendritic arborization and connections as compared to those in the developing brain.

Light and electron microscopy of DCX-labeled cells have provided evidence to support working hypotheses that address dendritic outgrowth for newborn granule cells. Shapiro et al. (2005) showed that cell bodies of DCX-labeled newly generated cells in the subgranular zone are mostly enveloped by the nonradial processes of radial glial cells (Figure 12.1). These processes form a cradle around

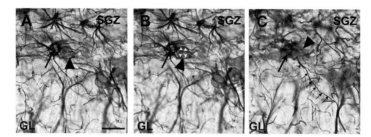

Figure 12.1. Light photomicrographs of double-labeled preparations showing DCX-positive cells (brown) and GFAP-positive astrocytes (purple) in the subgranular zone (SGZ). A–C show a through-focus series of a DCX-labeled cell (black arrowheads) that has a rudimentary process. A GFAP-immunolabeled astrocyte (large black arrows) is adjacent to this cell, and its fine GFAP-immunolabeled bundles (white arrowheads in **B**) wrap around the DCX-labeled cell. Note that this astrocyte has a radial process (small black arrows) extending through the GL in panel **C**. Another GFAP-positive radial process (white arrows in **B**) is adjacent to an apical dendrite of a DCX-labeled cell in the granule cell layer (GL). Scale bar = 10μm. Reprinted with permission from Shapiro et al. (2005). (See color Figure 12.1)

the cell body (Figure 12.2), as observed from serial section analysis of this pair (Shapiro et al. 2005). Plumpe et al. (2006) described a similar cradling of DCX-labeled cell bodies by GFAP-positive processes and indicated that most of the cradling astrocytes had a radial glial cell morphology, confirming the earlier report by Shapiro et al. (2005). When DCX-labeled cell bodies first show a labeled process, this process is observed to emanate from the pole of their cell body that is opposite the pole apposed to the cell body of the radial glial cell (Shapiro et al. 2005).

Electron microscopy confirmed this relationship (Figure 12.2B) and showed that the growing dendrite of DCX-labeled cells that are found at the base of the granule cell layer is apposed to the radial process of a radial glial cell (Shapiro et al. 2005). These growing dendrites have many mitochondria in their tips (Fig. 12.3), a characteristic previously described for growth cones (Sotelo and Palay 1968). To summarize at this point, the dendrites of newly generated granule cells arise from the cell body that is cradled by nonradial processes of radial glial cells, and then these dendrites grow along the radial processes of the radial glial cells. The appearance of many DCX-labeled dendrites apposed to the radial processes of radial glial cells in the granule cell layer confirm this relationship (Shapiro et al. 2005). Seki and Arai (1999) and Seki et al. (2007), using another marker for immature neurons, PSA-NCAM, showed a similar close relationship between the growing apical dendrite of newborn granule cells and the radial processes of radial glial cells in the granule cell layer. These observations are consistent with the hypothesis that the apical dendrite of newly generated granule cells is guided through the densely packed granule cell layer by growing along radial glial processes (Figure 12.4).

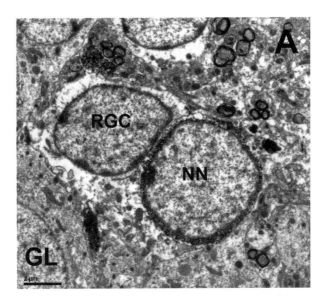

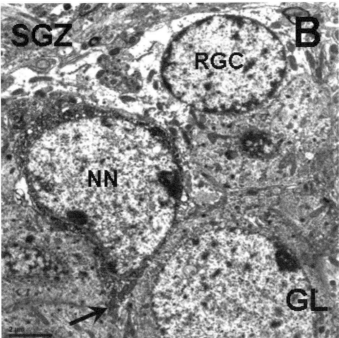

Figure 12.2. Electron micrographs of DCX-positive cells (NN) and astrocyte cell bodies (RGC) at the base of the granule cell layer (GL). **A** shows the one-to-one astrocyte to DCX-immunolabeled NN relationship with the astrocyte's processes cradling the NN. Bundles of glial filaments in both its cell body and processes identified the glial cell as an astrocyte. **B** shows a DCX-immunolabeled cell (NN) with a labeled apical process (large arrow) extending into the GL and an adjacent glial cell (RGC) with a watery cytoplasm. Note that the astrocyte is apposed to the basal surface of the DCX-labeled cell. Scale bars = 2μm. Reprinted with permission from Shapiro et al. (2005).

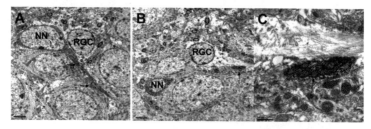

Figure 12.3. Electron micrographs of DCX-positive cells with apical processes and growth cones juxtaposed to astrocyte cell bodies and their radial processes in the granule cell layer. In **A**, the DCX-positive cell (NN) extends an apical process (arrows) that is apposed to a radial astrocyte (RGC). **B** shows another DCX-positive cell (NN) with an associated growth cone (arrow) apposed to the radial process of an astrocyte (RGC). **C** is an enlargement of the process indicated by a black arrow in **B** to demonstrate the presence of glial filaments within the radial process of the astrocyte and the many mitochondria (arrow) within the dendritic growth cone. Scale bars = 2μm in **A** and **B**, and 0.5μm in **C**. Reprinted with permission from Shapiro et al. (2005).

As stated above, once the growing dendrites from newly generated granule cells in the adult brain enter the molecular layer of the dentate gyrus, they encounter a mature and dense neuropil that provides another challenge for the growing dendrite. Electron microscopy of DCX-labeled dendrites in the molecular layer showed that they were smooth and lacked spines (Figure 12.5). In contrast, mature apical dendrites that were not labeled for DCX displayed spines with synapses (Shapiro et al. 2007b). The DCX-labeled dendrites were thinner in diameter than the unlabeled apical dendrites arising from mature granule cells (Fig. 12.5). The mean diameter of DCX-labeled dendrites was about 0.25μm whereas that for unlabeled apical dendrites found adjacent to DCX-labeled dendrites or nearby was approximately 1μm (Shapiro et al. 2007b). This latter finding is consistent with previous data on mature dendrites (Desmond and Levy 1984). In addition, the DCX-labeled dendrites branched in the molecular layer, and the branches of these dendrites, maintained about the same diameter as the main trunk from which they branched (Fig. 12.5). Based on the consistent finding of thin DCX-labeled dendrites in the molecular layer, it is hypothesized that thin dendrites can grow more efficiently through an established brain region's neuropil than a thicker one. The fact that the DCX-labeled dendrites and their branches are also thinner than the mature unlabeled dendrites provides a key to understanding how the dendrites of newly generated granule cells may mature. We suggest that these dendrites grow in a similar way as a tree grows, first having a thin trunk and thin branches, and then getting older and growing a thicker trunk and branches. This dendritic growth from newly generated granule cells in the adult contrasts with that in the developing brain, where massive sprouting of dendrites occurs from

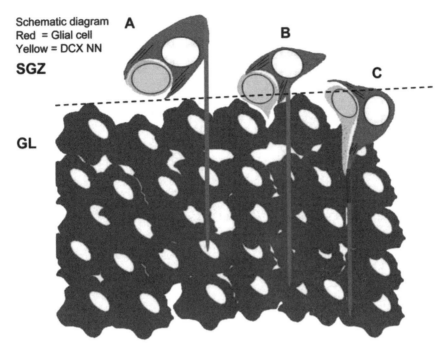

Figure 12.4. A schematic diagram shows the described one-to-one relationship in the adult dentate gyrus between a GFAP-expressing radial glia-like cell (red) and the DCX-labeled newly generated neuron (NN) (yellow). In **A**, an NN in the subgranular zone (SGZ) is cradled by the nonradial processes of a radial astrocyte. Note that the NN lacks processes and the majority of its surface is enveloped by this astrocyte that also sends a radial process through the granule cell layer (GL). In **B**, the NN displays a rudimentary apical process that projects into the GL. Note that the NN is still apposed by some of the nonradial processes of the GFAP-expressing radial glia-like cell. **C** shows a later stage in the development of an NN, where its apical dendrite extends into the GL. Note that this apical dendrite is apposed to the radial process of a radial astrocyte and this radial process provides a scaffold for the apical dendrite to extend. The blue cells represent mature granule cells in the GL. Reprinted with permission from Shapiro et al. (2005). (See color Figure 12.4)

all poles of the cell body of granule cells followed by pruning of this robust dendritic tree (Jones et al. 2003; Seress and Pokorny 1981).

Although most dendrites project into the granule cell layer from the apical portion of the cell, some dendrites may grow parallel or perpendicular to the granule cell layer and appear as basal dendrites (Ribak et al. 2004; Rao and Shetty 2004; Shapiro et al. 2005; Plumpe et al. 2006). In rodents, these basal dendrites appear to be transient in nature, as mature granule cells typically lack this feature (Seress and Pokorny 1981). It is pertinent to note that basal dendrites are not typically observed on most newborn neurons by the time their apical dendrites grow through the granule cell layer (Shapiro et al. 2007b). Because of their transient

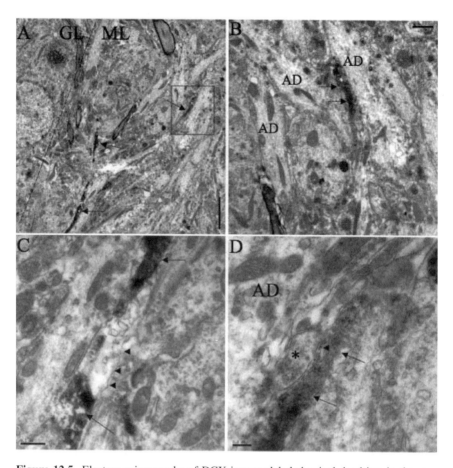

Figure 12.5. Electron micrographs of DCX-immunolabeled apical dendrites in the molecular layer (ML) showing synapses, glial apposition, and thin caliber diameters. **A** shows a low magnification image of a branching apical dendrite (arrows) as it emanates from the granule cell layer (GL). Note one branch lies just above the primary dendrite, whereas the other branch (in the box) is to the right. In **B**, the boxed area from **A** is enlarged to show the relative comparison between the thickness of the DCX-labeled dendrite (arrows) and the adjacent unlabeled apical dendrites (AD) from mature granule cells. Note how much thinner the DCX-labeled dendrite is. **C** is another example of a DCX-labeled dendrite (arrows) in the molecular layer, showing an adjacent astrocytic process (arrowheads) with its watery cytoplasm and vacuoles. In **D**, a small axon terminal (asterisk) with synaptic vesicles clustered at an active zone forms an immature synapse (arrowhead) with another DCX-labeled apical dendrite (arrows) in the molecular layer. An unlabeled apical dendrite (AD) is also shown. Scale bars = 1μm in **A** and **B**, 0.5μm in **C**, and 0.2μm in **D**. Reprinted with permission from Shapiro et al. (2007b).

nature and their appearance during the time when the newborn neuron migrates from the subgranular zone to the granule cell layer, this transient basal dendrite is hypothesized to be involved in migration along the radial glial scaffold.

SPATIOTEMPORAL PROFILE OF DENDRITIC OUTGROWTH

A few groups have described the rate of apical dendritic outgrowth from newly generated granule cells in the adult dentate gyrus, and the data obtained from the two different methods that were used yielded consistent findings (Zhao et al. 2006; Plumpe et al. 2006; Shapiro et al. 2007b). Following a single BrdU injection, Shapiro et al. (2007b) showed a rudimentary process emanating from a BrdU/DCX labeled cell as early as 4 hours after a BrdU injection (Figure 12.6). This rudimentary process could not be definitively classified as a dendrite. However, it should be noted that this process arose from the pole opposite the pole that apposed the BrdU-labeled cell that lacked DCX labeling (Fig. 12.6). Light microscopy of GFAP-positive radial glial-like cell bodies and adjacent DCX-labeled cell bodies showed this same point of origin for primitive dendrites (Shapiro et al. 2005). The data from the 4-hour time point also support the assumption that the DCX-labeled cell bodies with no processes were at the youngest stage of newly generated neurons (Shapiro et al. 2007b). Classically defined dendrites with dendritic growth cones displaying lamellipodia and filopodia were not found for the BrdU/DCX double-labeled cells until 24–48 hours following a single BrdU injection (Fig. 12.6). This finding is consistent with the change in distribution of the six morphological types described by Plumpe et al. (2006) during this same time interval. The labeling of growing dendrites with well-defined growth cones was previously described for DCX-positive cells in the dentate gyrus (Ribak et al. 2004; Rao and Shetty 2004). At later time points following a single BrdU injection (72–96 hr), one or two apical dendrites were observed to traverse the granule cell layer from these BrdU/DCX double-labeled granule cells (Fig. 12.6). This stage of dendritic growth coincides with the appearance of the "E" category of dendritic morphology described by Plumpe et al. (2006) at the 3-day time point for BrdU/DCX double-labeled cells. It should be noted that BrdU/DCX-labeled newly generated granule cells have extended their apical dendrites through the molecular layer by 4–5 days after their birth (Fig. 12.6).

Several differences exist between these two studies. First, Plumpe et al. (2006) describe the distribution of newly generated DCX-labeled cells into six dendritic categories at several time points following BrdU injections. Although they provide pie tables for their distribution at each stage examined, details about dendritic length are lacking. In contrast, Shapiro et al. (2007b) provide daily quantitative data on the mean apical dendritic length of BrdU/DCX-labeled cells. Also, these

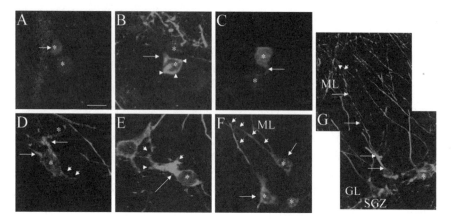

Figure 12.6. Confocal micrographs of BrdU-immunolabeled and DCX/BrdU double-immunolabeled cells at 4–96 hr after a single BrdU injection in adult rat dentate gyrus. In **A**, a pair of BrdU-labeled cells (asterisks) is shown at the 4 hr time point at the base of the granule cell layer. Note that the double-labeled cell (arrow) has a rudimentary DCX-labeled apical process. In **B**, another pair of BrdU-labeled cells (asterisks) at the base of the granule cell layer is shown at12 hr after BrdU injection. Note the thin shell of DCX-labeled perikaryal cytoplasm (arrowheads) and a rudimentary DCX-labeled apical process (arrow). In **C** and **D**, pairs of BrdU-labeled cells are shown (asterisks) from the 24 hr time point. In each case, one of the BrdU-labeled cells is double-labeled for DCX (arrow), whereas the other cell is not. In **C**, the double-labeled cell has a basal dendrite, but no apical dendrite is observed. In **D**, the double-labeled cell has two apical dendrites extending into the granule cell layer (arrows) and a basal process (arrowheads) that is curving toward the granule cell layer, as described for recurrent basal dendrites (Ribak et al., 2000). In **E**, a double-labeled cell (asterisk) is shown lying horizontally at the base of the granule cell layer from the 48 hr time point. Note that this cell has a thick apical process (arrow) with several branches displaying growth cones (arrowheads). In **F**, 3 BrdU-labeled cells (asterisks) are shown from the 72 hr time point, 2 of which are double-labeled with DCX (arrows) and the third that has a DCX-labeled process adjacent to it. Note that the 2 double-labeled cells have apical dendrites (arrowheads) that extend through the granule cell layer and into the molecular layer (ML) at this time point. In **G**, a BrdU/DCX double-labeled cell is shown from the 96 hr time point in the granule cell layer with its apical dendrite (arrows) extending into the ML and a terminal branching (arrowheads). Also, note that there is a second double-labeled cell (asterisk) located at the base of the granule cell layer (GL) adjacent to the subgranular zone (SGZ). Scale bar in **A** = 10μm for **A–E**, 15μm for **F**, and 20μm for **G**. Reprinted with permission from Shapiro et al. (2007b). (See color Figure 12.6)

data were used to generate an estimated growth rate over a period of 5 days following a single BrdU injection. A second difference is that Shapiro et al. (2007b) analyzed the percentage of BrdU/DCX-labeled granule cells with basal dendrites (Ribak et al. 2004; Rao and Shetty 2004) at each of these time points and showed that the percentage of newly generated cells with basal dendrites peaks at 3 days after they are born and then declines. It is pertinent to note that the apical dendrites undergo an increased growth rate after this same 3-day time point, tripling in length between 3 days and 4 days, then doubling in length between 4 days and 5 days.

Thus, Shapiro et al. (2007b) suggested that basal dendrites were retracting at approximately the same time point when apical dendrites undergo an increased dendritic growth rate.

It should be noted that labeling with DCX to examine dendritic outgrowth is only effective until the newly generated neuron differentiates to a certain stage of dendritic development, which appears to be about 2–3 weeks after the neuron is generated (Kempermann et al. 2003, 2004; Dayer et al. 2003). Another method can be used to follow the maturation and growth of dendrites from newly generated neurons beyond this stage of differentiation, and it is the use of retrovirus labeling.

The retrovirus labeling method for analyzing newly generated granule cells in the dentate gyrus was first applied by van Praag et al. (2002). The retrovirus carrying the green fluorescent protein (GFP) labels a subset of proliferating cells and reveals morphological details about them, including their dendrites and axons. Using this method, Zhao et al. (2006) reported that GFP-labeled cells had processes spanning the granule cell layer or were parallel to this layer at 3 days post-injection (dp) of the GFP retrovirus. GFP-labeled cells with apical dendrites spanning the granule cell layer were reported to be more common at 7 dp, a finding that is consistent with the results of Plumpe et al. (2006). By 10–14 dp, the GFP-labeled granule cells resembled the mature morphology of granule cells, except that their dendrites were short and displayed varicosities. Zhao et al. (2006) were able to precisely determine when spines appeared on the apical dendrites of GFP-labeled cells. They showed that a few of the examined cells had dendritic spines at 16 dp, but no GFP-labeled cells had spines at 15 dp. It should be noted that GFP-labeled cells at 21 dp had elaborate dendritic arbors and resembled the morphology of mature-looking neurons. In addition to these qualitative results, Zhao et al. (2006) also provided quantitative data to show that spine growth reaches a peak during the first 3–4 weeks for newly generated neurons in the adult brain. These findings with the GFP retrovirus labeling method provide important information about dendritic outgrowth and spine maturation that could not be obtained with the DCX labeling method due to the latter method's limited time period for labeling newly generated neurons. Combining the data from both the GFP retrovirus and BrdU/DCX labeling methods, it can be concluded that our understanding of the developmental profile of the dendrites of newly generated neurons in the adult dentate gyrus is well documented.

SYNAPSES ON THE APICAL DENDRITES OF NEWLY GENERATED GRANULE CELLS IN THE ADULT

The apical dendrites of newly generated neurons arise from cell bodies found in the subgranular zone or at the hilar border of the granule cell layer. These apical dendrites grow through the granule cell layer but are unable to be targeted for synapses in this layer because they grow along radial glial processes (Shapiro et al.

2005; Shapiro and Ribak 2006) and are ensheathed by them (Seki and Arai 1999; Mignone et al. 2004). Thus, the radial glial processes may be involved in blocking the formation of synapses on the portion of DCX-labeled apical dendrites within the granule cell layer. After growing through the granule cell layer, the DCX-labeled apical dendrites enter the molecular layer, where small axon terminals form immature synapses on their spiny surfaces (Shapiro et al. 2007b). Although the surface of DCX-labeled apical dendrites in the molecular layer is partially apposed by glial processes, adequate surface is exposed to the neuropil so that axon terminals are able to target these DCX-labeled dendrites (Fig. 12.5). Therefore, these data support the hypothesis that, after the apical dendrites of newly generated neurons grow through the granule cell layer, they are targeted for synaptogenesis. Other data from monkeys using a different marker for newly generated neurons, TUC-4, support this hypothesis (Ngwenya et al. 2006).

Findings with the GFP retrovirus labeling method have provided additional information about synaptogenesis on apical dendrites of newly generated neurons that the DCX labeling method could not provide (Toni et al. 2007). As stated above, dendritic spines on newly generated granule cells in the adult dentate gyrus were first shown at 16 dp using the GFP retrovirus labeling method (Zhao et al. 2006), and an examination of synapses for such GFP-labeled spines was performed at 30 dp (Toni et al. 2007). Toni et al. (2007) showed that about 75% of the dendritic spines at 30 dp had a bulbous tip and formed mature synapses, whereas the remaining 25% of spines displayed a fine tip that lacked synapses. In addition, they showed that about 64% of GFP-labeled dendritic spines synapsed with axonal boutons that were involved in another synapse, so-called multiple synapse boutons. By examining dendritic spines of newly generated granule cells at 180 dp, they concluded that the spines undergo a transition from being involved with multiple synapse boutons to being associated with a single synapse bouton (Toni et al. 2007). It should also be noted that, at 30 dp, newly generated neurons received axosomatic, axodendritic, and axospinous input. These data on synapses demonstrate conclusively that newly generated neurons in the adult brain become integrated into neuronal circuitry. It remains to be shown whether the immature synapses found on DCX-labeled dendritic shafts are transient or they become axospinous synapses.

AXONAL GROWTH OF NEWLY GENERATED GRANULE CELLS IN ADULT RATS

Two early studies showed that axons of newborn dentate granule cells grow into CA3 (Hastings and Gould 1999; Markakis and Gage 1999). In both studies, retrograde markers were combined with BrdU labeling to demonstrate that axons from newborn neurons were projecting to CA3. In addition, Hastings and Gould

(1999) analyzed the temporal outgrowth of axons from newborn granule cells and described their presence in CA3 of adult rats by 10 days after being born. More recently Zhao et al. (2006), using the GFP retrovirus labeling method, have analyzed the daily progression of axon growth into stratum lucidum of CA3. They showed that axons were not found in CA3a by 10 days after injection, although thin fibers were seen in the hilus at this time point. Between 11 days and 16 days after injection, the labeled axonal fibers projected farther and farther into the CA3 region (Zhao et al. 2006). Note that the projection of the axon into CA3 occurs prior to the appearance of dendritic spines that occurs 16 days after birth. These details provide important information about axonal outgrowth from newborn neurons in rats and mice.

More recently, findings were reported on the synapses made by the axons arising from newly generated granule cells in the adult dentate gyrus. Using viral-mediated expression of the GFP, Toni et al. (2008) showed axons of newly generated granule cells forming characteristic mossy fiber synapses with thorny excrescences in the CA3 area of the hippocampus. They examined three time points after injection of the GFP retrovirus. At the earliest time point, the labeled mossy fibers shared the postsynaptic thorny excrescence with an unlabeled mossy fiber. At the latest time point, almost all of the labeled mossy fibers synapsed with their own thorny excrescence. In addition, these labeled axons formed *en passant* boutons synapsing onto CA3 and hilar interneurons, and confirmed that newly generated neurons project to their appropriate targets in the hippocampus (Acsady et al. 1998). Therefore, adult-generated neurons accurately integrate into the adult hippocampal network, supporting the view that these cells may be involved in hippocampal function.

An important issue of axonal outgrowth still remains to be addressed. How do the axons of newborn granule cells traverse the neuropil of the hilus to reach stratum lucidum of CA3? As shown above for the dendrites of newly generated granule cells, they are guided through the granule cell layer by the radial processes of radial glial cells. It would be interesting to know if a similar lattice from astrocytes guides the outgrowing axon. Because the axons of granule cells form bundles and are unmyelinated, their membranes come into direct contact with each other in the hilus and stratum lucidum of CA3 (Laatsch and Cowan 1966) and some of these sites of apposition display gap junctions (Hamzei-Sichani et al. 2007). It has yet to be shown whether these gap junctions play a role in the outgrowth of axons from newly generated granule cells in the adult dentate gyrus.

SUMMARY AND FUTURE DIRECTIONS

This chapter provides a comprehensive review of our current state of knowledge of the development of newly generated granule cells in the adult dentate gyrus.

First, we showed that there are at least three progenitor cell types that can produce granule cells. It remains to be seen whether the type 2 and type 3 cells represent a continuum of transit amplifying cells (Seri et al. 2001; Filippov et al. 2003). Next, we described the dendritic growth of newly generated granule cells in adult rats, distinguishing between a transient basal dendrite and the definitive apical dendrite. Following, we reviewed the data on the spatiotemporal profile of dendritic outgrowth and the formation of synapses on the apical dendrites and dendritic spines of newly generated granule cells in the adult. The last topic involved the axonal outgrowth of newly generated granule cells and the synapses that they form. It remains to be seen how these axons are directed to grow through the hilus to reach their targets in CA3. Together, these data provide important aspects of the development of newly generated granule cells in the adult dentate gyrus. This detailed knowledge is especially important to address questions regarding the functional significance of these newborn neurons.

ACKNOWLEDGMENTS

The authors are grateful to the following collaborators who contributed significantly to one or several studies described in this review: Mathew J. Korn, Pooja Upadhyaya, Zhiyin Shan, and Dr. Andre Obenaus. We acknowledge the support from NIH grant R01-NS38331 (to C.E.R.) and NIH training grant T32-NS45540 (for L.A.S.).

REFERENCES

Acsady, L., Kamondi, A., Sik, A., Freund, T., Buzsaki, G. 1998. GABAergic cells are the major postsynaptic targets of mossy fibers in the rat hippocampus. *J Neurosci* 18: 3386–403.

Altman, J., Das, G. 1965. Autoradiographic and histological evidence of postnatal hippocampal neurogenesis in rats. *J Comp Neurol* 124:319–35.

Alvarez-Buylla, A., Seri, B., Doetsch, F. 2002. Identification of neural stem cells in the adult vertebrate brain. *Brain Res Bull* 57: 751–8.

Dayer, A.G., Cleaver, K.M., Abouantoun, T., Cameron, H.A. 2005. New GABAergic interneurons in the adult neocortex and striatum are generated from different precursors. *J Cell Biol* 168:415–27.

Dayer, A.G., Ford, A.A., Cleaver, K.M., Yassaee, M., Cameron, H.A. 2003. Short-term and long-term survival of new neurons in the rat dentate gyrus. *J Comp Neurol* 460:563–72.

De Marchis, S., Temoney, S., Erdelyi, F., Bovetti, S., Bovolin, P., Szabo, G., Puche, A.C. 2004. GABAergic phenotypic differentiation of a subpopulation of subventricular derived migrating progenitors. *Euro J Neurosci* 20:1307–17.

Desmond, N.L., Levy, W.B. 1984. Dendritic caliber and the 3/2 power relationship of dentate granule cells. *J Comp Neurol* 227:589–96.

Ehninger, D., Kempermann, G. 2008. Neurogenesis in the adult hippocampus. *Cell Tissue Res* 331:243–50.

Filippov, V., Kronenberg, G., Pivneva, T., Reuter, K., Steiner, B., Wang, L., Yamaguchi, M., Kettenmann, H., Kempermann, G. 2003. Subpopulation of nestin-expressing progenitor cells in the adult murine hippocampus shows electrophysiological and morphological characteristics of astrocytes. *Mol Cell Neurosci* 23:373–82.

Hamzei-Sichani, F., Kamasawa, N., Janssen, W., Yasumura, T., Davidson, K., Hof, P., Wearne, S., Stewart, M., Young, S., Whittington, M., Rash, J., Traub, R. 2007. Gap junctions on hippocampal mossy fiber axons demonstrated by thin-section electron microscopy and freeze-fracture replica immunogold labeling. *Proc Natl Acad Sci USA* 104:12548–53.

Hastings, N.B., Gould, E. 1999. Rapid extension of axons into the CA3 region by adult-generated granule cells. *J Comp Neurol* 413:146–54.

Horesh, D., Sapir, T., Francis, F., Wolf, S.G., Caspi, M., Elbaum, M., Chelly, J., Reiner, O. 1999. Doublecortin, a stabilizer of microtubules. *Human Mol Genetics* 8:1599–610.

Jones, S.P., Rahimi, O., O'Boyle, M.P., Diaz, D.L., Claiborne, B.J. 2003. Maturation of granule cell dendrites after mossy fiber arrival in hippocampal field CA3. *Hippocampus* 13:413–27.

Kaplan, M., Hinds, J. 1977. Neurogenesis in the adult rat: electron microscopic analysis of light radioautographs. *Science* 197:1092–4.

Kempermann, G., Gast, D., Kronenberg, G., Yamaguchi, M., Gage, F.H. 2003. Early determination and long-term persistence of adult-generated new neurons in the hippocampus of mice. *Develop* 130:391–9.

Kempermann G., Jessberger, S., Steiner, B., Kronenberg, G. 2004. Milestones of neuronal development in the adult hippocampus. *Trends Neurosci* 27:447–52.

Kempermann, G., Kuhn, H.G., Gage, F.H. 1997. More hippocampal neurons in adult mice living in an enriched environment. *Nature* 386:493–5.

Laatsch, R.H., Cowan, W.M. 1966. Electron microscopic studies of the dentate gyrus of the rat. I. Normal structure with special reference to synaptic organization. *J Comp Neurol* 128:359–96.

Lois, C., Alvarez-Buylla, A. 1994. Long-distance neuronal migration in the adult mammalian brain. *Science* 264:1145–8.

Markakis, E.A., Gage, F.H. 1999. Adult-generated neurons in the dentate gyrus send axonal projections to field CA3 and are surrounded by synaptic vesicles. *J Comp Neurol* 406:449–60.

Mignone, J., Kukekov, V., Chiang, A., Steindler, D., Enikolopov, G. 2004. Neural stem and progenitor cells in nestin-GFP transgenic mice. *J Comp Neurol* 469: 311–24.

Ngwenya, L., Peters, A., Rosene, D. 2006. Maturational sequence of newly generated neurons in the dentate gyrus of the young adult rhesus monkey. *J Comp Neurol* 498: 204–16.

Palmer, T.D., Willhoite, A.R., Gage, F.H. 2000. Vascular niche for adult hippocampal neurogenesis. *J Comp Neurol* 425:479–94.

Parent, J.M., Yu, T.W., Leibowitz, R.T., Geschwind, D.H., Sloviter, R.S., Lowenstein, D.H. 1997. Dentate granule cell neurogenesis is increased by seizures and contributes to aberrant network reorganization in the adult rat hippocampus. *J Neurosci* 17:3727–38.

Plumpe, T., Ehninger, D., Steiner, B., Klempin, F., Jessberger, S., Brandt, M., Romer, B., Rodriquez, G.R., Kronenberg, G., Kempermann, G. 2006. Variability of doublecortin-associated dendrite maturation in adult hippocampal neurogenesis is independent of the regulation of precursor cell proliferation. *BMC Neurosci* 7:77.

Rao, M.S., Shetty, A.K. 2004. Efficacy of doublecortin as a marker to analyse the absolute number and dendritic growth of newly generated neurons in the adult dentate gyrus. *Euro J Neurosci* 19:234–46.

Ribak, C.E., Korn, M.J., Shan, Z., Obenaus, A. 2004. Dendritic growth cones and recurrent basal dendrites are typical features of newly generated dentate granule cells in the adult hippocampus. *Brain Res* 1000:195–9.

Seki, T., Arai, Y. 1993. Highly polysialylated neural cell adhesion molecule (NCAM-H) is expressed by newly generated granule cells in the dentate gyrus of the adult rat. *J Neurosci* 13:2351–8.

Seki, T., Arai, Y. 1999. Temporal and spatial relationships between PSA-NCAM expressing, newly generated granule cells, and radial glia-like cells in the adult dentate gyrus. *J Comp Neurol* 410:503–13.

Seki, T., Namba, T., Mochizuki, H., Onodera, M. 2007. Clustering, migration, and neurite formation of neural precursor cells in the adult rat hippocampus. *J Comp Neurol* 502:275–90.

Seress, L., Pokorny, J. 1981. Structure of the granular layer of the rat dentate gyrus. *J Anat* 133:181–95.

Seri, B., Garcia-Verdugo, J., Collado-Morente, L., McEwen, B., Alvarez-Buylla, A. 2004. Cell types, lineage, and architecture of the germinal zone in the adult dentate gyrus. *J Comp Neurol* 478:359–78.

Seri, B., Garcia-Verdugo, J.M., McEwen, B.S., Alvarez-Buylla, A. 2001. Astrocytes give rise to new neurons in the adult mammalian hippocampus. *J Neurosci* 21:7153–60.

Shapiro, L.A., Korn, M.J., Shan, Z., Ribak, C.E. 2005. GFAP-expressing radial glia-like cell bodies are involved in a one-to-one relationship with doublecortin-immunolabeled newborn neurons in the adult dentate gyrus. *Brain Res* 1040:81–91.

Shapiro, L.A., Ng, K.L., Kinyamu, R., Whitaker-Azmitia, P., Geisert, E., Blurton-Jones, M., Zhou, Q., Ribak, C.E. 2007a. Origin, migration and fate of newly generated neurons in the adult rodent piriform cortex. *Brain Struct Funct* 212:133–48.

Shapiro, L.A., Ribak, C.E. 2006. Newly born dentate granule neurons after pilocarpine-induced epilepsy have hilar basal dendrites with immature synapses. *Epilepsy Res* 69:53–66.

Shapiro, L.A., Upadhyaya, P., Ribak, C.E. 2007b. Spatiotemporal profile of dendritic outgrowth from newly born granule cells in the adult rat dentate gyrus. *Brain Res* 1149:30–7.

Sotelo, C., Palay, S.L. 1968. The fine structure of the vestibular nucleus in the rat. I. Neurons and neuroglial cells. *J Cell Biol* 36:151–79.

Steiner, B., Klempin, F., Wang, L., Kott, M., Kettenmann, H., Kempermann, G. 2006. Type-2 cells as link between glial and neuronal lineage in adult hippocampal neurogenesis. *Glia* 58:805–14.

Toni, N., Teng, E.M., Bushong, E.A., Aimone, J.B., Zhao, C., Consiglio, A., van Praag, H., Martone, M.E., Ellisman, M.H., Gage, F.H. 2007. Synapse formation on neurons born in the adult hippocampus. *Nat Neurosci* 10:727–34.

Toni, N., Laplagne, D.A., Zhao, C., Lombardi, G., Ribak, C.E., Gage, F.H., Schinder, A.F. 2008. Neurons born in the adult dentate gyrus form functional synapses with target cells. *Nat Neurosci* 11:901–7.

van Praag, H., Kempermann, G., Gage, F.H. 1999. Running increases cell proliferation and neurogenesis in the adult mouse dentate gyrus. *Nat Neurosci* 2:260–5.

van Praag, H., Schinder, A.F., Christie, B.R., Toni, N., Palmer, T.D., Gage, F.H. 2002. Functional neurogenesis in the adult hippocampus. *Nature* 415:1030–4.

Zhao, C. 2007. Retrovirus-mediated cell labeling. In: *Adult Neurogenesis*, F.H. Gage, G. Kempermann, and H. Song, eds. (Cold Spring Harbor, NY: Cold Spring Harbor Laboratory Press), pp. 101–17.

Zhao, C., Teng, E.M., Summers, R.G. Jr., Ming, G.L., Gage, F.H. 2006. Distinct morphological stages of dentate granule neuron maturation in the adult mouse hippocampus. *J Neurosci* 26:3–11.

Chapter Thirteen

Functional Architecture of Directional Tuning in the Primate Motor Cortex During 3D Reaching

Hugo Merchant, Thomas Naselaris, Wilbert Zarco,
Ramón Bartolo, Luis Prado, Oswaldo Pérez,
and Juan Carlos Méndez

INTRODUCTION

The topographic organization of the primary motor cortex (M1) has been analyzed mainly in the context of its representation of muscles, joints, and body
parts (Andersen et al. 1975; Asanuma and Rosen 1972; Cheney and Fetz 1985;
Cheney et al. 1985; Donoghue et al. 1992; Fetz and Cheney 1978, 1980; Fischl
et al. 1999; Gould et al. 1986; Humphrey and Reed 1983; Huntley and Jones
1991; Kwan et al. 1978; Park et al. 2001; Penfield and Boldrey 1937; Penfield
and Rasmussen 1950; Schieber and Hibbard 1993; Strick and Preston 1978;
Waters et al. 1990). Throughout several decades of mapping studies, researchers
have used a variety of techniques for electrically activating regions of the motor
cortex and then have attempted to relate the activation sites with evoked muscle
contractions or movements of body parts around specific joints. Thus, the
somatotopic organization of M1 has been reported with different levels of resolution, not only in human subjects but also in a variety of other species. However, this historical emphasis on mapping somatotopic representations belies the
fact that M1 is not simply a map of the body's musculature. M1 maintains a
dynamic representation of higher-order features of movement, most notably the
direction of reaching (Caminiti et al. 1991; Georgopoulos et al. 1982, 1984,
1986). In fact, almost half of the cells in the arm region of the motor cortex show

an orderly variation in activity as a function of the movement direction, with a peak of activity in their preferred direction (PD), and progressively lower rates for movements farther and farther away from the PD (Figure 13.1) (Georgopoulos et al. 1982). This orderly variation of cell activity is characterized by the directional tuning curve that can be approximated by a cosine function. Consequently, the question addressed in this chapter is: What are the anatomical bases for directional tuning? Throughout this chapter we provide evidence regarding the micro- and macro-anatomical architecture of directional tuning in the motor cortex.

CORTICAL COLUMNS FOR PDs

Cytoarchitectural studies of the brain have revealed that the cortex is a highly organized structure (Mountcastle 1998; Douglas and Martin 2004). First, the cortex consists of six layers, and each layer has a distinct repertoire of cell types and a different input-output organization. Thus, the layers are arranged parallel to the cortical surface, forming a horizontal dimension of information processing. In addition, the neocortex has a vertical organization, in which narrow chains of heavily interconnected cells (approximately 50 neurons) extend vertically across all of the cellular layers, forming modules or minicolumns. Lorente de No (1949) was the first to describe the anatomical minicolumns. Many years later, studies that combined electrophysiological and neuroanatomical techniques demonstrated that neuronal functional units have, as a rule, a vertical pattern of organization (Mountcastle 1997). These findings led to the view that minicolumns form these functional units, which constitute the smallest information processing units of the neocortex (Mountcastle 1978). Furthermore, it is believed that minicolumns are further organized into functional modules of a higher order called cortical columns, each consisting of several minicolumns connected by short-range horizontal connections and representing all possible values of the variable encoded in the minicolumns.

Experimental evidence for a columnar organization of neuronal functional units was obtained by Mountcastle using single-cell recordings in the somatic sensory cortex of anaesthetized cats (Mountcastle 1957) and monkeys (Powell and Mountcastle 1959). It was found that the microelectrode penetrations made perpendicular to the cortical surface and parallel to the minicolumns encountered neurons with similar properties of peripheral receptive field position and submodality (nature of stimuli). In contrast, penetrations made parallel to the cortical surface and across different minicolumns traversed through 300- to 500-μm-sized regions, in each of which cells with identical properties were encountered. Such functional modular structures have also been described in other sensory areas of the cortex. For example, orientation columns have been found in the visual cortex (Hubel and Wiesel 1974, 1977) and iso-frequency columns in the auditory cortex

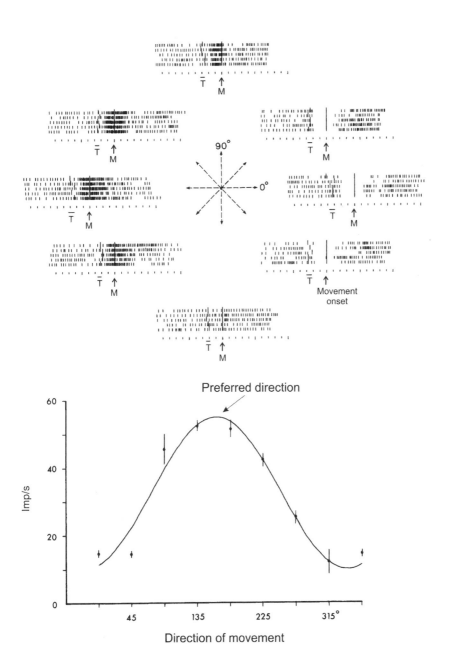

Figure 13.1. Modulation of a single cell discharge rate as a function of reaching direction. **Upper half:** rasters of the cell activity during five repetitions performed for each of the eight movement directions depicted in the center diagram. The activity is aligned with respect to movement onset (M). **Lower half:** directional tuning curve of the same cell. A cosine regression fitted to the mean discharge rate is shown as a continuous line. Modified from Georgopoulos et al. (1982).

(Merzenich and Brugge 1973; Morel et al. 1993). However, little is known about whether a similar modular organization exists in the motor cortical areas. Earlier work in this field relied on the effect of intracortical microstimulation in the primary motor cortex to activate muscles (Asanuma and Rosen 1972) or elicit motion about a joint (Kwan et al. 1978). Again, it was found that the microstimulation at different depths on electrode penetrations made perpendicular to the cortical surface produced the contraction of the same group of muscles, whereas penetrations that ran parallel to the cortical surface produced a different pattern of muscle contractions (Asanuma and Rosen 1972). Nevertheless, it was only recently that a systematic evaluation of the columnar organization of dynamic aspects of movement was performed in M1. Most notably, the group of Apostolos Georgopoulos embarked on a methodical characterization of the functional architecture of preferred directions at different spatial scales.

Early studies using arm movements in 2D space (Georgopoulos et al. 1984) indicated that the preferred directions of cells recorded in the exposed part of the motor cortex tended to be similar, whereas the preferred directions of cells recorded along the anterior bank of the central sulcus (CS) tended to change in blocks. These qualitative patterns suggested a columnar organization of the PD, with modular properties that were similar to those of the primary sensory cortices. An analysis of the relations between the spread of the PDs along a penetration and the angle formed between the penetration and the anatomical columns in the motor cortex revealed a high positive correlation ($r = 0.756$; $P < 0.01$), providing further support for the hypothesis of a columnar organization of the PD (Georgopoulos et al. 1984). Finally, a quantitative method to detect functional cortical modules using data from a 3D reaching task revealed that cells with similar PDs tended to segregate into vertically oriented minicolumns 50–100μm wide and at least 500μm high. Specifically, this method quantified the density of pairs of cells as a function of the angular difference in their PDs and their recording distance (Figure 13.2) (Amirikian and Georgopoulos 2003). These data were obtained for two orthogonal dimensions in the cortex; one was parallel (Fig. 13.2c,d) and the other perpendicular (Fig. 13.2a,b) to the cortical layers. The distribution of directionally tuned cells in these dimensions was nonuniform and highly structured. Besides the minicolumn organization observed in the analysis in the dimension perpendicular to the cortical layers, it was found that minicolumns with similar PDs were repeated every ~200μm in the horizontal dimension (Amirikian and Georgopoulos 2003). Furthermore, nonoverlapping columns representing nearly opposite PDs were approximately 350μm apart. Therefore, these studies have provided strong support for the notion of a columnar organization of PDs in the motor cortex.

As a final commentary, it is important to state that the columnar organization of PDs in the motor cortex is a statistical property of the cortical tissue that depends on the analysis of large databases and a careful determination of the microelectrode trajectories in the exposed part and the bank of the CS, as we describe below.

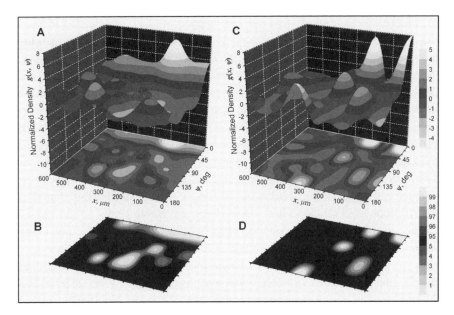

Figure 13.2. Neuronal density fields computed for two mutually orthogonal dimensions: perpendicular (**A,B**) and parallel (**C,D**) to the cortical surface. **A** and **C**, 3D landscape of the density $g(x, \psi)$ of pairs of cells recorded at a spatial distance x and showing an angular deviation ψ between their PDs. **B** and **D**, 2D contour map showing the probability $p(x, \psi)$ that the neuronal density field, produced by a uniformly random sample, was less than the density field generated from actual penetrations. Color scales are shown to the right. Modified from Amirikian and Georgopoulos (2003). (See color Figure 13.2)

METHODOLOGICAL INTERLUDE

In order to determine the short- and long-range organization of PDs in the motor cortex, we first designed a procedure for identifying the locations of recording sites visited by an array of 16 electrodes. We view the multielectrode approach as a complement to existing techniques for cortical mapping such as optical imaging (OI) (Arieli and Grinvald 2002; Blasdel 1992; Fung et al. 1998; Grinvald et al. 1988, 1991). Although OI has proven to be indispensable for the study of cortical maps, OI cannot access the neural response of cells in the deep layers of the cortex or in cortical regions buried in a sulcus such as the CS. Therefore, in our situation microelectrode recording was extremely advantageous.

Unlike OI, microelectrode recording possesses no intrinsic means of identifying the location at which activity is sampled. In principle, it should be possible to reconstruct the trajectory of an electrode if one knows the point at which it was inserted into the cortex, the angle it makes with respect to the cortical surface, and the total distance the electrode has traveled. In the past, the approach has been to use stereotaxic coordinates to identify the insertion point of the recording or stimulating electrode. To find out what happens to the electrode after it enters the cortex, researchers have relied on readings from the microdrive used to push the electrode and, in many cases, on the creation of electrolytic lesions. These lesions can be identified in sectioned tissue and used to infer the final depth and penetration angle of the electrode. This procedure has limitations that make it inadequate when the experimental goal is to map large areas of the cortex in three dimensions, because the lesioning technique cannot be overused. In order to overcome these restrictions, we used electrodes coated with lipophilic fluorescent dyes that leave tracks marking their trajectory through the cortex (DiCarlo et al. 1996). In fact, we successfully reconstructed all the coated-electrode trajectories, with the certainty that the dyes caused no cortical damage beyond that caused by the electrode itself (DiCarlo et al. 1996; Honig and Hume 1989).

The reconstructed tracks were used to estimate the parameters of a simple geometrical model that generates coordinates for each recording site (Figure 13.3, right panel). We also introduced a coordinate transformation that takes into account the convoluted structure of the cortex near sulci to conveniently visualize recording-site locations in a rectilinear representation (Fig. 13.3, left panel). This method relies on analysis of Nissl-stained sections of the recorded area and takes into consideration the orientation of anatomically defined cortical columns (Fig. 13.3, left panel). It also allows for a convenient way to identify the cortical layers in which the recording sites are located (Naselaris et al. 2005). Finally, we measured different sources of error for this procedure, and the experimental results from recordings in the motor cortex of macaque monkeys showed that the estimation error of each recording site was less than 100µm (Naselaris et al. 2005).

We used this methodology for the PD mapping study. The specific experimental procedure was as follows. All neural data were collected while monkeys worked on the 3D center-out task developed by Georgopoulos and colleagues (Schwartz et al. 1988). Monkeys reached using the left hand toward 8 targets located near the corners of a cube. All movements were made from the same starting position, located at the center of the cube, which was at the shoulder's level of the monkey's reaching arm. Between 5 and 8 experimental trials in each of the movement directions were available for each cell recorded. All recordings were obtained from the arm region of the M1. The recorded area was within a region that extended 3–4mm along the CS, and 7–12mm in the direction perpendicular to the CS. Once the top of the cortex was identified, electrodes were advanced at 150µm increments until they reached the white matter. Raw extracellular potentials were recorded at each site with a sampling frequency of 60 kHz, and high-pass filtered at 0.5 kHz. After the experiment, the monkey was sacrificed, and the recorded area of the cortex was blocked and sectioned every 50µm. Registered digital fluorescence and Nissl-stained images of each slice were used to reconstruct the trajectories of the electrodes passing through the cortex, as described above (Naselaris et al. 2005, 2006a).

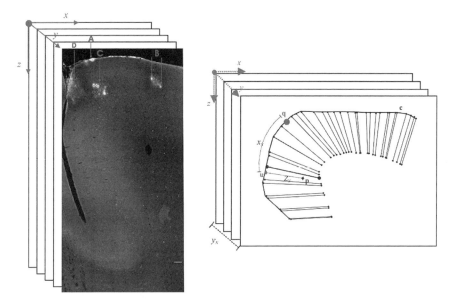

Figure 13.3. Left panel: electrode trajectory parameters are measured using fluorescence imaging: grayscale image of a sagittal section through the CS. Axes of the extrinsic coordinate system used to express recording site coordinates are depicted as blue arrows labeled x, y, and z. Black borders surrounding the image indicate its position within a stack of similar images. Marks made by dye-coated electrodes from several penetrations appear as bright white blobs. **A**: insertion point for an electrode. **B**: marks made by 2 coated electrodes at the corners of the same array. **C**: red circles show intersection of the current slice and all 16 reconstructed electrode trajectories from a single penetration. **D**: in some cases, diffusion of the fluorescent dye away from corner electrodes outlined the full region covered by the 16-electrode array. Scale bar = 0.5mm.
Right panel: unfolded coordinates are derived from measurements taken in each Nissl slice: unfolded coordinates of each recording site are a function of the measurements (X_N, Y_N, Z_N) shown here with dashed lines. The black diamond–labeled p indicates the position within a slice of a single recording site. The dashed line segment extending from the recording site is parallel to the nearest labeled anatomical column (thick black line; other columns shown by thin black lines). The small black dot labeled u is the intersection of this line segment with the cortical surface c. X_N measures the distance along c between u and q, the crown of the CS (large red dot). Z_N measures the distance between u and p within the plane of section. Y_N measures the distance from the most medial sagittal slice. For comparison, axes of the extrinsic coordinate system are shown as blue arrows labeled x, y, and z. Used with permission and modified from Naselaris et al. (2005). (See color Figure 13.3)

Electrode penetrations passed from the exposed surface of the precentral gyrus, through the crown, and into the anterior bank of the CS. Finally, the recording sites were transformed into a "flattened" coordinate system that had the effect of unfolding the cortical surface about the crown of the CS and projecting each recording site along the anatomical columns.

SHORT-SCALE TANGENTIAL ORGANIZATION OF PDs

Another prominent feature of the functional architecture of the cortex is the existence of a tangential organization of a particular behavioral variable. For example, in the primary visual cortex the columns of orientation preference change continuously as a function of the horizontal cortical location. In fact, as revealed by microelectrode measurements, a single 180°-cycle of orientation change encompasses 500–700μm of cortex (Hubel and Wiesel 1974). This portion of tissue was called an orientation column, because it includes minicolumns with all possible orientations. Later experiments using optical imaging revealed a more complete picture of the 2D topography of the cortical tangential arrangement (Bonhoeffer and Grinvald 1991; Blasdel 1992), including: (1) the singularities or pinwheels in the horizontal orientation gradients, (2) the existence of linear zones (bounded by pinwheels) within which iso-orientation regions form parallel slabs, and (3) the presence of linear zones that tend to cross the borders of ocular dominance stripes at right angles; pinwheels tend to align with the centers of ocular dominance stripes.

Consequently, the next question with respect to the functional architecture of PDs was: What is the tangential organization of PDs in the motor cortex? In this regard, the study of Amirikian and Georgopoulos (2003) analyzed the PD differences as a function of the displacement of recording sites along single electrodes, and they obtained evidence for short-range correlations and columnar organization. However, the data used in these studies did not allow for direct observation of the layout of PDs across the tangential dimension of the cortex. Hence, we used the multielectrode mapping methodology described above to determine the approximate location of the recording sites on a flattened cortical surface, as projected along anatomical columns. Of 2,385 recording sites analyzed, 985 (41.3%) were directionally tuned. The horizontal map of PDs for the two monkeys is shown in Figure 13.4, where it is evident that each PD is represented at multiple, widely distributed sites on the motor cortical surface (Georgopoulos et al. 2007a). In this map, each PD is colored according to its presence in one of the octants that partition the surface of the sphere into eight equal areas (Fig. 13.4).

It is clear that the map of PDs is quite complex, and it is difficult to establish a tangential organization with the naked eye (Fig. 13.4). Therefore, we investigated the possible regularity in the representation of the PD as follows. On a given directionally tuned site, we fit a circular grid consisting of 30μm annuli, extending up to 1,200μm from the center. Then, for every annulus, we counted the number of sites recorded from and the number of sites with similar directional tuning to the center site, as determined by a correlation analysis of the firing rates between pairs of cells during the reaching motion in each of the eight directions. The average angle between the PDs of significantly correlated sites ($P < 0.05$, $n = 8$, $df = 6$) was 24.8°. This process was repeated for every directionally tuned recording site to derive average estimates of the prevalence of similar PDs, determined as the

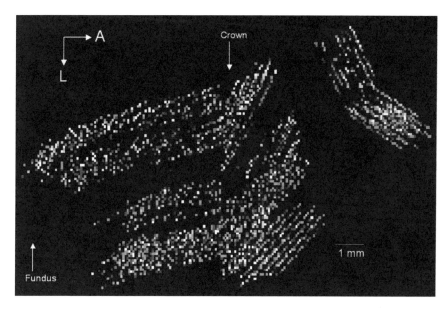

Figure 13.4. Location on the flattened motor cortical surface of the preferred directions of directionally tuned sites. The octant of the unit sphere to which a preferred direction belongs is color-coded depending on the sign of the directional cosines [x, y, z]. (Modified from Georgopoulos et al. 2007.) A, anterior; L, lateral. (See color Figure 13.4)

fraction of these sites over the total recorded in an annulus. As expected, the total number of recording sites increased with distance away from the center of the grid as the area of the annulus increased (Georgopoulos et al. 2007a). By contrast, the proportion of similarly tuned sites fell exponentially with distance, indicating a local enrichment of similar PDs. In fact, a decreasing power function gave a significant fit to the data. Finally, the residuals of the power-function fitting (detrended data) were subjected to spectral analysis to check for and identify possible spatial periodicities in the fluctuation of similarly tuned cells. The resulting fractions were detrended, because periodicities cannot be properly assessed from a series of data in the presence of linear or curvilinear trends. The resulting periodogram (Figure 13.5a) revealed two striking peaks at periods of 240µm and 86µm (Georgopoulos et al. 2007a). A finer-grain analysis of higher spatial frequencies using a 10µm annulus revealed additional significant power at periods of 30µm and 60µm (Fig. 13.5b). These results suggest: (1) a minicolumn width of approximately 30µm, (2) clustering of two to three minicolumns with similar directions, and (3) a regular repetition of minicolumns with similar directions every 240µm. An analysis of the spatial distribution of nontuned, multiunit sites revealed quite the opposite: no significant periodicities.

A tentative model of the map of PDs in the motor cortex is shown in Figure 13.6a, in which a given PD is represented by a filled circle. There are two additional

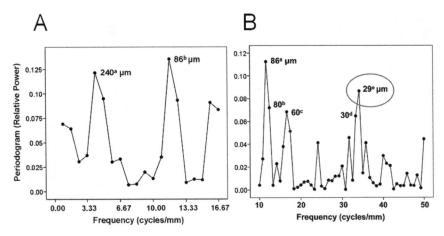

Figure 13.5. (**A**) Normalized periodogram of detrended observed data using a circular grid of 30μm annulus. The period of statistically significant points is displayed next to the points. The levels of statistical significance of the labeled points were as follows: a, P = 0.032; b, P = 0.017. (**B**) Normalized periodogram of detrended original data using a circular grid of 10μm annulus. The levels of significance of the labeled points were as follows: a, P = 0.004; b, P = 0.018; c, P = 0.027; d, P = 0.03; e, P = 0.01. Modified from Georgopoulos et al. (2007a).

aspects of this model of a 240μm radius column. First, there was a wide representation of the PDs within each column. In fact, we found a wide distribution in the angular difference (azimuth and elevation) between the PD observed at the center of the circle and that observed at a given site within the circle. Second, there was a radial gradient of PDs; they became more and more dissimilar from that at the center of the circle as the distance increased away from the center, up to the radius of the circle (120μm). These two findings lend strong, independent support to our model (Fig. 13.6a) (Georgopoulos et al. 2007a). In addition, they provide approximate quantitative estimates of some key mapping parameters, as follows. Assuming a tangential area of a minicolumn (r = 15μm) of 707μm^2 and a tangential area of a column (r = 120μm) of 45,230μm^2, there are 64 (45,230/707) minicolumns in a column, within which the unit sphere of PDs is mapped with a resolution of approximately 360°/64 = 5.62° solid angle.

LARGE-SCALE TANGENTIAL ORGANIZATION OF PDs

In the classic Hubel and Wiesel (1977) description of the organization of the primary visual cortex, repeating modules, or hypercolumns, encode all the parameters needed to represent a small portion of a visual stimulus. Within each hypercolumn, all the information about the orientation, spatial frequency, and drift direction of

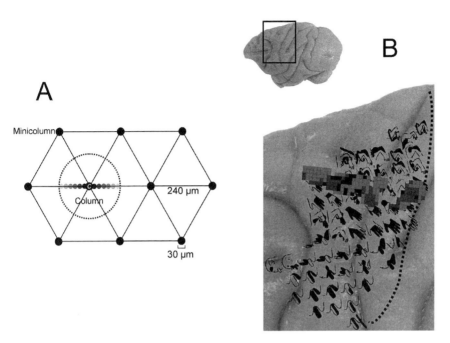

Figure 13.6. (**A**) Schematic model of short-range tangential organization of preferred directions in the motor cortex. The letter *c* inside a black circle denotes a minicolumn at the center of a 240μm column, depicted as a dashed circle. Inside the column there is a gradient (in gray scale) of minicolumns, whose PDs become farther and farther away from the PD in *c*. The other black circles are minicolumns with the same preferred direction. (**B**) Model of the motor cortical hypercolumns with a surface area of 3 mm², with bimodial (red), unimodal (blue), or uniform (black) local PD distribution superimposed on the somatotopic organization of the primary motor cortex, taken from the original maps of Woolsey et al. (1952). (See color Figure 13.6)

image components is encoded by overlapping groups of neurons organized in variable-specific modules of different dimensions (Bonhoeffer and Grinvald 1991; Hubel and Wiesel 1977; Swindale et al. 2000). Thus, these hypercolumns tile the cortical surface, making interlacing maps of response properties. The last mapping issue that we addressed for PDs in the motor cortex was precisely to determine the large-scale horizontal topography. With that purpose, we reanalyzed the motor cortical PD map shown in Fig. 13.4 in light of the two main properties of the PD distribution: (1) the broad distribution of PDs across the directional continuum and (2) the enrichment for forward- and backward-reaching directions (Naselaris et al. 2006a). Hence, the nonuniform structure of the PD distribution leads naturally to questions about the spatial distribution of PDs. Given what is known about somatotopic organization in M1, it is possible that two peaks in the global distribution are generated by PDs that are clustered together in distinct, spatially separated cortical regions. Another possibility is that the features of the global distribution are replicated locally, so that the distribution of PDs in any local region of M1 may have the same properties as the distribution of PDs taken from across all regions of M1.

To distinguish between these possibilities, we examined the surface map of PDs. We first determined a functionally meaningful size for a "local region" of cortex. For that we estimated the size of the local region in which the full complement of PDs is represented by counting the number of empty octants within a radially expanding circular border centered on each recording site on the map. The result of this analysis (Figure 13.7) indicates that the median radius of the cortical patch containing all octants is about 1mm. Thus we can assert that PD distributions in local regions with a radius of ≤1mm replicate the structure of the global distribution in their covering of the sphere. In what follows, we will use the term "local region" to refer to any contiguous patch of cortex with a surface area of 3mm^2 (Naselaris et al. 2006b).

Having determined the size of the local region required to cover all octants of the sphere, we analyzed local distributions from across the recorded area to determine whether the enrichment of forward- and backward-reaching directions that is seen globally is also present locally. We examined distributions of PD populations within square-shaped, overlapping local regions with a side of 1.6mm, spaced at 400μm intervals (surface area = 2.5mm^2). Statistical tests were applied in series to classify each local distribution as uniform, unimodal, or bimodal, using a mixture model that estimated the significance of two modes in the PD distribution. Figure 13.8 shows the map of local distribution types (Naselaris et al. 2006b). The maps demonstrate a preponderance of nonuniform local distributions (monkey 1: 70%; monkey 2: 86%), with the majority of local regions being bimodal (monkey 1: 53%; monkey 2: 53%).

Finally, the primary direction(s) estimated in each nonuniform local region is shown under an equal-area projection in Figure 13.9. It is evident from this figure that the local primary directions cluster in the forward and backward directions, similar to the global primary directions.

Overall, the results suggest that the motor cortex may be considered as an assemblage of overlapping hypercolumns with a surface area of about 3mm^2. Within these hypercolumns the diversity of cells' PDs is sufficient to represent not only any given direction of reach, but more importantly, in most of such modules we found an enrichment for forward- and backward-reaching, replicating the global distribution of PDs. Furthermore, considering the columns of 240μm described above, we can suggest that within a hypercolumn, the PDs are organized into columns with an arrangement that appears to have a periodic structure. Interestingly, the hypercolumn topography can be linked to the somatotopic organization in M1. Let us first mention some important properties of the distributed nature of the motor cortical somatotopy. Assessment of the anatomical convergence

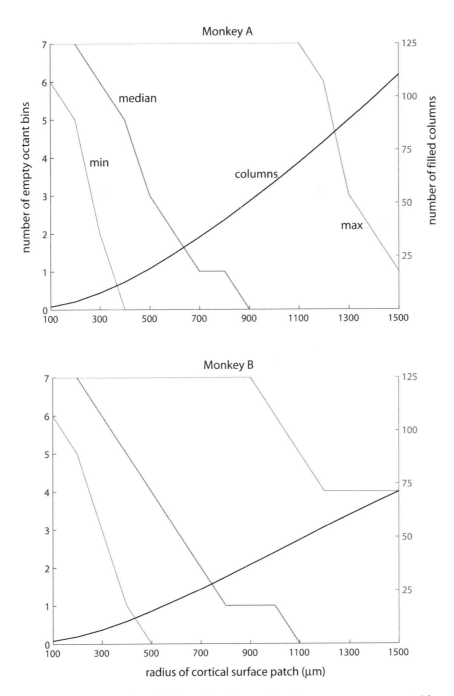

Figure 13.7. Spatial scale of PD dispersion. The number of empty octants was counted for the set of PDs within a circular region of a given radius (abscissa) centered at each recording site. Minimum, median, and maximum number of empty octants (left axis) as a function of radius is shown by the green, blue, and red lines, respectively. Black line shows the average number of column-sized (80μm diameter) patches within each circular region that contained a recording site (right axis). Used with permission and modified from Naselaris et al. (2006b). (See color Figure 13.7)

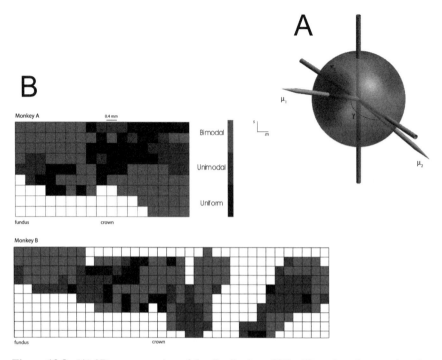

Figure 13.8. (A) 3D representation of the distribution of PDs. The sphere is rotated so that the forward pole appears in the foreground. The perspective is that of an observer facing the monkey; thus the hemisphere to the viewer's right of the blue meridian corresponds to reaching directions to the monkey's left. Gray cylinders extend from the up/down and left/right poles. Green arrows extending from the surface show the direction of the two modes (μ_1 and μ_2) the dashed circle surrounding the forward mode is the corresponding dispersion (κ_1), and γ is the angle between the two modes. These values were obtained from a mixture model for the global distribution of PDs (modified from Naselaris et al. 2006a). (B) Surface maps of local PD distributions. This map was constructed by partitioning the cortical surface into overlapping squares spaced at 400μm intervals with a side of 1.6mm. The distribution of PDs in each region is classified as uniform (black), unimodal (blue), or bimodal (red). Used with permission and modified from Naselaris et al. (2006b). (See color Figure 13.8)

(Andersen et al. 1975; Darian-Smith et al. 1990; Jankowska et al. 1975) and divergence (Shinoda et al. 1981) of cortico-spinal inputs and the application of sensitive tools (such as spike-triggered averaging) for revealing connections between M1 neurons and muscle activity have helped to define two main aspects of distributed somatotopy: (1) single cells in M1 make weighted contributions to multiple muscles, typically three (Cheney et al. 1985; Donoghue et al. 1992; McKiernan et al. 1998; Park et al. 2001; Shinoda et al. 1981), and (2) a single muscle is represented in a repeated fashion at multiple locations across M1 (Asanuma and Rosen 1972; Donoghue et al. 1992; Gould et al. 1986; Kwan et al. 1978). Thus, considering

Monkey A   ## Monkey B

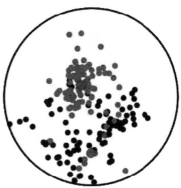

Figure 13.9. Distribution of local primary directions. A mixture model was fitted to the distribution of PDs in each local region defined as nonuniform. Primary directions from each of these local regions are shown under an equal-area projection, where red dots indicate the forward hemisphere and black dots the backward hemisphere. Primary directions for the global distribution are shown as large green dots. Used with permission and modified from Naselaris et al. (2006b). (See color Figure 13.9)

the divergent nature of the somatotopic organization, it is quite probable that cells inside a hypercolumn will have access to a group of muscles. Under this scenario, each cell could make a contribution to an arm reach in the direction of its own PD by making a differentially weighted contribution to the activation of the muscles accessible to the local region. The divergence of somatotopic representation thus provides an ideal substrate for translating the directional signal generated by a local region (Georgopoulos 1996; Lewis and Kristan 1998). In addition, considering the map of the motor homunculus, the existence of hypercolumns containing all of the possible PDs and the global distributive property of PDs will be an ideal combinatorial substrate for controlling the direction of movement using different parts of the body musculature, as presented in the model of Fig. 13.6b.

DIRECTIONAL TUNING AND THE INTRINSIC PROPERTIES OF THE M1 CIRCUITS

Numerous studies have reported that sensory, motor, and cognitive information can be represented in the central nervous system by neurons that are tuned to distinct behavioral parameters. Needless to say, directional tuning in M1 is a clear example of this coding scheme. In addition, it has been demonstrated that pyramidal cell tuning in the visual and auditory systems depends on a balance of thalamocortical excitatory inputs and local circuit inhibition (Wehr and Zador 2003; Ma and Suga 2004). For example, narrow orientation tuning in the visual cortex is generated by both an enhancement near the preferred orientation caused by specific inputs from the lateral geniculate nucleus and cortico-cortical amplification, and by global suppression supplied by cortical inhibition (Shapley et al. 2003; Ferster and Miller 2000). Hence, we propose that the regular, bell-shaped directional tuning curve is primarily the result of strong excitatory thalamic input to a particular column, followed by a mixture of excitatory and inhibitory inputs mediated by local interneurons acting in the tangential dimension. This idea is supported by the findings that: (1) the onset latency of cell activity is shortest for movements in the PD and progressively longer with movements increasingly distant from it (Georgopoulos et al. 1982), and (2) movements well away from the PD are often associated with abrupt cessation of activity, suggestive of inhibitory effects (Georgopoulos et al. 1982). Furthermore, unpublished observations from our group investigated how directional tuning of putative pyramidal cells is sharpened by inhibition from neighboring interneurons. First, different functional and electrophysiological criteria were used to identify putative pyramidal and interneuronal subtypes in a large database of motor cortical cells recorded during performance of the 3D center-out task. Then we analyzed the relation between the magnitude of inhibition and the tuning width, and a significant decrease of the latter as a function of the former was found in a population of putative pyramidal cells. In fact, the coupling of inhibition-narrow tuning was observed before and during movement execution, indicating an important dynamic role of inhibition during movement control. Overall, these results suggest that local inhibition is involved in sculpting the directional specificity of a group of putative pyramidal neurons in the motor cortex.

Finally, another line of evidence in support of the local shaping of PDs in M1 comes from electrophysiological studies that described the impact of recurrent collaterals of pyramidal axons and the associated interneurons on the inhibition of motor cortical pyramidal neurons (Stefanis and Jasper 1964, 1965). Specifically, Stefanis and Jasper (1964) recorded the motor cortical excitatory postsynaptic potentials and inhibitory postsynaptic potentials elicited by electrical stimulation of the pyramidal tract, and they described the existence of strong recurrent inhibition probably mediated by local interneurons that were driven by the pyramidal collaterals. Hence, these findings strengthen the idea that recurrent collateral inhibition plays a fundamental role in the spatial sharpening of the focus of excitation in M1.

FINAL CONSIDERATIONS

Directional tuning has been a hallmark in cortical encoding since the 1980s. Not only the idea that high-order spatial features of movement are represented in M1 (Georgopoulos et al. 1982), but also the implementation of a population code that could integrate the information of tuned cells to predict and properly decode movement trajectories (Georgopoulos et al. 1986), were revolutionary contributions to motor control. Recent papers have emphasized that directional tuning is more related to dynamic (force, joint torques) rather than to kinematic (direction and velocity) aspects of the reaching movement (Todorov 2000). Nevertheless, despite the discussion of its corresponding reference frame (internal or external; Georgopoulos et al. 2007b; Kakei et al. 1999), the present results indicate that directional tuning in M1 has a specific and complex anatomical origin.

The development of methodological tools that allowed the appropriate estimation of the position of multiple recording sites throughout long cortical trajectories was a fundamental element for the mapping of PDs at different spatial scales. Thus, several lines of evidence support the notion of columnar organization of directional tuning in M1. Minicolumns of an approximate diameter of 30μm were demonstrated using different methodologies (Fig. 13.6a) (Amirikian and Georgopoulos 2003; Georgopoulos et al. 2007a). In addition, minicolumns with similar directions show a regular repetition every 240μm, forming columns that include all directions. In fact, inside a column of 240μm there is a gradient of PDs: they become increasingly dissimilar from the center PD, until the peripheral limit of the column is reached (Fig. 13.6a). The smooth tuning curves might be generated by both an enhancement near the preferred orientation caused by specific thalamic and cortico-cortical amplification, and by global suppression supplied by cortical inhibitory interneurons inside the directional columns. Finally, hypercolumns with a surface area of 3mm^2 contain enough columns and minicolumns to represent locally the global-bimodal distribution of PDs in the motor cortex. These hypercolumns probably interact with the map of the motor homunculus, providing an ideal combinatorial substrate for controlling the direction of movement using different parts of the body musculature (Fig. 13.6b).

The topographic organization of PDs is probably subjected to behaviorally dependent plasticity. The motor cortex has a clear capacity for massive reorganization (Sanes and Donoghue 2000). Motor-cortical plasticity has been demonstrated using a variety of techniques, including intracortical microstimulation (Nudo et al. 1996), slice preparations (Hess and Donoghue 1994), functional magnetic resonance imaging (Karni et al. 1995), and transcranial magnetic stimulation (TCMS) (Classen et al. 1998; Pascual-Leone et al. 1995). Collectively, work on motor-cortical plasticity has demonstrated that the cortical representation of movements and movement sequences associated with the learning and production of a stereotyped motor task is enlarged as a result of the learning. Hence, it will not be surprising that the modular organization of PDs can be reorganized at all minicolumn, column, and hypercolumn levels. Indeed, in a recent study in which focal TCMS was applied to the representation of the thumb in the motor cortex, it was found that intensive practice in one thumb movement direction could change the representation of other directions in M1 (Classen et al. 1998).

In conclusion, the functional architecture of PDs should be taken into account to design more efficient multielectrode arrays and subdural electrocorticogram probes for brain–machine interfaces (BMI). The sudden increase in studies using neuroprosthetics as a potential aid for people with severe motor disabilities should consider the anatomical organization of PDs in the motor cortex. Indeed, our finding suggests that the surface area spanned by an array of electrodes in BMIs needs be at most about $3mm^2$. In addition, a desirable location for recording electrodes in these systems should be near the crown of the CS, because this is the area where uniform PD distributions were obtained (Fig. 13.8) and where BMI decoding procedures will be more efficient.

ACKNOWLEDGMENTS

We thank Apostolos P. Georgopoulos for all his aid regarding this chapter. We also thank Dorothy Pless for proofreading the manuscript and Raul Paulín for his technical assistance. Supported in part by PAPIIT: IN209305 and FIRCA: TW007224-01A1.

REFERENCES

Amirikian B and Georgopoulos AP. Modular organization of directionally tuned cells in the motor cortex: is there a short-range order? *Proc Natl Acad Sci USA* 100:12474–9, 2003.

Andersen P, Hagan PJ, Phillips CG, and Powell TP. Mapping by microstimulation of overlapping projections from area 4 to motor units of the baboon's hand. *Proc R Soc Lond B Biol Sci* 188:31–6, 1975.

Arieli A and Grinvald A. Optical imaging combined with targeted electrical recordings, microstimulation, or tracer injections. *J Neurosci Methods* 116:15–28, 2002.

Asanuma H and Rosen I. Topographical organization of cortical efferent zones projecting to distal forelimb muscles in the monkey. *Exp Brain Res* 14:243–56, 1972.

Blasdel GG. Orientation selectivity, preference, and continuity in monkey striate cortex. *J Neurosci* 12:3139–61, 1992.

Bonhoeffer T and Grinvald A. Iso-orientation domains in cat visual cortex are arranged in pinwheel-like patterns. *Nature* 353:429–31, 1991.

Caminiti R, Johnson PB, Galli C, Ferraina S, and Burnod Y. Making arm movements within different parts of space: the premotor and motor cortical representation of a coordinate system for reaching to visual targets. *J Neurosci* 11:1182–97, 1991.

Cheney PD and Fetz EE. Comparable patterns of muscle facilitation evoked by individual corticomotoneuronal (CM) cells and by single intracortical microstimuli in primates: evidence for functional groups of CM cells. *J Neurophysiol* 53:786–804, 1985.

Cheney PD, Fetz EE, and Palmer SS. Patterns of facilitation and suppression of antagonist forelimb muscles from motor cortex sites in the awake monkey. *J Neurophysiol* 53:805–20, 1985.

Classen J, Liepert J, Wise SP, Hallett M, and Cohen LG. Rapid plasticity of human cortical movement representation induced by practice. *J Neurophysiol* 79:1117–23, 1998.

Darian-Smith C, Darian-Smith I, and Cheema SS. Thalamic projections to sensorimotor cortex in the macaque monkey: use of multiple retrograde fluorescent tracers. *J Comp Neurol* 299:17–46, 1990.

De Nó, Lorente R. Cerebral cortex: Architecture, intracortical connections, motor projections. In: *Physiology of the Nervous System*, Fulton, F.J. (ed.), New York: Oxford University Press, 1949:289–330.

DiCarlo JJ, Lane JW, Hsiao SS, and Johnson KO. Marking microelectrode penetrations with fluorescent dyes. *J Neurosci Methods* 64:75–81, 1996.

Donoghue JP, Leibovic S, and Sanes JN. Organization of the forelimb area in squirrel monkey motor cortex: representation of digit, wrist, and elbow muscles. *Exp Brain Res* 89:1–19, 1992.

Douglas RJ and Martin KAC. Neuronal circuits in the neocortex. *Annu Rev Neurosci* 27:419–51, 2004.

Ferster D and Miller KD. Neural mechanisms of orientation selectivity in the visual cortex. *Annu Rev Neurosci* 23:441–71, 2000.

Fetz EE and Cheney PD. Muscle fields of primate corticomotoneuronal cells. *J Physiol* (Paris) 74:239–45, 1978.

Fetz EE and Cheney PD. Postspike facilitation of forelimb muscle activity by primate corticomotoneuronal cells. *J Neurophysiol* 44:751–72, 1980.

Fischl B, Sereno MI, Tootell RB, and Dale AM. High-resolution intersubject averaging and a coordinate system for the cortical surface. *Hum Brain Mapp* 8:272–84, 1999.

Fung SH, Burstein D, and Born RT. In vivo microelectrode track reconstruction using magnetic resonance imaging. *J Neurosci Methods* 80:215–24, 1998.

Georgopoulos AP. On the translation of directional motor cortical commands to activation of muscles via spinal interneuronal systems. *Brain Res Cogn Brain Res* 3:151–5, 1996.

Georgopoulos AP, Kalaska JF, Caminiti R, and Massey JT. On the relations between the direction of two-dimensional arm movements and cell discharge in primate motor cortex. *J Neurosci* 2:1527–37, 1982.

Georgopoulos AP, Kalaska JF, Crutcher R, Caminiti R, and Massey JT. The representation of movement direction the motor cortex: single cell and population studies. In: *Dynamic Aspects of Neocortical Functions*, Edelman, G.M. (ed.), New York: Wiley, 1984.

Georgopoulos AP, Merchant H, Narselaris T, and Amirikian B. Mapping of the preferred direction in the motor cortex. *Proc Natl Acad Sci USA* 104:11068–72, 2007a.

Georgopoulos AP, Narselaris T, Merchant H, and Amirikian B. Contrasting interpretations of the non-uniform distribution of preferred directions within primary motor cortex. Reply to Kurtzer and Herter. *J Neurophysiol* 97:4391–2, 2007b.

Georgopoulos AP, Schwartz AB, and Kettner RE. Neuronal population coding of movement direction. *Science* 233:1416–9, 1986.

Gould HJ 3rd, Cusick CG, Pons TP, and Kaas JH. The relationship of corpus callosum connections to electrical stimulation maps of motor, supplementary motor, and the frontal eye fields in owl monkeys. *J Comp Neurol* 247:297–325, 1986.

Grinvald A, Frostig RD, Lieke E, and Hildesheim R. Optical imaging of neuronal activity. *Physiol Rev* 68:1285–1366, 1988.

Grinvald A, Frostig RD, Siegel RM, and Bartfeld E. High-resolution optical imaging of functional brain architecture in the awake monkey. *Proc Natl Acad Sci USA* 88: 11559–63, 1991.

Hess G and Donoghue JP. Long-term potentiation of horizontal connections provides a mechanism to reorganize cortical motor maps. *J Neurophysiol* 71:2543–7, 1994.

Honig MG and Hume RI. Dil and diO: versatile fluorescent dyes for neuronal labelling and pathway tracing. *Trends Neurosci* 12:333–40, 1989.

Hubel DH and Wiesel TN. Sequence regularity and geometry of orientation columns in the monkey striate cortex. *J Comp Neurol* 158:267–93, 1974.

Hubel DH and Wiesel TN. Ferrier lecture. Functional architecture of macaque monkey visual cortex. *Proc R Soc Lond B Biol Sci* 198:1–59, 1977.

Humphrey DR and Reed DJ. Separate cortical systems for control of joint movement and joint stiffness: reciprocal activation and coactivation of antagonist muscles. *Adv Neurol* 39:347–72, 1983.

Huntley GW and Jones EG. Relationship of intrinsic connections to forelimb movement representations in monkey motor cortex: a correlative anatomic and physiological study. *J Neurophysiol* 66:390–413, 1991.

Jankowska E, Padel Y, and Tanaka R. Projections of pyramidal tract cells to alpha-moto-neurones innervating hind-limb muscles in the monkey. *J Physiol* 249:637–67, 1975.

Kakei, S, Hoffman DS, and Strick, PL. Muscle and movement representations in the primary motor cortex. *Science* 285:2136–9, 1999.

Karni A, Meyer G, Jezzard P, Adams MM, Turner R, and Ungerleider LG. Functional MRI evidence for adult motor cortex plasticity during motor skill learning. *Nature* 377:155–8, 1995.

Kwan HC, MacKay WA, Murphy JT, and Wong YC. Spatial organization of precentral cortex in awake primates. II. Motor outputs. *J Neurophysiol* 41:1120–31, 1978.

Lewis JE and Kristan WB Jr. A neuronal network for computing population vectors in the leech. *Nature* 391:76–9, 1998.

Ma X and Suga N. Lateral inhibition for center-surround reorganization of the frequency map of bat auditory cortex. *J Neurophysiol* 92:3192–9, 2004.

McKiernan BJ, Marcario JK, Karrer JH, and Cheney PD. Corticomotoneuronal postspike effects in shoulder, elbow, wrist, digit, and intrinsic hand muscles during a reach and prehension task. *J Neurophysiol* 80:1961–80, 1998.

Merzenich MM and Brugge JF. Representation of the cochlear partition on the superior temporal plane of the macaque monkey. *Brain Res* 50:275–96, 1973.

Morel A, Garraghty PE, and Kaas JH. Tonotopic organization, architectonic fields, and connections of auditory cortex in macaque monkeys. *J Comp Neurol* 335:437–59, 1993.

Mountcastle VB. Modality and topographic properties of single neurons of cat's somatic sensory cortex. *J Neurophysiol* 20:408–34, 1957.

Mountcastle VB. An organizing principle for cerebral function. In: Edelman, G.M. and Mountcastle, V.B. (eds.), *The Mindful Brain*. Cambridge: MIT Press, 1978:7–50.

Mountcastle, VB. The columnar organization of the neocortex. *Brain* 120:701–22, 1997.

Mountcastle, VB. *Perceptual Neuroscience: The Cerebral Cortex*. Cambridge: Harvard University Press, 1998.

Naselaris T, Merchant H, Amirikian B, and Georgopoulos AP. Spatial reconstruction of trajectories of an array of recording microelectrodes. *J Neurophysiol* 93:2318–30, 2005.

Naselaris T, Merchant H, Amirikian B, and Georgopoulos AP. Large-scale organization of preferred directions in the motor cortex I: Motor cortical hyperacuity for forward reaching. *J Neurophysiol* 96:3231–6, 2006a.

Naselaris T, Merchant H, Amirikian B, and Georgopoulos AP. Large-scale organization of preferred directions in the motor cortex II: Analysis of local distributions. *J Neurophysiol* 96:3237–47, 2006b.

Nudo RJ, Milliken GW, Jenkins WM, and Merzenich MM. Use-dependent alterations of movement representations in primary motor cortex of adult squirrel monkeys. *J Neurosci* 16:785–807, 1996.

Park MC, Belhaj-Saif A, Gordon M, and Cheney PD. Consistent features in the forelimb representation of primary motor cortex in rhesus macaques. *J Neurosci* 21:2784–92, 2001.

Pascual-Leone A, Nguyet D, Cohen LG, Brasil-Neto JP, Cammarota A, and Hallett M. Modulation of muscle responses evoked by transcranial magnetic stimulation during the acquisition of new fine motor skills. *J Neurophysiol* 74:1037–45, 1995.

Penfield W and Boldrey E. Somatic motor and sensory representation in the cerebral cortex of man as studied by electrical stimulation. *Brain* 37:389–443, 1937.

Penfield W and Rasmussen T. *The Cerebral Cortex of Man*. New York: Macmillan, 1950.

Powell TPS and Mountcastle VB. Some aspects of the functional organization of the cortex of the postcentral gyrus of the monkey: a correlation of findings obtained in a single unit analysis with cytoarchitecture. *Bull Johns Hopkins Hosp* 105:133–62, 1959.

Sanes JN and Donoghue JP. Plasticity and primary motor cortex. *Annu Rev Neurosci* 23:393–415, 2000.

Schieber MH and Hibbard LS. How somatotopic is the motor cortex hand area? *Science* 261:489–92, 1993.

Schwartz AB, Kettner RE, and Georgopoulos AP. Primate motor cortex and free arm movements to visual targets in three-dimensional space. I. Relations between single cell discharge and direction of movement. *J Neurosci* 8:2913–27, 1988.

Shapley R, Hawken M, and Ringach DL. Dynamics of orientation selectivity in the primary visual cortex and the importance of cortical inhibition. *Neuron* 38:689–99, 2003.

Shinoda Y, Yokota J, and Futami T. Divergent projection of individual corticospinal axons to motoneurons of multiple muscles in the monkey. *Neurosci Lett* 23:7–12, 1981.

Stefanis C and Jasper H. Intracellular microelectrode studies of antidromic responses in cortical pyramidal tract neurons. *J Neurophysiol* 27:828–54, 1964.

Stefanis C and Jasper H. Recurrent collateral inhibition in pyramidal tract neurons. *J Neurophysiol* 27:855–77, 1965.

Strick PL and Preston JB. Multiple representation in the primate motor cortex. *Brain Res* 154:366–70, 1978.

Swindale NV, Shoham D, Grinvald A, Bonhoeffer T, and Hubener M. Visual cortex maps are optimized for uniform coverage. *Nat Neurosci* 3:822–6, 2000.

Todorov E. Direct cortical control of muscle activation in voluntary arm movements: a model. *Nat Neurosci* 3:391–8, 2000.

Waters RS, Samulack DD, Dykes RW, and McKinley PA. Topographic organization of baboon primary motor cortex: face, hand, forelimb, and shoulder representation. *Somatosens Mot Res* 7:485–514, 1990.

Wehr M and Zador AM. Balanced inhibition underlies tuning and sharpens spike timing in auditory cortex. *Nature* 426:442–6, 2003.

Woolsey CN, Settlage PH, Meyer DR, Sencer W, Hamuy TP, and Travis AM. Patterns of localization in precentral and "supplementary" motor areas and their relation to the concept of a premotor area. *Res Pub Assoc Res Nerv Ment Dis* 30:238–64, 1952.

Chapter Fourteen

Neural Codes for Perceptual Decisions

Ranulfo Romo, Adrián Hernández, Luis Lemus,
Rogelio Luna, Antonio Zainos, Verónica Nácher,
Manuel Alvarez, Yuriria Vázquez, Silvia Cordero,
and Liliana Camarillo

INTRODUCTION

A difficult and enduring problem in neuroscience is the elucidation of how sensory experiences arise from activity of the brain. A major component of this problem involves understanding how brain circuits represent sensory features. Pioneering investigations in several sensory systems have shown how neural activity represents the physical parameters of the sensory stimuli both in the periphery and central areas of the brain (Adrian 1928; Hubel and Wiesel 1998; Mountcastle et al. 1967; Talbot et al. 1968). These investigations have paved the way for new questions that are more closely related to cognitive processing. For example, what components of neuronal activity evoked by a sensory stimulus are directly related to perception (Parker and Newsome 1998; Romo and Salinas 2001, 2003)? Where and how in the brain is sensory information stored in memory (Brody et al. 2003; Romo et al. 1999)? Where and how in the brain do the neuronal responses that encode the sensory stimuli translate into responses that encode a perceptual decision (Gold and Shadlen 2007; Romo and Salinas 2001, 2003; Schall 2001)?

These questions have been investigated in behavioral tasks by which the sensory stimuli are under precise quantitative control and the subject's psychophysical performances are quantitatively measured (Newsome et al. 1989; de Lafuente and Romo 2005; Hernández et al. 1997). One of the main challenges of this approach is that even the simplest cognitive tasks engage a large number of cortical areas, and each one might render the sensory information in a different way (de Lafuente and Romo 2006; Romo et al. 2003, 2004). Also, the sensory information might be combined in these cortical areas with other types of stored signals representing, for example, past experience and future actions (Hernández et al. 2002; Lemus et al. 2007; Romo et al. 2002, 2003, 2004). Thus, a central issue in neuroscience is the isolation of the neural codes associated with these processes.

The underlying idea is that if neural codes for such stimuli are readily identifiable, then determining the individual functional roles of those brain areas should become less difficult. Recent studies have provided new insights into this problem using a somatosensory discrimination task. In particular, these studies have shown the neural codes that are related to sensation, working memory, and decision making in a somatosensory discrimination task. Here we review the evidence supporting these conjectures.

PSYCHOPHYSICS AND NEUROPHYSIOLOGY OF VIBROTACTILE DISCRIMINATION

We have studied the extracellular activity of single neurons of diverse cortical areas (Figure 14.1) while trained monkeys executed a highly simplified vibrotactile

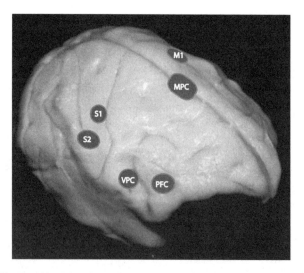

Figure 14.1. Picture of brain surface of one of the monkeys used to investigate the neuronal response properties of diverse cortical areas during the vibrotactile discrimination task. Recordings were made in primary somatosensory cortex (S1; areas 3b and 1); secondary somatosensory cortex (S2); ventral premotor cortex (VPC); prefrontal cortex (PFC); medial premotor cortex (MPC); and primary motor cortex (M1).

discrimination task (Figure 14.2). In this two-alternative, forced-choice task, subjects must compare the frequency of two vibratory stimuli applied sequentially to their fingertips and then use their free hand to push one of two response buttons to indicate which stimulus was of higher or lower frequency. The discrimination task, although apparently simple, is designed so that it can only be executed correctly when a minimum of neuronal operations or cognitive steps is performed: encoding the two stimulus frequencies, maintaining the first stimulus frequency (f1) in working memory, comparing the second stimulus frequency (f2) with the memory trace of f1, and, finally, executing a motor response to report discrimination (Hernández et al. 1997). Thus, the discrimination task allows us to investigate a wide range of essential processes associated with this task.

A simple testable hypothesis is that the sequential events associated with the vibrotactile discrimination task are represented in the neuronal activity of a widely

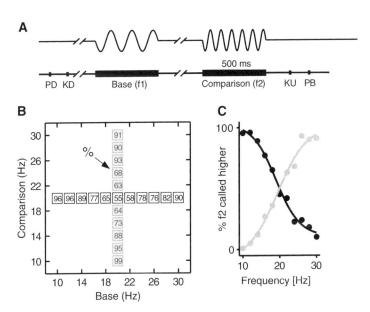

Figure 14.2. Discrimination task. (**A**) Sequence of events during discrimination trials. The mechanical probe is lowered, indenting the glabrous skin of one digit of the hand (PD); the monkey places his free hand on an immovable key (KD); the probe oscillates vertically, at the base frequency; after a delay, a second mechanical vibration is delivered at the comparison frequency; the monkey releases the key (KU) and presses one of two push-buttons (PB) to indicate whether the comparison frequency was higher or lower than the base. (**B**) Stimulus set used to estimate psychometric thresholds. Each box indicates a base frequency/comparison frequency stimulus pair used; the number inside the box indicates overall percent correct trials for that base/comparison pair. (**C**) Psychometric curves computed from (**B**). Adapted from Romo et al., 1998, 2000.

distributed system, beginning in the primary somatosensory (S1) cortex and ending in the motor cortices, where the motor commands are triggered to report this cognitive operation. It is unlikely that the ascending inputs to the S1 cortex encode the essential neuronal computations required to solve this task. Their role could simply be to transmit a neural copy of vibrotactile stimuli, in which the stimulus location and features are safely encoded and transmitted to the S1 cortex. Based on these premises, we sought the neuronal activity in the S1 cortex and cortical areas central to it that might be associated with the different components of the vibrotactile discrimination task. We assumed that, in the neuronal responses, the stimulus parameters could be quantified and interpreted according to the task demands.

NEURAL CODING OF VIBROTACTILE STIMULI IN THE S1 CORTEX

Mountcastle and colleagues recorded S1 responses in behaving monkeys trained to detect and discriminate the frequencies of flutter stimuli (Mountcastle et al. 1990). The results support previous findings (Mountcastle et al. 1969). First, it was found that quickly adapting (QA) neurons of the S1 cortex (areas 3b and 1), like their afferent fibers, fire periodically, in phase with mechanical oscillations. Second, their firing rates seem to change little in the flutter range (this conclusion was based, however, on data from only 17 neurons). Third, psychophysical performance matched the inferred performance based on the discriminability of the periodic interspike intervals (Mountcastle et al. 1990). It followed that, as proposed before, stimulus frequency could not be encoded by S1 firing rates; stimulus frequency had to be encoded temporally, in the serial order of evoked spikes (Mountcastle et al. 1969, 1990; Talbot et al. 1968).

In support of this proposal, using flutter stimuli, Merzenich and colleagues compared psychophysical data from monkeys to S1 recordings in separate experiments from the same animals (Recanzone et al. 1992). The comparison was consistent with a temporal coding mechanism, and firing rates were not seen to vary with stimulus frequency (however, the range of frequencies tested was quite narrow, and animals were anaesthetized). Merzenich and colleagues made another important observation: spike timing associated with the sine wave was much more precise in trained animals compared to untrained monkeys (Recanzone et al. 1992). Thus, based on these results, a psychophysical observer should exploit the periodic spike timing evoked in the QA neurons of the S1 cortex for sensory discrimination.

Arguments in favor of the proposal reviewed above could be strengthened if a large number of neurons was studied, and if neurons were studied in behaving animals during vibrotactile discrimination. To this end, we trained monkeys to discriminate between flutter stimulus frequencies and recorded many neurons with QA properties in areas 3b and 1 of the S1 cortex (Hernández et al. 2000; Salinas et al. 2000; Luna et al. 2005). Each recorded neuron with QA properties was studied during the discrimination task. There were three major results. First, the majority of neurons from the S1 cortex were phase-locked to the input stimulus frequency (Figure 14.3A,B); however, almost a third of QA neurons modulated their firing rates as a function of the stimulus frequency (Figure 14.4A,B) (Hernández et al. 2000; Salinas et al. 2000; Luna et al. 2005). The second important finding was that QA neurons that modulate their firing rates were affected by the task condition; that is, they increased their transmitted information about the stimulus frequency during task performance (Salinas et al. 2000). Third, only those neurons that varied their firing rates as a function of the stimulus frequency were affected in error trials (Salinas et al. 2000).

These findings question a unique role of periodic, spike timing in discrimination of flutter stimuli and suggest that a firing rate code cannot be discarded (Salinas et al. 2000). But, apart from this, what do these findings suggest? They suggest the presence of two subpopulations of QA neurons in the S1 cortex that behave differently in response to a periodic mechanical stimulus (Hernández et al. 2000; Salinas et al. 2000; Luna et al. 2005). These two subpopulations might be arranged in hierarchical fashion: QA neurons that respond periodically might be closer to the input stimulus, and those that modulate their firing rates might integrate the responses of the periodic neurons and transform them into a rate code (Hernández et al. 2000). Such last-order neurons of the QA circuit could distribute the neural representation to those structures anatomically linked to the S1 cortex, in order to solve the sensory discrimination task. However, further studies are needed to see whether this is so.

NEURONAL CORRELATE OF VIBROTACTILE DISCRIMINATION IN THE S1 CORTEX

A more direct test for the role of periodicity in vibrotactile discrimination is measuring the discrimination capabilities of these subtypes of QA neurons associated with the psychophysical performance (Fig. 14.3C,D and Fig. 14.4C,D). A second test is to prove whether the evoked neural activity during discrimination in the S1 cortex co-varies with sensory performance, and whether the temporal order of the spikes is important for sensory discrimination. These are incisive tests to validate the meaning of the neural encoding of the flutter stimuli in the S1 cortex.

The vibrotactile discrimination task requires the comparison of the second stimulus frequency against the first (Hernández et al. 1997). As indicated above, we found two types of responses in QA neurons of the S1 cortex: one that is periodically entrained by the stimulus frequency, and a second that, although not periodically entrained, has average firing rates during the stimulus period that are modulated as a function of the stimulus frequency (Hernández et al. 2000;

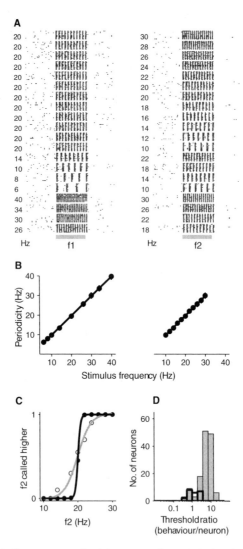

Figure 14.3. Periodic responses of a QA neuron of area 1 during the discrimination task. (**A**) Raster plots. Each row of ticks represents a trial, and each tick represents an action potential. Trials were randomly delivered. Gray horizontal lines indicate the first (f1) and the second (f2) stimulus. (**B**) Periodicity (mean ± S.D.) as a function of the first (f1) and second stimulus (f2) frequencies. (**C**) Relationship between psychometric and neurometric discrimination functions. This is plotted as the probability that the second stimulus is judged higher than the first; data and sigmoidal fits (χ^2 test, P < 0.001) for eleven pairs of stimulus frequencies in which the base frequency was 20 Hz. Gray and black lines represent psychometric and neurometric functions, respectively. (**D**) Thresholds ratios (psychometric/neurometric thresholds) calculated from neurons with periodicity (gray bars). Open bars represent the threshold ratios between psychometric and neurometric thresholds calculated from a small number of neurons with modulations in their firing rate. Adapted from Hernández et al. (2000).

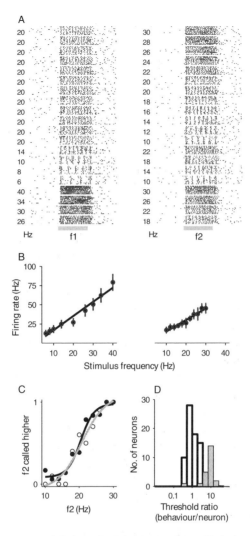

Figure 14.4. Firing rate modulation of a QA neuron of area 3b during the discrimination task. Same format as Fig. 14.3. (**A**) Raster plots; (**B**) mean firing rate (± S.D.) as a function of the stimulus frequency; (**C**) relationship between psychometric and neurometric discrimination functions; (**D**) threshold ratios calculated between psychometric and neurometric thresholds for each neuron, which varied the firing rate as a function of the stimulus frequency (open bars). Gray bars represent the threshold ratios between psychometric and neurometric thresholds calculated from a small number of neurons that show periodicity. Adapted from Hernández et al. (2000).

Salinas et al. 2000; Luna et al. 2005). To investigate which of these two representations is associated with the psychophysical performance, we determined the probability that an observer (a cortical region central to the S1 cortex) could distinguish the difference between the two stimuli (Hernández et al. 2000; Salinas et al. 2000; Luna et al. 2005). This could be based on a comparison of the neuronal response distributions of the second stimulus frequency made against the neuronal response distributions of the first stimulus frequency. According to this, the observer could use a simple rule: If the number of spikes during the second stimulus is higher than during the first stimulus, then the second stimulus is higher than the first. The same rule can be used when considering the periodicity values: If the periodicity (estimated as the frequency with greatest power in a Fourier transform of the spiking responses) during the second stimulus period is higher than during the first stimulus, then the second stimulus is higher than the first. The effect of this type of rule is equivalent to determining the area under the curve receiver operating characteristic (ROC) (Green and Swets, 1966) generated by the neuronal response distributions for each pair of stimulus frequencies, using both periodicity and firing rate values (Hernández et al. 2000; Luna et al. 2005). The areas under each of these two ROC curves are an estimate of the proportion of correct trials that an optimal observer would obtain by comparing numbers of spikes or periodicity. In pairs of stimulus frequencies in which the neuronal response distributions during the second stimulus are much higher than the neuronal distributions of the first stimulus, ROC values are close to 1; if the neuronal response distributions during the second stimulus are much lower than the neuronal response distributions of the first stimulus, ROC values are close to 0; for overlapping distributions, intermediate ROC values are found. The ROC values were then used to compute neurometric functions. Psychophysical and neuronal discrimination thresholds are calculated as half the difference between the stimulus frequency identified as higher than the standard in 75% of trials, and that frequency identified as higher in 25% of the trials. These are read directly from the logistic functions expressed in terms of Hz. Using this analysis, we are in the position to address the question of which of the two representations is meaningful for frequency discrimination.

Neurometric functions based on periodicity (Fig. 14.3C,D) or firing rate (Fig. 14.4C,D) of single S1 neurons were directly compared to the psychometric thresholds (Hernández et al. 2000). The results of this analysis show that neurometric threshold values based on periodicity are far lower than psychometric thresholds (Fig. 14.3D). This is not the case when neurometric thresholds based on firing rate are compared to the psychometric thresholds (Fig. 14.4D). They are very close to the psychometric thresholds. The goal of computing neurometric functions was not only to reveal the relationship between the neuronal responses of the S1 cortex to the mechanical stimulus, but also to discern whether these neural signals account for the psychometric behavior. However, what is then the functional meaning of the periodic neural signal in the S1 cortex? One possible role is that they simply represent the temporal structure of the stimulus and that monkeys do not use this exquisite representation for frequency discrimination. This would be the case if, for example, discrimination were based on the mean number of spikes (or bursts) fired by the population of QA neurons as a function of the stimulus frequency. Consistent with this idea, we found that QA neurons in the S1 cortex whose firing rates are modulated by the stimulus frequencies and their neurometric thresholds based on firing rates are closely similar to the monkey's psychophysical thresholds (Hernández et al. 2000). However, these correlations do not prove they are sufficient for discrimination (Romo et al. 1998, 2000).

One experiment, which could give an insight about the functional meaning of the periodic spike structure of the evoked activity in the S1 cortex, is testing whether monkeys could discriminate the difference between the two stimuli when periodicity is broken. If monkeys failed to discriminate the difference in mean frequency between the two stimuli, this would strengthen the proposal that discrimination of flutter stimuli depends on the periodic structure of the spike trains evoked in the S1 cortex (Figure 14.5). However, monkeys were able to extract the mean frequency from the nonperiodic signals and the psychophysical measures were almost identical with the periodic stimuli (Romo et al. 1998).

We then studied QA neurons in each of two conditions: while monkeys discriminated between periodic stimuli, and while monkeys discriminated between aperiodic stimuli (Hernández et al. 2000). Due to the aperiodic stimulus design, even highly stimulus-entrained neurons do not carry information about stimulus frequency in their periodicity (Fig. 14.5A,B). Clearly, neurometric thresholds based on the firing rate were again closely associated with the psychometric thresholds (Fig. 14.5C,D). As in the periodic condition, a psychophysical observer could exploit firing rate for frequency discrimination of aperiodic stimuli. These results suggest that an observer could solve this task with a precision similar to that of the monkey, based only on the firing rate produced during the stimulus periods.

There are, however, some further unexplored possibilities. For example, QA neurons of the S1 cortex typically respond to each stimulus pulse with a discrete burst of spikes. Encoding of vibrotactile stimuli could therefore be based on the number or rate of events, by which each event is defined as a burst instead of being defined as a single spike. An observer counting bursts would obtain a good estimate of the count of stimulus pulses, and this estimate would be independent of variability in the number of spikes fired in response to each pulse. Indeed, there is experimental evidence suggesting that bursting activity could efficiently encode the stimulus features (Reinagel et al. 1999; Martínez-Conde et al. 2000; Kepecs et al. 2002; Krahe and Gabbiani 2004). But whether bursting actually contributes directly to the psychophysical behavior is not known. Finally, the

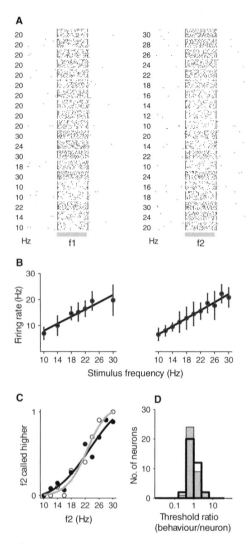

Figure 14.5. Firing rate modulation of a QA neuron of area 1 during the discrimination of aperiodic stimuli. Same format as Fig. 14.3, but both base (f1) and comparison (f2) frequencies (mean frequencies) lack periodicity. (**A**) Raster plots; (**B**) mean firing rate (± S.D.) as a function of the stimulus frequency; (**C**) relationship between psychometric and neurometric discrimination functions; (**D**) threshold ratios calculated between psychometric and neurometric thresholds for each neuron during the discrimination of periodic stimulus frequencies (open bars). Gray bars represent threshold ratios between psychometric and neurometric thresholds during the discrimination of aperiodic frequencies. Adapted from Hernández et al. (2000).

temporal window on which vibrotactile discrimination is based has not been determined. In our previous experiments, stimulus periods were always 500 milliseconds long. Under those conditions, the use of a code based on counting events and the use of a code based on the rate of events could not be distinguished.

To distinguish among all these alternatives, we conducted new combined psychophysical and neurophysiological experiments in the vibrotactile discrimination task (Luna et al. 2005). We reasoned that if an observer uses firing rate, bursting rate, or a measure of periodicity, then increases or decreases in the duration of either of the two stimuli used in each trial of the task should not lead to a systematic bias in discrimination, in either one of the two possible directions. (In contrast, under this hypothesis, stimulus duration could affect the sensory signal-to-noise ratio and therefore affect the psychometric threshold.) Alternatively, if the observer uses a strategy based on the total number of spikes or bursts fired in response to each stimulus, then manipulation of the stimulus duration should systematically bias performance, with longer stimuli being perceived as having been of higher frequencies than they actually were. We found that when the duration of one of the two stimuli was changed by 50% relative to the other stimulus, monkeys indeed biased their discrimination performance (Luna et al. 2005). Monkeys treated shortened stimuli as if the applied stimulus frequency had been slightly but significantly lower than it actually was; conversely, monkeys treated lengthened stimuli as if the applied frequency had been slightly but significantly higher than it actually was. These effects were observed with both periodic and aperiodic stimuli. We then sought an explanation for these psychophysical biases by recording QA neurons of the S1 cortex while the monkeys performed in variable stimulus–length conditions (Luna et al. 2005). We found that the effects can be qualitatively explained if one assumes that the neural signal used by the observer to solve the task is an integral of either spikes or bursts over a time window that concentrates most of its mass within the first 250 milliseconds of the stimulus, but also has a small tail into later parts of the stimulus. Finally, examining trial-by-trial co-variations of weighted counts of spikes and weighted counts of bursts, we found that only the weighted count of spikes co-varied with performance on a trial-by-trial basis.

In summary, firing rates that vary as functions of stimulus frequency are seen in multiple areas activated during the task, in particular in the S1 cortex, and there is evidence that these rate variations have a significant impact on behavior. Clearly, the brain must be able to extract at least some information from the precise timing of S1 spikes evoked during the task; for instance, humans can easily distinguish periodic stimuli from aperiodic. However, we found no indication that the high periodicity found in the S1 cortex contributes to frequency discrimination, although this possibility is hard to rule out entirely.

ARTIFICIAL INDUCTION OF ACTIVITY IN THE S1 CORTEX UNDERLYING VIBROTACTILE DISCRIMINATION

How can we be sure that the activity recorded in the S1 cortex is actually related to perception and behavior? Intracortical microstimulation is a powerful technique capable of establishing a causal link—not just a correlation—between the activity of localized neuronal populations and specific cognitive functions (Britten and van Wezel 1998; de Lafuente and Romo 2005; Romo et al. 1998, 2000; Salzman et al. 1990). For flutter discrimination, this approach has provided the most compelling evidence that all of the cognitive processes of the task may be triggered directly by the QA circuit in the S1 cortex, and it has also allowed us to explore questions about the neural code for flutter stimuli (Romo et al. 1998, 2000). Importantly, the S1 cortex is organized in modules of neurons sharing the same receptive field and mechanoreceptor submodality (Mountcastle 1957; Powell and Mountcastle 1959; Sur et al. 1984). The experiments described below were aimed to drive a column(s) of the S1 cortex—mostly of the QA type—in a way that matched the dynamic responses recorded when mechanical stimuli were applied to a patch of skin on the fingertips.

Initially, the idea was to manipulate the comparison stimulus only (Romo et al. 1998). The monkeys first learned to discriminate the frequencies of two sinusoidal vibrations delivered successively to the fingertips. Once they mastered the task, neurophysiological recordings were made in area 3b of the S1 cortex, which allowed the identification of clusters of QA neurons. An applied microstimulation current spreads around a certain cortical area, activating many neighboring units. Thus, a key for the success of microstimulation experiments is that the microelectrode must be located in the midst of a functionally homogeneous cluster of neurons. Fortunately, area 3b is indeed organized into modules of units with similar properties, or columns (Sur et al. 1984). So, having identified a set of QA neurons, the comparison stimulus was substituted with microstimulation in half of the trials. Artificial stimuli consisted of periodic current bursts delivered at the same comparison frequencies as mechanical stimuli. Microstimulation sites in the S1 cortex were selected to have QA neurons with receptive fields on the fingertip at the location of the mechanical stimulating probe. Remarkably, the monkeys discriminated the mechanical (base) and electrical (comparison) signals with performance profiles indistinguishable from those obtained with mechanical stimuli only (Figure 14.6A), so the artificially induced sensations probably resembled natural flutter quite closely (Romo et al. 1998).

Going back to the question of whether periodicity is crucial for frequency discrimination, we applied aperiodic microstimulation patterns that mimicked the random trains of mechanical pulses discussed earlier (Fig. 14.6B). The same mean frequencies were used in this condition—20 Hz still corresponded to 10 current

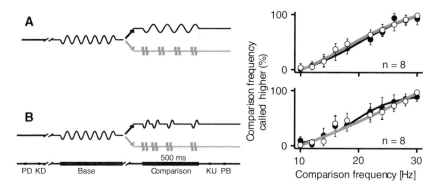

Figure 14.6. Psychophysical performance in frequency discrimination with natural, mechanical stimuli and with artificial, electrical stimuli injected into clusters of quickly adapting (QA) neurons of area 3b. **Left**: these diagrams show two types of trials that were interleaved during the experiments. In half of the trials, the monkeys compared two mechanical vibrations delivered on the skin. In the other half, one or both stimuli could be replaced by electrical frequencies microinjected into clusters of QA neurons of area 3b. **Right**: these curves show the animals' performance in the different situations, illustrated on the left. Filled and open circles indicate mechanical and electrical stimuli, respectively. In (**A**) and (**B**), the y-axis corresponds to the percentage of times the monkeys called the second stimulus frequency (x-axis) higher than the first (20 Hz). (**A**) Psychophysical performance using periodic stimuli; the comparison stimulus could be either mechanical or electrical frequencies. (**B**) Psychophysical performance when the comparison stimulus could be either aperiodic, mechanical, or electrical stimulus frequencies. PD, indentation of the glabrous skin by the mechanical probe; KD, detection of indentation; KU, detection of the end of the comparison stimulus; PB, the monkeys pressed one of two push-buttons to indicate whether the second stimulus frequency was higher or lower than the first. Adapted from Romo et al. (1998).

bursts delivered in 500 milliseconds—but the bursts were separated by random time intervals. Everything else proceeded as before, with mechanical and stimulation trials interleaved, as indicated in Figure 14.6B. From the very first trials, the animals were able to discriminate both mechanical and electrical aperiodic signals (Fig. 14.6B), with practically the same performance level reached with mechanical, periodic vibrations (Romo et al. 1998).

Because of the design of the paradigm, comparison of the second stimulus is made against a memory trace of the first one (Hernández et al. 1997). Having shown that the monkeys could use an artificial stimulus during the comparison, we wondered whether they would be able to memorize and use an electrical stimulus delivered during the base period (Romo et al. 2000). In this case, in half of the trials the base stimulus consisted of electrical microstimulation at a frequency equal to f1 (Figure 14.7), with the electric current again being injected into QA neurons. The frequency pairs and event sequence during the task were the same as in previous experiments with natural stimuli; we stress this because careful design of the stimulus sets was particularly crucial here, to ensure that the monkeys paid attention to the base stimulus and stored it in working memory (Romo et al. 1999). The monkeys' psychophysical behavior was again indistinguishable from that observed with only natural stimuli (Fig. 14.7), showing that the signals evoked by mechanical and artificial stimuli could be stored and recalled with approximately the same fidelity (Romo et al. 2000). Finally, we also investigated whether monkeys could perform the entire task on the basis of purely artificial stimuli. In most sessions in which the two mechanical stimuli were replaced by microstimulation patterns, monkeys were able to reach discrimination levels close to those measured with mechanical stimuli delivered to the fingertips. This demonstrates that activation of QA neurons is sufficient to drive all the cognitive processes involved in the task with little degradation in performance (Romo et al. 2000).

A couple of additional observations derived from these experiments are also noteworthy. First, early experiments with primary afferents had demonstrated that the flutter sensation is specifically mediated by QA fibers (Ochoa and Torebjörk 1983; Vallbo and Johanson 1984; Vallbo 1995), but this was more difficult to test at the level of the S1 cortex (Romo et al. 1998). When microstimulation was applied to clusters of neurons identified as having slowly adapting (SA) properties (Figure 14.8A), the monkeys could barely discriminate, if at all (Romo et al. 2000). As the electrode was advanced to the border between SA and QA clusters, performance became somewhat better (Fig. 14.8B), and it reached its usual degree of accuracy when QA properties became most evident in the recordings (Fig. 14.8C) (Romo et al. 2000). Hence, QA and SA units are still functionally segregated in the S1 cortex, consistent with previous observations (Sur et al. 1984).

In some sessions, we were able to introduce three microelectrodes into a cluster of QA neurons in area 3b that shared the same receptive field (Romo et al.

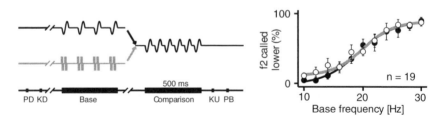

Figure 14.7. Psychophysical performance when the base stimulus could be periodic, mechanical, or electrical stimulus frequencies injected into clusters of quickly-adapting QA neurons in area 3b. The same protocols and labels as in Fig. 14.6, but here the base mechanical stimulus frequency was substituted by electrical stimulus frequencies. The y-axis corresponds to the percentage of times the monkeys called the comparison stimulus (20 Hz) lower than base stimuli at the frequency specified in the x-axis. Adapted from Romo et al. (2000).

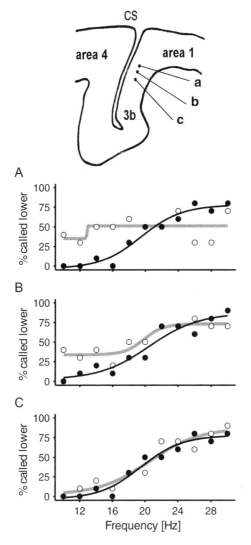

Figure 14.8. Psychophysical performance elicited by microstimulating at the base stimulus frequency in three different sites of area 3b. Same protocol and labels as in Fig. 14.6 (**A–C**) Data collected in three separate runs during the same electrode penetration; (**A**) psychophysical performance when microstimulation was applied in the center of a cluster of slowly adapting (SA) neurons; (**B**) psychophysical performance when microstimulation was applied in the border between QA and slowly adapting (SA) neurons; (**C**) psychophysical performance when microstimulation was applied in a cluster of QA neurons. Adapted from Romo et al. (2000).

2000). We knew that the most anterior microelectrode was placed in the superficial layers, because another microelectrode was placed in front of it and recorded units in primary motor cortex that were driven by spontaneous or passive movements of the fingers and lacked cutaneous receptive fields. We thought that the most posterior microelectrode was placed in the lower layers, and the remaining three microelectrodes were in the middle layers. In separate runs, the frequency pairs and event sequence were the same in both mechanical and microstimulation trials, except that in the microstimulation trials the first mechanical stimuli were substituted with a train of current pulses delivered at the frequency of the mechanical stimulus they were substituting. Figure 14.9 shows that discrimination is triggered by microstimulating each of the three different clusters. Thus, activation of any part of the cluster of neurons (probably a QA column) with similar functional properties is sufficient to trigger discrimination in this task (Romo et al. 2000).

The results obtained in the microstimulation experiments show that the relationship between the neuronal responses and the animal's behavior in the flutter discrimination task are not simple coincidences (Romo et al. 1998, 2000). Monkeys were able to discriminate the stimulus frequencies either delivered to the fingertips or artificially injected into a cluster of QA neurons. The specificity of QA stimulation for frequency discrimination is suggested by the fact that SA stimulation did not produce discrimination (Romo et al. 2000). Interestingly, it has been shown that activity in a single cutaneous afferent fiber could produce localized somatic sensations (Ochoa and Torebjörk 1983; Macefield et al. 1990; Vallbo 1995), and frequency microstimulation of QA afferents linked to Meissner's corpuscles produced the sensation of flutter (Vallbo 1995). These observations strongly support the notion that the activity initiated in specific mechanoreceptors is read by the S1 cortex; this reading is then widely distributed to those anatomical structures that are linked to the S1 cortex (Romo and Salinas 2001). The whole sequence of events associated with this sensory discrimination task must depend on this distributed neural signal (Brody et al. 2003; Hernández et al. 2002; Romo and Salinas 2003; Romo et al. 1999, 2002, 2004).

DECODING SENSORY PROCESSES FROM NEURONAL ACTIVITY ACROSS CORTICAL AREAS

In the vibrotactile stimulus range used here (5–50 Hz), mean responses of some S1 neurons (about 30% of the sampled population) typically increase as a monotonic function of the increasing stimulus frequency (Hernández et al. 2000; Luna et al. 2005; Salinas et al. 2000). For example, during the f1 period, the firing rate can be approximated to a lineal function: firing rate = $a1 \times f1 + b$, where $a1$ and b are constants. The coefficient $a1$ is the slope of the rate frequency function,

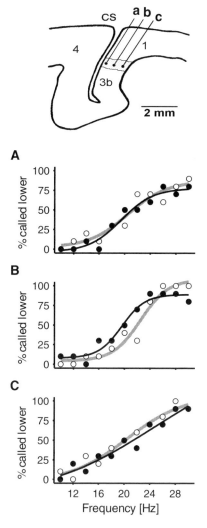

Figure 14.9. Psychophysical performance elicited by microstimulating at the base stimulus frequency in three independent microelectrodes in three different sites of a cluster of QA neurons of area 3b. Protocols and labels as for Fig. 14.6. CS, central sulcus. Adapted from Romo et al. (2000).

and it is a measure of how strongly a neuron is driven by changes in frequency (in this case, f1). To get an idea of modulation strength, a value of 1 means that the rate increases by 1 spike per second when frequency increases by 1 Hz. This means that the firing rates of some S1 neurons usually increase with increasing stimulus frequency. Figure 14.10A shows the slope distributions derived from S1 responses. As illustrated in these plots, this analysis can also be extended to the

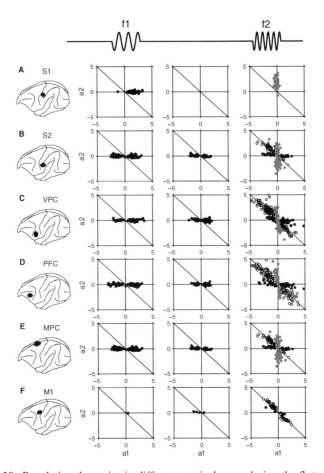

Figure 14.10. Population dynamics in different cortical areas during the flutter discrimination task. Each data point represents one neuron. For each neuron, responses were fit to the equation: firing rate = a1 × f1 + a2 × f2 + b. The coefficients a1 and a2 were computed from responses at different times during the task. Points that fall on the a1 = 0 axis represent responses that depend on f1 only (black dots); points that fall on the a2 = 0 axis represent responses that depend on f2 only (gray dots); points that fall on the a2 = –a1 line represent responses that are functions of f2 –f1 (open circles). The data shown are significantly different from (0,0) in at least one of the epochs analyzed. (**A**) S1 responses during the first stimulation period (f1; left), the inter-stimulus period (delay; middle), and the second stimulation period (f2; right). These neurons were active only during stimulation; most of them increased their rates with increasing frequency (positive a1 and a2). (**B**) S2 neurons respond to f1 (left) and exhibit a modest but significant amount of delay activity (middle). Positive and negative coefficients indicate rates that increase and decrease as functions of frequency, respectively. During the initial part of f2 (right), neurons may have significant a1 coefficients (black dots) or may respond exclusively to f2 (gray dots), as computed from the first 200 ms after stimulus onset. Later on, the coefficients cluster around the line a2 = –a1 (open circles dots), as computed from the last 300 ms before stimulus offset. Brain diagram shows region of approach to S2, which is hidden in the lateral sulcus. (**C–F**) Data from prefrontal cortex (PFC), ventral premotor cortex (VPC), medial premotor cortex (MPC), and primary motor cortex (M1) are calculated as in (**B**). Modified from Hernández et al. (2000, 2002), Salinas et al. (2000), Romo et al. (2002, 2004), and from unpublished data from Romo et al. for PFC and M1.

delay period between the f1 and f2 periods. Clearly, none of the S1 neurons that were modulated as a function of the increasing f1 show a modulation of this type during the delay period. This suggests that S1 neurons do not encode f1 during the working memory component of the task.

The responses during f2, during which the comparison process takes place, could be an arbitrary linear function of both f1 and f2. This could be approximated by this equation: firing rate = a1 × f1 + a2 × f2 + b. Fitting this equation to neuronal responses and plotting a2 as a function of a1 allows a quantification of the neurons' response dependence on the f1 and f2. Responses that are a function of f2–f1 are of particular importance for our ordinal comparison task, because correct responses depend only on the sign of f2–f1: f2 > f1 or f2 < f1. However, the analysis shows that S1 neurons do not show the comparison process during the f2 period (Fig. 14.10A). They increase their firing rate as a function of the increasing f2, suggesting that the computation between the memory referent of f1 and the current f2 input may occur in an area(s) central to the S1 cortex.

The same analysis used to decode f1 and f2 can also be applied to the neuronal responses of areas central to the S1 cortex. This is an important issue, because it might be possible to quantitatively show sensory information processes in these areas. For example, in secondary somatosensory (S2) cortex variations in firing rate similar to those in the S1 cortex are also observed; however, about 40% of the neurons have negative slopes during the f1 period (Romo et al. 2002, 2003; Salinas et al. 2000). The firing rates of these neurons decrease as a linear function of the increasing stimulus frequency, whereas the remainders have positive slopes and fire more strongly to the increasing stimulus frequency (Fig. 14.10B). All areas central to the S2 cortex that have been examined so far (except for M1) and that are active in the vibrotactile discrimination task show similar monotonic responses and similar proportions of positive and negative slopes (Fig. 14.10C–F). These areas are the ventral premotor cortex (VPC), prefrontal cortex (PFC), and the medial premotor cortex (MPC) (Brody et al. 2003; Hernández et al. 2002; Romo et al. 2002, 2003, 2004). The responses seem to proceed in a serial fashion, with shorter latencies in the S1 cortex than in the S2 cortex, the PFC, the VPC, and the MPC (Romo et al. 2004). Whether this reflects serial or parallel processing is not clear. There is strong evidence that the S2 cortex is driven by the S1 cortex (Burton et al. 1995; Pons et al. 1987), but it is not clear whether the S2 cortex drives the PFC, the VPC, and the MPC. Some anatomical studies suggest that the S2 cortex is connected with these areas, but more studies are needed to establish whether this is so (Cipolloni and Pandya 1999; Disbrow et al. 2003; Godschalk et al. 1984). Thus, the f1 representation in the S1 cortex (Fig. 14.10A) is transformed in the S2 cortex (Fig. 14.10B) in a dual representation (positive and negative slopes), which is also observed in areas of the frontal lobe (Fig. 10C–F). According to these results, the areas of the frontal lobe that process sensory information could also be considered as parts of the somatosensory system.

DECODING MEMORY PROCESSES FROM NEURONAL ACTIVITY ACROSS CORTICAL AREAS

One of the key features of the vibrotactile discrimination task is that it requires short-term memory storage of information about f1. Because we did not find any trace of f1 in the S1 cortex, we wondered where and how the f1 trace is held in the brain. The first neural correlate about this process was found in the PFC (Brody et al. 2003; Romo et al. 1999), an area involved in working memory. The inferior convexity of the PFC contains neurons that increase their firing rate in a frequency-dependent manner during the delay period (Fig. 14.10D). The dependence of firing rate on f1 is monotonic, exactly as observed for the f1 periods in those areas central to the S1 cortex (S2, PFC, VPC, and MPC). This mnemonic representation is not static, in the sense that the intensity of the persistent activity varies throughout the delay period. Some of the PFC neurons carry information about f1 during the early component of the delay period, others only during the late part of the delay period, and still others persistently throughout the entire delay period. These findings suggest that distinct neuronal populations coexist in the PFC and they carry information of f1 at different times. The data may also indicate that the PFC circuit is composed of a chain of neurons that dynamically hold the f1 information (Brody et al. 2003; Miller et al. 2003; Romo et al. 1999).

An important observation regarding the working memory systems is that other cortical areas hold information about f1. The VPC (Fig. 14.10C) also encodes information about f1 during the delay period, exactly as it does in the PFC (Romo et al. 2004). Also, some S2 neurons show a similar type of monotonic encoding (Fig. 14.10B), but only during the early part of the delay period, suggesting the presence of working memory signals in the S2 cortex (Salinas et al. 2000). Whether these S2 neurons are the ones that drive PFC and VPC neurons during the delay period or whether the S2 neurons that respond during the f1 periods are the ones that activate the mnemonic circuits is not known.

One wonders about this mnemonic coding scheme. Is there any distinction about the functional role of these mnemonic neurons found in these cortical areas? There are a couple of additional observations that may shed light on this question, and they come from recordings in the MPC (Hernández et al. 2002). First, the MPC contains neurons that encode f1 during the late part of the delay period, just before the presentation of f2. Again, this occurs with similar monotonic responses and similar proportions of positive and negative slopes. Second, the dynamics of these neurons are similar to those from the PFC and the VPC that encode f1 during the late part of the delay period (Brody et al. 2003; Romo et al. 1999, 2004). This would suggest a coding mnemonic scheme according to the task demands. Information about f1 must be available during the f2 period for the comparison with the f2 input that persistent late neurons might provide. Persistent and late neurons are therefore well positioned to compute the comparison process.

DECODING COMPARISON PROCESSES FROM
NEURONAL ACTIVITY ACROSS CORTICAL AREAS

Reaching a decision in the vibrotactile discrimination task requires the comparison between the memory trace of f1 and the current sensory input of f2. We sought evidence of this operation in the S1 cortex, but as already indicated, the activity of these neurons does not combine f1 and f2 during the comparison period; they encode only information of f2. Where and how is this neuronal operation executed? A simple inspection of the neuronal activity in areas central to the S1 cortex indicated that the responses during the f2 period are quite complex (Fig. 14.10). For example, some S2 neurons encoded f2 in their firing rates similarly as for f1 (positive and negative slopes). But, surprisingly, many S2 neurons responded differentially during the comparison f2 > f1 or f2 < f1 trials during correct discriminations (Romo et al. 2002). These differential responses were even more abundant in areas of the frontal lobe (PFC, VPC, MPC, and M1) examined in this task (Hernández et al. 2002; Romo et al. 2004). The question is whether the responses during f2 depended on f1—even though f1 had been applied 3 seconds earlier—or they simply reflected their association with the motor responses. We ruled out the presence of a simple differential motor activity associated with the push-button presses by testing these neurons in a control task in which the same vibrotactile stimuli were used, but animals had to follow a visual cue to produce the motor responses. In this condition all neurons reduced the differential activity, indicating that the differential activity observed during the comparison period depends on the actual computation between f1 and f2 and does not reflect a purely motor response aimed to press one of the two push-buttons (Hernández et al. 2002; Romo et al. 2002, 2004).

If the neuronal discharges during the comparison period are the product of the interaction between f1 and f2, then the trace of f1 and the current f2 could be observed during the comparison period before the discharges indicated the motor decision responses. To further quantify these interactions between f1 and f2 and beyond it, we used the multivariate regression analysis described already. The analysis revealed the contributions of f1 and f2 during the comparison period for the S2, PFC, VPC, and MPC neurons (Fig. 14.10B–E). This is clearly shown in the successive time windows by plotting the coefficients a1 and a2 and the absolute difference between the two (a1 = –a2) during the entire sequence of the vibrotactile task (Figure 14.11). This allows appreciating the time dynamics of the neurons' response dependence on f1 and f2 for each of the cortical areas that are active during the vibrotactile discrimination task. This comparative analysis shows that the decision-making process is widely distributed through the cortex, although with various strengths across these areas (Romo et al. 2004). The comparison signal evolves into a signal, which is consistent with the motor choice, but this is again stronger in some areas than in others. But it is widespread nonetheless.

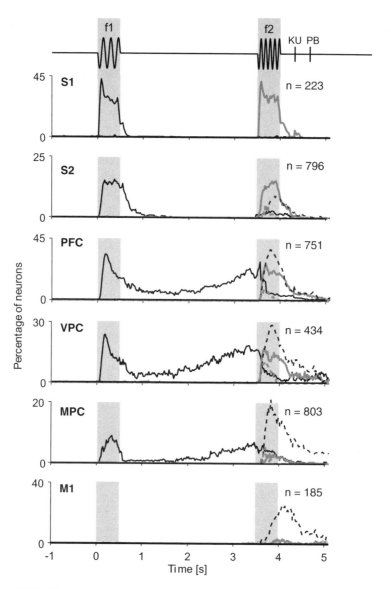

Figure 14.11. Dynamics of population responses of six cortical areas during the vibrotactile discrimination task. Coefficient values of a1 (black line), a2 (gray line), and as a function of the interaction between a1 and a2 (discontinuous black line) indicate those neurons that show f2 > f1 or f2 < f1. The responses are expressed as percentage of the total number of neurons (n) that had task-related responses. S1, primary somatosensory cortex; S2, secondary somatosensory cortex; PFC, prefrontal cortex; VPC, ventral premotor cortex; MPC, medial premotor cortex; M1, primary motor cortex. Original data from S1, S2, MPC, PVC, and M1 were previously published (Hernández et al. 2000, 2002; Romo et al. 2002, 2004), and data from PFC are unpublished results (Romo et al.).

The resulting motor signal is also observed in M1, but M1 does not seem to participate in the sensory, memory, and comparison components of the task (Fig. 14.10F
and 14.11). Also, the differential signal in M1 is considerably delayed in comparison to the S2 cortex, the PFC, the VPC, and the MPC (Romo et al. 2004).
The results suggest that the comparison between stored and ongoing sensory
information takes place in a distributed fashion. But, in their activity, do these
neurons predict the motor decision report?

DECODING DECISION PROCESSES FROM NEURONAL
ACTIVITY ACROSS CORTICAL AREAS

Responses during correct trials alone do not allow us to determine to what extent
the comparison-dependent responses observed in the S2 cortex and frontal lobe
are correlated with the sensory evaluation or with the monkey's action choice
itself (Figs. 14.10 and 14.11). To answer these questions, we sorted the responses
for each neuron into hits and errors and calculated a choice probability index
(Green and Swets 1966; Britten et al. 1996; Hernández et al. 2002; Romo et al.
2002, 2004). This method quantified for each f2, f1 pair whether responses during error trials were different from responses during correct trials (Figure 14.12).
If the responses were exclusively stimulus-dependent, they should show little or
no difference between error and correct trials. In contrast, if the responses were
linked to the monkey's choice, then the responses should vary according to which
button the monkey chose to press. In principle, this represents the probability
with which an observer of a neuron's response to a given (f1, f2) pair would accurately predict the monkey's choice. We found that the closer a neuron's responses
to correct trials were purely f2–f1 dependent, the higher the separation between
responses to correct and error trials, as quantified by a higher choice probability.
We also found that the choice probability indices increased during the course of
the f2 period. This was quite evident for those neurons that had f2–f1 responses,
but not for those neurons that responded to f2 only. This tendency was observed
for each area examined central to the S1 cortex (Romo et al. 2004). We illustrate
these processes for subgroups of VPC neurons in Figure 14.12. An interesting
finding was that the neuronal population that carried f1 information during the
delay period also shows large choice probability (above 0.5) values just before
the comparison period (Fig. 14.12). We suggest that this activity is related to the
working memory component of the task, as opposed to the decision component
of the task. If trial-by-trial variations of f1 encoding during the working memory
period correlate with trial-by-trial variations in performance, this will then be
reflected in the choice probability index. The choice probability analysis shows that
responses from the S2 cortex and the frontal cortex reflect the active comparisons
between f1 and f2 and the motor choice that is specific to the context of the vibrotactile discrimination task.

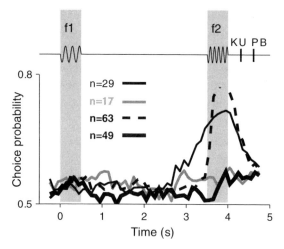

Figure 14.12. Correlation between neuronal and behavioral responses. Choice probability indices for ventral premotor cortex (VPC) neurons as functions of time for three different groups of neurons. Results are averaged over (f1, f2) pairs. **Black line:** neuronal responses that depended on f1 during the delay period and on f2–f1 during the comparison period; **gray line:** responses that depended only on f2 during the comparison period; **black discontinuous line:** neuronal responses that depended on f1 during the delay period and on f2–f1 during the comparison period; **thick line:** neuronal responses that had large choice probability indices (black line and black discontinuous line) but that tested in a control task in which animals had to follow a visual cue to produce the motor response. Modified from Romo et al. (2004).

POSTPONING THE DECISION REPORT

The vibrotactile discrimination task described above simulates a behavioral condition in which a perceptual decision based on a sensory evaluation is immediately reported through a voluntary action. However, depending on the behavioral demands, a perceptual decision can be postponed for later report. If postponed, it must be stored in working memory. But, what is stored in the memory circuits: the final decision itself, or the sensory information on which the decision is based? We investigated this question by recording from single neurons in the MPC, an area involved in decision making and motor choice (Hoshi and Tanji, 2004; Hernández et al. 2002; Romo et al. 1993, 1997), while trained monkeys discriminated the difference in frequency between consecutive vibrotactile stimuli, f1 and f2. Crucially, monkeys were asked to report discrimination after a fixed delay period between the end of f2 and a cue that triggered the beginning of the motor report. This delay period thus separates the comparison between the two stimuli from the motor response. Notice that the postponed decision report in this task is different from the processes involved in purely working memory tasks, in which the relevant process is holding the sensory cue until a cue triggers the behavioral report (Funahashi et al. 1989; Fuster 1973; Muhammad et al. 2006). In our task, monkeys must hold f1 in working memory and must compare the current sensory input f2 to the memory trace of f1, and must postpone the decision until a sensory cue triggers the motor report. We found that during the post-discrimination delay period, MPC neurons encode not only the differences between stimuli that correspond to the monkey's two possible choices but also past information on which the decision is based (Figure 14.13A). These responses could switch back and forth with remarkable flexibility across the post-discrimination period, from encoding the original information on which the decision is based to encoding the monkey's two possible choices (Fig. 14.13B). Moreover, MPC responses appear to participate directly in the monkey's decision-making process, as quantified by high choice probability indices obtained during the post-discrimination report period (Figure 14.14). Thus, maintaining in working

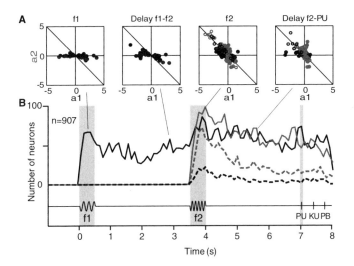

Figure 14.13. Dynamics of MPC population responses during the postponed decision report. (**A**) Values of a1 and a2 coefficients for all neurons' selected times (200 ms) in (**B**). For each point, at least one coefficient is significantly different from zero. Different plots are for various times in (**B**). n, number of neurons. (**B**) Number of neurons with significant coefficients as a function of time. Black and gray lines correspond to a1 and a2, respectively. Gray discontinuous line corresponds to neurons with both significant a1 and a2 coefficients of opposite signs but significantly different magnitudes; these are partially differential responses. Black discontinuous line corresponds to neurons with both significant a1 and a2 coefficients of opposite signs and statistically equal magnitude; these are fully differential or categorical responses encoding f2–f1. The dynamics of these coefficients was analyzed using a sliding window of 200 ms duration moving in steps of 100 ms. PU, probe up; KU, key up; PB, push-button. Adapted from Lemus et al. (2007).

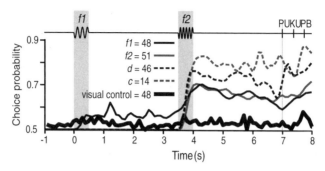

Figure 14.14. Correlation between neuronal and behavioral responses during the postponed decision report. Choice probability indices as a function of time. **Black line:** neurons that encoded information about f1; **gray line:** neurons that carried information about f2; **black discontinuous line:** partially differential neurons that carried information about f1 and f2 (**D**); **gray discontinuous line:** fully differential neurons that carried information about f2–f1 only (**C**); **thick black line:** neurons that had large choice probability indices and were tested in a control task in which animals received the same stimulus pairs but had to follow a visual cue to produce the motor choice response. Adapted from Lemus et al. (2007).

memory the original stimulus information on which the decision is based could serve to continuously update the postponed decision report in this task.

This result might be somewhat surprising in view of previous studies showing that a categorical decision consistent with the motor choice develops immediately after a sensory evaluation is completed (de Lafuente and Romo 2005; Shadlen and Newsome 1996, 2001). This could be explained by fundamental differences between these tasks. For example, decision reports in these tasks (de Lafuente and Romo 2005; Shadlen and Newsome 1996, 2001) are based on the evaluation of one single sensory quantity that varies from trial to trial, whereas in our task, discrimination is based on the evaluation of two quantities that vary also from trial to trial: one being the current sensory input f2, and the other, the memory trace of f1 (Hernández et al. 2002; Romo et al. 2002, 2004). In our task, however, some of the partially and fully differential responses that develop around the offset of f2 are consistent with those findings, because these predicted the monkey's motor choice. The question is why, during the postponed decision report period, information about the stimuli on which the decision is based is still present. As mentioned above, it is possible that the perceptual decision is revised or updated as long as there is time for it to be reconsidered. Our results are consistent with this interpretation, because most of the single neuron responses switched back and forth during the post-discrimination period, from encoding the original information on which the decision is based to encoding the monkey's two possible choices.

These results also have implications regarding the organization of the recurrent neuronal circuits thought to underlie working memory (Goldman-Rakic 1995; Fuster 1997; Miller et al. 2003). It is possible, for instance, that the neurons that store information about the stimuli during the postponed decision report period are linked to the neurons that compute the difference between stimulus frequencies and, thus, the motor choice (Goldman-Rakic 1995; Machens et al. 2005). Although a substantial number of the neurons that initially carried only sensory information later developed a differential signal that predicted the motor choice, such a link is difficult to prove. Another point to consider is that the MPC may be part of a larger network subserving working memory (Cisek 2006; Goldman-Rakic 1995; Fuster 1997; Machens et al. 2005; Miller et al. 2003). This is consistent with the fact that responses similar to those reported here have been recorded in the ventral premotor cortex and in the prefrontal cortex (unpublished results). Thus, these frontal circuits appear to be important nodes in the readout of sensory information from working memory at the service of action selection, two important ingredients in decision making. In fact, all these circuits are anatomically linked to sensory, memory, and motor circuits (Rizzolatti and Lupino 2001). Thus, these frontal circuits appear critically suited to integrate and reorganize all the elements associated with decision making in this task. Furthermore, they reflect the flexibility needed when a perceptual decision must be either immediately reported or postponed for later report.

GENERAL DISCUSSION

The evidence in this chapter suggests that the comparison between stored and ongoing sensory information takes place in a distributed fashion. It also suggests that there is a continuum between sensory- and motor-related activities. For example, f1 is encoded in multiple cortical areas. Such encoding seems to proceed in a serial fashion from the S1 cortex to the S2 cortex, the PFC, the VPC, and then to the MPC. Although the strength of this signal varies across these areas, all of those except for the S1 cortex store f1 at different times during the working memory component of the task. This is consistent with the proposal that there is a large cortical network that dynamically stores sensory information during working memory (Fuster 1997). During the comparison period, f2 is processed similarly by the same cortical areas. The comparison between the stored sensory information of f1 and the current sensory input of f2 is observed in the S2 cortex, the PFC, the VPC, and the MPC, again with various strengths across the cortical areas. This comparison signal evolves into a signal that is consistent with the motor choice; this is again stronger in some areas than in others, but it is widespread nonetheless. The resulting motor signal is also observed in M1, but it does not seem to participate in the sensory, memory, and comparison components of the task.

This comparative analysis shows that, in the vibrotactile task, the S1 cortex is predominantly sensory and M1 is predominantly motor, but otherwise there is broad overlap in response characteristics across all other cortical areas studied.

The difference between the S2 cortex, the PFC, the VPC, and the MPC might best be characterized as shifts in the distributions of response types (Figs. 14.10 and 14.11). For example, compare the PFC, the VPC, and the MPC: their response latencies were significantly different, with the f1 and f2 signals beginning slightly earlier in the PFC and the VPC than in the MPC (Romo et al. 2004). The percentages of neurons that encoded each component of the discrimination task were also different. These findings suggest that the premotor areas may coordinate the sensory, memory, and decision components of the task, but that these processes are first coordinated in the S2 cortex and the PFC. This result, however, should be interpreted cautiously, because recordings were made in different animals and the same population from each cortical area may vary from animal to animal.

An interesting finding worth detailed discussion is the existence of neural populations with opposite responses or, more precisely, of populations with opposite-sign tuning curves (positive and negative slopes). One of the simplest ways in which neurons could encode the frequency of vibratory stimuli is by means of a tuning curve in which particular firing rate values encoded particular stimulus frequencies, determined by any arbitrary function (Romo et al. 2003). Then, if all neurons of a given area had similar responses, pooling of individual responses could provide an accurate estimate of the stimulus frequency (the fidelity of this estimate would be determined by the correlation values among neurons) (Parker and Newsome 1998). Instead of this simple coding scheme, the results showed that, in all areas central to the S1 cortex, there is not a single, but a dual stimulus encoding. Given that the slopes are of opposite signs (antagonistic responses), pooling the activity of these two groups of neurons would not give any useful information about the stimulus frequency. Therefore, well-structured cortical circuits are necessary to keep the information of each separated population. As we have seen, this dual encoding is preserved along the processing levels, from the S2 cortex, the PFC, the VPC, and the MPC. What is the role of this dual representation?

It has been shown that responses of individual S2 neurons provide less information about the stimulus frequency than individual responses of S1 neurons (Romo et al. 2003; Salinas et al. 2000). Unlike the S1 cortex, where the information provided by individual neurons is enough to explain the monkeys' discrimination thresholds, neurometric curves obtained from individual responses of S2 neurons are well below the discrimination threshold of monkeys (Romo et al. 2003). Is sensory information degraded as it flows from the S1 cortex to the S2 cortex? At first glance, this may seem to be the case. However, combining the responses of neurons with opposite slopes could compensate for the loss of information. Indeed, we have shown that it is possible to recover the information apparently lost between the S1 cortex and the S2 cortex by means of a subtraction operation between pairs of neurons with opposite tuning curves (Romo et al. 2003). This operation, which can be thought of as a contrast enhancement mechanism, is particularly useful when neurons show positive correlation coefficients: subtracting the activity of two positively correlated neurons cancels correlated random modulations. Thus, the existence of neuronal populations with opposite signs constitutes a mechanism for representing sensory information along the successive processing stages of cortex, even though significant levels of positive correlation exist among the activity of the neurons. Importantly, this encoding scheme has also been found in the cortices of monkeys that require behavioral decisions based on sensory evaluation.

CONCLUDING REMARKS

The highly simplified sensory discrimination task used here requires perceiving a stimulus, storing it in working memory, combining the stored trace with the current sensory stimulus, and producing a decision that is communicated to the motor apparatus. The entire sequence of the task is reflected in the activity of neuronal populations from several cortical areas of the parietal and frontal lobes. Our results indicate that neurons from areas central to the S1 cortex do not simply wait for a signal encoding decision; rather, they participate at every step of its generation by combining working memory and sensory inputs. This process is carried out by two complementary neuronal responses. This dual representation is found in all areas central to the S1 cortex examined in this task, and might serve to compute optimally the entire perceptual process of the task. This coding scheme has also been found in some cortices of monkeys performing tasks that require behavioral decisions based on a comparison operation. An important problem posed by these findings is whether each neuronal correlate found in each cortical area actually has an impact in the perceptual task. Perhaps, microstimulation experiments of the type carried out in the S1 cortex are necessary to prove whether this is so.

ACKNOWLEDGMENTS

The research of R. Romo was supported in part by an International Research Scholars Award from the Howard Hughes Medical Institute and grants from CONACYT and DGAPA-UNAM.

REFERENCES

Adrian, E.D. (1928) *The basis of sensation. The action of the sense organs.* London: Christophers.

Britten, K.H., Newsome, W.T., Shadlen, M.N., Celebrini, S., and Movshon, J.A. (1996) A relationship between behavioral choice and the visual responses of neurons in macaque MT. *Vis Neurosci* 13:87–100.

Britten, K.H., and van Wezel, R.J. (1998) Electrical microstimulation of cortical MST biases heading perception in monkeys. *Nat Neurosci* 1:59–63.

Brody, C.D., Hernández, A., Zainos, A., and Romo R. (2003) Timing and neural encoding of somatosensory parametric working memory in macaque monkey. *Cereb Cortex* 13: 1196–207.

Burton, H., and Fabri, M. (1995a) Ipsilateral intracortical connections of physiologically defined cutaneous representations in areas 3b and 1 of macaque monkeys. *J Comp Neurol* 355:508–38.

Burton, H., Fabri, M. and Alloway, K. (1995b) Cortical areas within the lateral sulcus connected to cutaneous representations in areas 3b and 1: a revised interpretation of the second somatosensory area in macaque monkeys. *J Comp Neurol* 355:539–62.

Cipolloni, P.B., and Pandya, D.N. (1999) Cortical connections of the frontoparietal opercular areas in the rhesus monkey. *J Comp Neurol* 403:431–58.

Cisek, P. (2006) Integrated neural processes for defining potential actions and deciding between them: a computational model. *J Neurosci* 26:9761–70.

de Lafuente, V. and Romo, R. (2005) Neuronal correlates of subjective sensory experience. *Nat Neurosci* 12:1698–1703.

de Lafuente, V. and Romo, R. (2006) Neural correlate of subjective sensory experience gradually builds up across cortical areas. *Proc Natl Acad Sci USA* 10:1266–71.

Disbrow, E.A., Litinas, E., Recanzone, G.H., Padberg, J., and Krubitzer, L. Cortical connections of the second somatosensory area and the parietal ventral area in macaque monkeys. *J Comp Neurol* 462:382–99.

Funahashi, S., Bruce, C.J. and Goldman-Rakic, P.S. (1989) Mnemonic coding of visual space in the monkey's dorsolateral prefrontal cortex. *J Neurophysiol* 61:331–49.

Fuster, J.M. (1973) Unit activity in prefrontal cortex during delayed-response performance: neuronal correlates of transient memory. *J Neurophysiol* 36:61–78.

Fuster, J. (1997) Network memory. *Trends Neurosci* 20:451–9.

Godschalk, M., Lemon, R.N., Kuypers, H.G., and Ronday, H.K. (1984) Cortical afferents and efferents of monkey postarcuate area: an anatomical and electrophysiological study. *Exp Brain Res* 56:410–24.

Goldman-Rakic, P.S. (1995) Cellular basis of working memory. *Neuron* 14:477–85.

Gold, J.I., and Shadlen, M.N. (2007) The neural basis of decision making. *Annu Rev Neurosci* 30:535–74.

Green, D.M., and Swets, J.A. (1966). *Signal detection theory and psychophysics.* New York: Wiley.

Hernández, A., Salinas, E., Garcia, R., and Romo, R. (1997). Discrimination in the sense of flutter: new psychophysical measurements in monkeys. *J Neurosci* 17:6391–400.

Hernández, A., Zainos, A., and Romo, R. (2000). Neuronal correlates of sensory discrimination in the somatosensory cortex. *Proc Natl Acad Sci USA* 97:6091–6.

Hernández, A., Zainos, A., and Romo, R. (2002). Temporal evolution of a decision-making process in medial premotor cortex. *Neuron* 33:959–72.

Hoshi, E., and Tanji, J. (2004) Differential roles of neural activity in the supplementary and presupplementary motor areas: from information retrieval to motor planning and execution. *J Neurophysiol* 92:3482–9.

Hubel, D.H., and Wiesel, T.N. (1998) Early exploration of the visual cortex. *Neuron* 20: 401–12.

Kepecs, A., Wang, X.J., and Lisman, J. (2002) Bursting neurons signal input slope. *J Neurosci* 22:9053–62.

Krahe, R., and Gabbiani, F. (2004) Burst firing in sensory systems. *Nat Rev Neurosci* 5:13–24.

Lemus, L., Hernández, A., Luna, R., Zainos, A., Nácher, V., and Romo, R. (2007) Neural correlates of a postponed decision report. *Proc Natl Acad Sci USA* 104:17174–9.

Luna, R., Hernández, A., Brody, C.D., and Romo, R. (2005) Neural codes for perceptual discrimination in primary somatosensory cortex. *Nat Neurosci* 8:1210–9.

Macefield, G., Gandevia, S.C., and Burke, D. (1990) Perceptual responses to microstimulation of single afferents innervating joints, muscles and skin of the human hand. *J Physiol* 429:113–29.

Machens, C.K., Romo, R., and Brody, C.D. (2005) Flexible control mutual inhibition: A neural model of two-interval discrimination. *Science* 307:1121–1224.

Martínez-Conde, S., Mckinik, S.L., and Hubel, D.H. (2000) The function of bursts of spikes during visual fixation in the awake primate lateral geniculate nucleus and primary visual cortex. *Proc Natl Acad Sci USA* 99:13920–5.

Miller, P., Brody, C.D., Romo, R., and Wang, X-J. (2003) Recurrent network model of somatosensory parametric memory in the prefrontal cortex. *Cereb Cortex* 13:1208–18.

Mountcastle, V.B. (1957) Modality and topographic properties of single neurons of cat's somatic sensory cortex. *J Neurophysiol* 20:408–34.

Mountcastle, V.B., Steinmetz, M.A., and Romo, R. (1990) Frequency discrimination in the sense of flutter: psychophysical measurements correlated with postcentral events in behaving monkeys. *J Neurosci* 10:3032–44.

Mountcastle, V.B., Talbot, W.H., Darian-Smith, I., and Kornhuber, H.H. (1967) Neural basis of the sense of flutter-vibration. *Science* 155:597–600.

Mountcastle, V.B., Talbot, W.H., Sakata, H., and Hyvärinen, J. (1969) Cortical neuronal mechanisms in flutter-vibration studied in unanesthetized monkeys. Neuronal periodicity and frequency discrimination. *J Neurophysiol* 32:452–84.

Muhammad, R., Wallis, J.D., and Miller, E.K. (2006) A comparison of abstract rules in the prefrontal cortex, premotor cortex, inferior temporal cortex, and striatum. *J Cog Neurosci* 18:974–89.

Newsome, W.T., Britten, K.H., and Movshon, J.A. (1989) Neural correlates of a perceptual decision. *Nature* 341:52–4.

Ochoa, J., and Torebjörk, E. (1983) Sensations evoked by intraneural microstimulation of single mechanoreceptor units innervating the human hand. *J Physiol* 342:633–54.

Parker, A.J., and Newsome, W.T. (1998) Sense and the single neuron: probing the physiology of perception. *Annu Rev Neurosci* 21:227–77.

Pons, T.P., Garraghty, P.E., Friedman, D.P., and Mishkin, M. (1987) Physiological evidence for serial processing in somatosensory cortex. *Science* 237:417–20.

Powell, T.P.S., and Mountcastle, V.B. (1959) Some aspects of the functional organization of the cortex of the postcentral gyrus of the monkey: a correlation of findings obtained in a single unit analysis with cytoarchitecture. *Bull Johns Hopkins Hosp* 105:133–62.

Recanzone, G.H., Merzenich, M.M., and Schreiner, C.E. (1992) Changes in the distributed temporal response properties of SI cortical neurons reflect improvements in performance on a temporally based tactile discrimination task. *J Neurophysiol* 67:1071–91.

Reinagel, P., Godwin, D., Sherman, M., and Koch, C. (1999) Encoding of visual information by LGN bursts. *J Neurophysiol* 81:2558–69.

Rizzolatti, G., and Lupino, G. (2001) The cortical motor system. *Neuron* 31:889–901.

Romo, R., Brody, C.D., Hernández, A., and Lemus, L. (1999) Neuronal correlates of parametric working memory in the prefrontal cortex. *Nature* 399:470–3.

Romo, R., Hernández, A., and Zainos, A. (2004) Neuronal correlates of a perceptual decision in ventral premotor cortex. *Neuron* 41:165–73.

Romo, R., Hernández, A., Zainos, A., Brody, C.D., and Lemus, L. (2000) Sensing without touching: psychophysical performance based on cortical microstimulation. *Neuron* 26:273–8.

Romo, R., Hernández, A., Zainos, A., Lemus, L., and Brody, C.D. (2002) Neuronal correlates of decision-making in secondary somatosensory cortex. *Nat Neurosci* 5:1217–25.

Romo, R., Hernández, A., Zainos, A., and Salinas, E. (1998) Somatosensory discrimination based on cortical microstimulation. *Nature* 392:387–90.

Romo, R., Hernández, A., Zainos, A., and Salinas, E. (2003) Correlated neuronal discharges that increase coding efficiency during perceptual discrimination. *Neuron* 38:649–57.

Romo, R., Merchant, H., Zainos, A., and Hernández, A. (1997) Categorical perception of somesthetic stimuli: psychophysical measurements correlated with neuronal events in primate medial premotor cortex. *Cereb Cortex* 7:317–26.

Romo, R., Ruiz, C., Crespo, P., Zainos, A., and Merchant, H. (1993) Representation of tactile signals in primate supplementary motor cortex. *J Neurophysiol* 70:2690–4.

Romo, R., and Salinas, E. (2001) Touch and go: Decision-making mechanisms in somatosensation. *Annu Rev Neurosci* 24:107–37.

Romo, R., and Salinas, E. (2003) Flutter discrimination: neural codes, perception, memory and decision making. *Nat Rev Neurosci* 4:203–18.

Salinas, E., Hernández, A., Zainos, A., and Romo, R. (2000) Periodicity and firing rate as candidate neural codes for the frequency of vibrotactile stimuli. *J Neurosci* 20:5503–15.

Salzman, D., Britten, K.H., and Newsome, W.T. (1990) Cortical microstimulation influences perceptual judgements of motion direction. *Nature* 346:174–7.

Schall, J.D. (2001) Neural basis of deciding, choosing and acting. *Nat Rev Neurosci* 2: 583–91.

Shadlen, M.N., and Newsome, W.T. (1996) Motion perception: seeing and deciding. *Proc Natl Acad Sci USA* 93:628–33.

Shadlen, M.N., and Newsome, W.T. (2001) Neural basis of a perceptual decision in the parietal cortex (area LIP) of the rhesus monkey. *J Neurophysiol* 86:1916–36.

Sur, M., Wall, J.T., and Kaas, J.H. (1984) Modular distribution of neurons with slowly adapting and rapidly adapting responses in area 3b of somatosensory cortex in monkeys. *J Neurophysiol* 51:724–44.

Talbot, W.H., Darian-Smith, I., Kornhuber, H.H., and Mountcastle, V.B. (1968) The sense of flutter-vibration: comparison of the human capacity response patterns of mechanoreceptive afferents from the monkey hand. *J Neurophysiol* 31:301–34.

Vallbo, A.B. (1995) Single-afferent neurons and somatic sensation in humans. In: Gazzaniga, MS, editor. *The cognitive neurosciences*. Cambridge: MIT Press, pp. 237–52.

Vallbo, A.B., and Johansson, R.S. (1984) Properties of cutaneous mechanoreceptors in the human hand related to touch sensations. *Hum Neurobiol* 3:3–14.

Chapter Fifteen

Human Neural Stem Cell–Mediated Repair of the Contused Spinal Cord: Timing the Microenvironment

Brian J. Cummings, Mitra J. Hooshmand,
Desirée L. Salazar, and Aileen J. Anderson

INTRODUCTION

Spinal cord injury (SCI) is a debilitating and devastating condition that affects approximately 11,000 new people in the United States each year, with estimates of individuals currently suffering from this injury reaching 250,000 in the United States alone (Ackery et al. 2004). With a high incidence in the younger population, SCI results in enormous financial and physical costs for affected individuals, their families, and society as a whole (Tator et al. 1993; Ackery et al. 2004). For the past 15 years, pharmacological treatment of SCI has primarily relied on the use of steroids, such as methylprednisolone, and other anti-inflammatory agents (Baptiste and Fehlings 2006; Sipski and Pearse 2006). However, this approach has recently lost favor in light of limited improvements and risk of infection. A more comprehensive understanding of the basic biological mechanisms in experimental models of spinal cord injury (SCI) could suggest alternative therapeutic targets.

Understanding of the pathophysiology and potential points of therapeutic intervention for human SCI has been shaped strongly by the results of studies performed in laboratory animals. Accordingly, appropriate selection of relevant models and utilization of reproducible, standardized, and consistent methods will be essential for clinical translation. In this regard, three animal models of SCI have been central to investigating SCI mechanisms and treatments: contusion, compression, and transection (Grill 2005).

Contusion injuries are the most common type of spinal injury in humans (>49% of cases). In animal models, contusion injuries are induced by exposing the spinal cord to a mechanical trauma while the dura is maintained intact (Jakeman et al. 2000; Stokes and Jakeman 2002; Young 2002; Scheff et al. 2003). Contusion injuries have become widely accepted in the field of SCI as clinically relevant experimental models. Histopathology of the injured spinal cord in these models is generally assessed using defined parameters including white and gray matter loss, white and gray matter sparing, and total lesion volume.

ASSESSMENT OF FUNCTIONAL RECOVERY IN ANIMAL MODELS OF SCI

A number of instruments are available to assess locomotor recovery in rodents following SCI. Due to the range of possible outcomes following SCI, from complete hindlimb paralysis to normal locomotion with slightly impaired trunk stability or paw position, a single instrument cannot differentiate with equal sensitivity across such a broad spectrum of recovery. Open-field locomotion in spinal injured rats can be assessed using the Basso, Beattie, and Bresnahan locomotor rating scale, the BBB (Basso et al. 1995). This test can assess a wide variety of spinal injuries resulting in impairments ranging from partial joint movement, to weight supported standing, through coordinated walking and trunk stability.

Similarly, the Basso Mouse Scale (BMS) was developed for open-field locomotor assessment to account for the unique recovery pattern seen in mice (Engesser-Cesar et al. 2005; Basso et al. 2006). Both the BBB and BMS are designed to assess gross recovery levels across the full range of recovery, but can be less sensitive at specific levels of recovery, in part due to the ordinal nature of the scale. This issue may be particularly limiting when discriminating between animals that have achieved some degree of coordination between forelimbs and hindlimbs.

Other instruments to evaluate forelimb and hindlimb function include grid walking (Kunkel-Bagden et al. 1993; Prakriya et al. 1993), rope climbing (Z'Graggen et al. 1998), inclined plane (Rivlin and Tator 1977), kinematic analysis (Gimenez y Ribotta et al. 1998), gait analysis (including CatWalk) (Hamers et al. 2006), measures of ground reaction forces (Muir and Whishaw 1999), and the horizontal ladder beam (Cummings et al. 2007).

ACUTE, SUBACUTE, AND CHRONIC PHASES POST-SCI

Strategies for repair after SCI are dependent on the characterization of the progression of degenerative and regenerative processes, and on the identification of therapeutic windows for intervention. Classification of acute, subacute, and chronic time points is somewhat nebulous in both rodent models and the human clinical SCI setting. The acute period after SCI in humans is often defined based on the period of initial hospitalization, extending for days and perhaps weeks, after the traumatic injury (Fawcett et al. 2007). In contrast, in animal models of SCI this phase is generally equated with the period during which neuroprotective strategies would have the potential for efficacy, and it is therefore defined based on histological assessment of traumatic cell death and degeneration, extending from the time of initial insult to 2–3 days post-SCI.

The subacute and chronic stages are more challenging to define, but it has been suggested that a relatively stable host microenvironment in which the spinal cord undergoes little to no physiological and functional change could be reasonably classified as chronically injured (Houle and Tessler 2003). Assessment of neurological measures to rate functional change in cervical-injured individuals suggests that spontaneous recovery occurs for up to 6 months following SCI but remains relatively stable 6–12 months post-injury (Fawcett et al. 2007). A chronic time frame in a clinical setting would therefore hypothetically begin 6 months following SCI. In rodents, changes in spinal cord pathology (defined as lesion size, circuitry reorganization, and endogenous repair capacity) following contusion SCI have been shown to continue for at least 3 weeks (Hill et al. 2001), whereas behavioral recovery in moderately contused rats reaches a plateau approximately 2–3 weeks post-SCI (Basso et al. 1995). A chronic time frame in an animal model setting could therefore be defined as at least 4 weeks post-SCI.

Based on the definition above, the subacute period would, by default, be classified as any time point falling between acute and chronic on this continuum (Fawcett et al. 2007). As discussed below, studies in our laboratory address mechanisms of recovery in mice following what we will define here as acute (0-dpi [days post-injury]), subacute (9-dpi), and chronic (30-dpi) time points after SCI.

THE DYNAMIC SCI NICHE: ACUTE TO CHRONIC CHANGES IN THE MICROENVIRONMENT POST-SCI

The environment in the spinal cord following initial mechanical trauma is dynamic, including both primary injury and secondary degenerative processes. In the acute period, hours to days post-SCI, the blood–brain barrier is disrupted, even in closed contusion or compression models. This leads to the rapid invasion into the CNS of blood and serum components including thrombin, heme, circulating antibodies, chemokines/cytokines, and complement components (Anderson 2002). Additionally, constituents of the cellular immune response are rapidly recruited to the site of damage, particularly polymorphonuclear neutrophils followed by macrophages/microglia (Popovich and Jones 2003; Jones et al. 2005). The role of the inflammatory response to SCI is complex, contributing to control of infection, clearance of debris, and possibly modulation of endogenous host regeneration and oligodendrocyte progenitor cells (OPCs) and neurogenesis over the subacute and chronic stages post-SCI (Anderson 2002; Foote and Blakemore 2005a; Foote and Blakemore 2005b; Rus et al. 2006; Schwartz et al. 2006). Concurrently, glutamate is released from central nervous system (CNS) cells directly damaged by the initial trauma, contributing to a wave of excitotoxic, ischemic, and oxidative secondary death of both neurons and oligodendrocytes (Kigerl et al. 2006; Belegu et al. 2007).

In the subacute period, within days to weeks post-SCI, astrocytes become hypertrophic and reactive, upregulating glial fibrillary acidic protein (GFAP) and proliferating in an attempt to protect the CNS by repairing the disrupted blood–brain barrier (Faulkner et al. 2004; Sofroniew 2005). Over a period of several weeks, delayed apoptosis of white matter oligodendrocytes extends out rostrally and caudally from the injury epicenter, resulting in increased axonal demyelination distal from the initial lesion site (Crowe et al. 1997). During this period, a glial scar that includes growth-inhibitory molecules such as chondroitin-sulfate proteoglycans (CSPGs) is formed (Davies et al. 1997; Fitch et al. 1999; Silver and Miller 2004).

The physical and molecular properties of the glial scar contribute to an environment that is not permissive for neurite outgrowth and it inhibits axonal regeneration (Fawcett and Asher 1999; Chen et al. 2002; Fawcett 2006). This inhibitory environment is further confounded by the presence of myelin-associated inhibitors of regeneration (MAIs) (Chaudhry and Filbin 2007; Gonzenbach and Schwab 2008), which have also recently been reported to exert effects on stem cell migration and fate (Zhao et al. 2007; Syed et al. 2008; Wang et al. 2008). Finally, during this subacute period, depending on the species, either a fibronectin-rich matrix (mice) or a fluid-filled cystic cavity (rats and a majority of humans) develops at the site of trauma (Stokes and Jakeman 2002; Inman and Steward 2003).

There have been few studies in animal models or human SCI patients assessing variables such as inflammation, cell death, scar or lesion remodeling, or other events in chronic conditions. The few studies that have been completed suggest that there may be a chronic contribution of inflammatory, and possibly other processes, to continued remodeling of the injured cord as a part of ongoing degenerative events, regenerative events, or both (Fleming et al. 2006; Nguyen et al. 2008). Investigation of the dynamics of the host microenvironment after SCI may improve identification of successful therapeutic targets for SCI, as well as the optimal clinical timing for their application based on cell type.

TARGETS AND TIMING FOR SCI INTERVENTION

Potential points of intervention for SCI are defined by the acute, subacute, and chronic stages of pathogenesis. Conventional treatment strategies have focused on three main targets: (1) minimizing the initial lesion and loss of neurons and oligodendrocytes by neuroprotective intervention, for example, via administration of trophic factors, antioxidants, anti-inflammatories, etc.; (2) promoting functional circuitry reorganization by providing trophic factors to increase host sprouting/ regeneration; and (3) promoting functional circuitry reorganization by modulating the inhibitory microenvironment via removal of the proteoglycan scar or blockade of MAIs or MAI signaling. In this regard, anti-inflammatory agents (Bethea et al. 1999), steroids (Wells et al. 2003), as well as infusion of trophic factors such as GDNF (Cheng et al. 2002), BDNF, and NT-3 (Namiki et al. 2000) have been shown to exert neuroprotective roles when administered early following injury. Similarly, administration of chondroitinase ABC to digest CSPGs in the injured rat cord has been shown to result in behavioral recovery associated with regeneration of corticospinal, raphespinal, and spinothalamic tract axons (Bradbury et al. 2002; Ikegami et al. 2005; Fawcett 2006; Kim et al. 2006). Additionally, studies using either neutralizing antibodies directed against Nogo, a myelin-associated inhibitor of neurite outgrowth, or blockade of the neuronal receptors for MAIs or their downstream signaling pathways have demonstrated regeneration of corticospinal tract fibers in injured rats (Brosamle et al. 2000; Fournier et al. 2003; Ji et al. 2006).

CELL TRANSPLANTATION AS A THERAPEUTIC INTERVENTION FOR SCI

Several additional points of intervention are afforded through cell transplantation approaches. These include: (1) promoting remyelination of spared axons, either through transplantation of alternative myelinating cell populations (Schwann cells or olfactory ensheathing cells) or transplantation of stem or progenitor cell populations with the capacity to replace oligodendrocytes lost after injury; (2) promoting restoration of disrupted circuitry via transplantation of stem or progenitor cell populations that could contribute to formation of bridge or bypass connections, reconnecting severed projection pathways; and (3) initiating neuronal replacement via transplantation of stem cell–derived neural progenitor populations (e.g., motor neurons or interneurons), which could have applications for specific types of SCI, for example, cervical trauma in which loss of motor neuron pools at the level of damage produces key deficits in function (such as tricep control).

A wide array of cell transplantation strategies, including transplantation of stem cell populations, have been tested for the potential to promote recovery in animal models of SCI. These include, but are not limited to, olfactory ensheathing cells (Lu et al. 2002; Keyvan-Fouladi et al. 2003; Ramer et al. 2004; Sasaki et al. 2006), bone marrow stromal cells (Hofstetter et al. 2002; Swanger et al. 2005), Schwann cells (Pearse et al. 2004; Hill et al. 2006), genetically modified fibroblasts

(Liu et al. 2002; Murray et al. 2002; Tobias et al. 2003; Nothias et al. 2005), embryonic-derived neural/glial stem cells (McDonald et al. 1999; Liu et al. 2000; Keirstead et al. 2005), and fetal/adult neural stem cells (NSCs) (Cummings et al. 2005; Karimi-Abdolrezaee et al. 2006; Kamei et al. 2007; Tarasenko et al. 2007; Yan et al. 2007). Many of these studies have focused selectively on successful cell transplantation, whereas few have addressed cell differentiation and the mechanisms of recovery following engraftment. Yet understanding the mechanisms by which cell-based therapies may affect SCI will be critical for understanding how these cells affect functional recovery in a clinically relevant way.

ALTERNATIVE MECHANISMS OF CELL-MEDIATED REPAIR

Though the presumptive strategy behind transplantation of stem cell populations for SCI has been cell replacement via integration of myelinating cells or new neurons, it is increasingly clear that transplanted cells can and do have a variety of effects on the host microenvironment. Genetically modified fibroblasts, olfactory ensheathing cells, Schwann cells, and NSCs have been reported to promote host axonal regeneration (Liu et al. 1999; Liu et al. 2002; Keyvan-Fouladi et al. 2003; Tobias et al. 2003; Heine et al. 2004; Hill et al. 2004; Ishii et al. 2006). Transplantation of OPCs after SCI has been reported to promote white matter sparing (Bambakidis and Miller 2004). Similarly, implantation of a polymer scaffold containing NSCs in contused rat spinal cord has been shown to reduce tissue loss and glial scarring (Teng et al. 2002), and transplantation of GFP-labeled glial-restricted progenitors (GRPs) has been shown to reduce astroglial scarring and CSPG deposition as early as 8 days post-transplant (Hill et al. 2004). Similar modifications altering the permissiveness of the post-SCI microenvironment and promotion of regeneration have been reported for GRPs (Davies et al. 2006).

In addition to modulation of the scar, stem cells may also provide the host microenvironment with trophic factors or a permissive guidance substrate that could play a role for both neuroprotection and regeneration, or alter the recruitment of endogenous precursor populations that could contribute to repair. OPCs derived from human embryonic stem cells have recently been reported to express a number of neurotrophins, including TGF-β and BDNF in vitro (Zhang et al. 2006). BDNF, GDNF, and NGF have been demonstrated to be present in higher amounts in NSC-transplanted animals compared to vehicle controls following a lesion to the spinal cord motor neuron pools (Yan et al. 2004). Immortalized NSCs have also been shown to secrete a variety of neurotrophins, both in vitro and in vivo (Lu et al. 2003). Additionally, transplantation of adult neural precursors in combination with fibroblasts into the contusion SCI cavity has been shown to enhance the regeneration of host axons, which were reported to align longitudinally in association with transplanted GFAP-positive precursors (Pfeifer et al. 2004). Finally, recruitment of host Schwann cells by transplanted Schwann cells has been suggested to play a significant role in remyelination in some animal models of SCI (Hill et al. 2006).

Critically, modulation of the host microenvironment by transplanted cell populations may extend beyond direct effects within the CNS, as both neural stem cells/precursors and mesenchymal stem cells have been shown to modulate the host immune response to injury and disease (Pluchino et al. 2005; Ziv et al. 2006; Einstein et al. 2007; Gerdoni et al. 2007). Collectively, the current literature supports multiple mechanisms by which engrafted stem cells could either directly integrate with the host or indirectly affect the host microenvironment following CNS injury.

NEURAL STEM CELLS AND SCI

NSCs are multipotent stem cells that are lineage-restricted to generate three populations of CNS cells: neurons, oligodendrocytes, and astrocytes. This population of stem cells can be derived from rodent and human embryonic, fetal, and adult tissue. NSCs have numerous potential applications for repair/regeneration of various neurodegenerative diseases, including Parkinson's disease, Alzheimer's disease, Huntington's disease, stroke, traumatic brain injury, and SCI. NSC transplantation could promote recovery by multiple mechanisms, including: (1) differentiation into neurons and oligodendrocytes and integrating with the host circuitry, (2) release of factors that modify the host microenvironment, and (3) via a combination of mechanisms 1 and 2. In the following sections, we focus on specific microenvironment and cell-intrinsic factors that may contribute to the therapeutic potential of NSCs in the CNS.

INFLUENCE OF THE MICROENVIRONMENT ON CELL FATE AND POTENTIAL FOR REPAIR

Transplantation of NSCs into normal CNS tissue results in region-specific differentiation, suggesting that factors in the transplantation niche contribute to fate selection. NSCs transplanted into neurogenic regions of the brain such as the hippocampus exhibit differentiation to neurons and oligodendrocytes, whereas NSCs transplanted into less neurogenic regions of the brain such as the cerebellum or striatum exhibit preferential differentiation to astrocytes (Gage et al. 1995; Brustle et al. 1998; Flax et al. 1998; Fricker et al. 1999; Herrera et al. 1999; Chow et al. 2000; Shihabuddin et al. 2000; Cao et al. 2001). Similarly, it appears that local cues within the spinal cord selectively promote glial differentiation of transplanted multipotent NSCs. Adult NSCs differentiate into neurons after engraftment into the dentate gyrus of the hippocampus, but they are unable to exhibit neurogenic potential when transplanted into the adult intact spinal cord, where they demonstrate predominantly astrocytic differentiation (Shihabuddin et al. 2000). Together, these data suggest that the microenvironment into which cell populations are transplanted affects the fate of engrafted cells.

The restrictive cues that limit the differentiation potential of transplanted cells remain to be elucidated, but they appear to be augmented in the injured spinal cord. Many studies have demonstrated that when neural cell populations are transplanted acutely (Chow et al. 2000; Vroemen et al. 2003; Hill et al. 2004) or subacutely (Cao et al. 2002; Macias et al. 2006) after SCI, the engrafted cells either remain undifferentiated or primarily differentiate into glia. The mechanisms regulating glial lineage restriction after SCI are not well understood, and there has been a lack of empirical testing to determine whether variations in cell fate potential across different studies reflect aspects of the host niche or intrinsic properties of different cell populations and/or derivation methods.

INFLUENCE OF CELL-INTRINSIC PROPERTIES ON POTENTIAL FOR REPAIR

Although local signals within the host niche could affect stem cell fate and influence recovery, it is also possible that the intrinsic properties of transplanted cells influence these processes and the resultant capacity for neurorepair. Both the heterogeneity and differentiation capabilities of NSCs could be affected by the method used to derive and culture the cells prior to transplantation. Currently, two main approaches have been established for culturing NSCs: (1) as a monolayer of substrate-anchored cells (Richards et al. 1992; Palmer et al. 1999), and (2) as neurospheres (Reynolds and Weiss 1992). When cultured under conditions that do not promote differentiation, NSCs grown as monolayers can retain their multipotent capacity and give rise to neural precursor/progenitor populations (Pollard et al. 2006; Babu et al. 2007; Daadi et al. 2008). When expanded as neurospheres, NSCs represent a heterogeneous population of both multipotent neural stem cells and more restricted progenitors (Kim et al. 2006). It is possible that cells grown as monolayers versus neurospheres would behave differently in an in vivo setting.

In addition to the culturing techniques, the source of transplanted NSCs (i.e., murine vs. human, embryonic vs. fetal) adds another variable to the interpretation of SCI studies addressing cell fate in vivo. Diversity in source of original cell populations, methods of isolation, and preparation of cells all make it difficult to compare starting populations between studies. In the remainder of this chapter, we focus exclusively on studies from our lab using human CNS-derived neural stem cells (HuCNS-SC) isolated from the fetal brain and propagated as neurospheres, conducted in collaboration with StemCells, Inc. HuCNS-SCs are unique as a human NSC population because these lines are prospectively isolated based on fluorescence-activated cell sorting for a CD133+ and CD24-/lo population (Uchida et al. 2000). This process theoretically selects for an NSC-enriched population; accordingly, these cells exhibit approximately a 2,000-fold enhancement in neurosphere initiating capacity. It is unknown whether the cell-intrinsic properties of NSCs prospectively isolated by this or similar methods differ from other NSC populations. However, it is possible that selection for specific markers could alter either the response of the cells to the microenvironment or, conversely, the effect of the microenvironment on the cells.

TIMING THE MICROENVIRONMENT

Transplantation studies following SCI are often performed within 7–14 days post-injury (dpi), a period that has been referred to as the "window of opportunity" (Okano 2002). However, the basis for a therapeutic window lacks supporting empirical data in which multiple transplantation times with the same cell population have been tested and mechanisms of host recovery compared. Thus, one issue we have investigated in detail is the effect of the injured niche over time on stem cell survival, fate, and ability to promote recovery of locomotor function.

Below, we present a subset of studies from our laboratory that focus on the injured microenvironment using identical methodology and cell source, while varying the time post-injury at which HuCNS-SC are transplanted. This allows for a direct comparison of time in relationship to NSC survival, differentiation, and potential to promote functional recovery. This series of studies used female NOD-scid mice. NOD-scid mice are constitutively immunodeficient, lacking a normal T-cell, B-cell, and complement response. As such, NOD-scid mice provide an excellent experimental model in which the potential of transplanted human cell populations to engraft and promote histological and locomotor recovery can be assessed in the absence of confounds due to a xenograft rejection response (Greiner et al. 1998).

In our studies, NOD-scid mice received a moderate contusion injury and transplantation with HuCNS-SC in either the acute, subacute, or chronic phase post-SCI. Animals received a total of 1μl of cell suspension at 75,000 cells/μl, injected into the parenchyma above and below the contusion epicenter (250nl at each of four injection sites), as described previously (Cummings et al. 2005, 2006).

SUBACUTE TRANSPLANTATION OF HuCNS-SCs

In our initial studies using HuCNS-SC in a 9-dpi paradigm, we found successful engraftment in all HuCNS-SC–transplanted animals (Figure 15.1C). Engrafted cells transplanted at vertebral level T9 migrated rostrally to T6 and caudally to T12. Migration past these levels was not investigated, and no evidence of migration toward the SCI epicenter was observed. A subset of HuCNS-SC integrated within the host circuitry and terminally differentiated into myelinating oligodendrocytes and synapse-forming neurons, based on immuno-electron microscopy. Based on double immunofluorescence labeling and confocal microscopy, approximately 64% of differentiated human cells expressed the oligodendrocytic marker CC-1/APC, whereas 25% expressed the neuronal marker ß-tubulin III. Surprisingly, less than 3% expressed the astrocytic marker GFAP. Though HuCNS-SC migrated in both the white and gray matter, the morphology of cells located in these regions was distinct and consistent with oligodendrocyte and neuronal differentiation, respectively (Fig. 15.1D).

HuCNS-SCs promoted locomotor recovery on open-field testing (BBB/BMS) and on the horizontal ladder beam. A number of studies have shown evidence for integration of transplanted cell populations within the host based on anatomical and/or physiological analyses (Cummings et al. 2005; Keirstead et al. 2005; Karimi-Abdolrezaee et al. 2006; Yan et al. 2007). However, whether survival of integrated cells was required for maintenance of recovery of function had not been previously investigated. We tested this possibility using selective ablation of engrafted HuCNS-SC with diphtheria toxin, which abolished locomotor improvements (Cummings et al. 2005), suggesting that integration of HuCNS-SC within the mouse host was responsible for recovery.

This initial study did not investigate additional possible mechanisms of functional recovery induced by HuCNS-SCs, such as promotion of tissue sparing, reduction of glial scarring, or enhancement of host regeneration. Nor were the number of engrafted cells quantified. In a subsequent analysis of animals transplanted subacutely (9-dpi), stereological quantification revealed an average of 145,000 HuCNS-SCs in transplanted animals (Hooshmand et al. 2005, 2006). Unbiased stereological determination of lesion volume, tissue sparing, glial scarring (as assessed by GFAP or CSPG), sprouting of host serotonergic fibers, and angiogenesis detected no significant differences between control animals and animals transplanted with HuCNS-SCs on any of these parameters. Additionally, linear regression analysis of the number of engrafted HuCNS-SCs versus the number of errors on a horizontal ladder beam task revealed a negative correlation between these variables, suggesting that increased engraftment was directly related to a reduction in errors in this quantitative measure of locomotor recovery (Hooshmand et al. 2006, 2008). Taken together, these data support the hypothesis that subacute HuCNS-SC transplantation after SCI mediates functional recovery

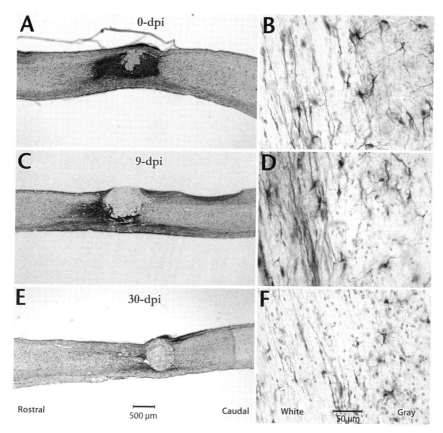

Figure 15.1. (A–F): Survival, migration, and site-specific differentiation of HuCNS-SCs in the injured mouse spinal cord. Photomicrographs of spinal cord 12 weeks (0-dpi) or 16 weeks (9-dpi and 30-pdi) post-transplantation immunostained for a human cytoplasmic marker (SC121, brown DAB, StemCells, Inc.) and counterstained with methyl green to reveal host mouse cells. Scale bar for **A, C,** and **E** = 500μm; scale bar for **B, D,** and **E** = 50μm. All images are orientated the same as indicated in **E** or **F** (**A, C, E,** rostral to the left; **B, D, E,** white matter to the left). (**A**) Low-power parasagittal image from an acute (0-dpi) transplant demonstrating many SC121 immunopositive human cells (brown) migrated toward the lesion epicenter as well as rostral and caudal from the injection sites. Human cells within the epicenter were predominantly GFAP-positive astrocytes (not shown). (**B**) High-power image of SC121 immunopositive human cells (brown) at a site distal to the lesion demonstrates that human cells were morphologically distinct depending on locus within either white matter or gray matter in an acute transplant. (**C**) Low-power parasagittal image demonstrating SC121 immunopositive cells (brown) migrated away from the lesion epicenter in a subacute (9-dpi) transplant. (**D**) High-power image of SC121 immunopositive human cells (brown) with the morphological appearance of oligodendrocytes in white matter and neuronal phenotypes in gray matter in a subacute transplant. (**E**) Low-power parasagittal image demonstrating SC121 immunopositive cells (brown) migrated away from the lesion epicenter in a chronic (30-dpi) transplant. (**F**) High-power image of SC121 immunopositive human cells (brown) with the morphological appearance of oligodendrocytes in white matter and neuronal phenotypes in gray matter. (See color Figure 15.1)

by cellular integration with the host and not via overt modification of the host microenvironment.

ACUTE TRANSPLANTATION OF HuCNS-SCs

The host microenvironment (including both cellular and molecular cues) is different acutely after SCI compared to subacute time points. Given the beneficial effects observed for HuCNS-SCs in the subacute paradigm (9-dpi), we next asked whether transplantation of HuCNS-SCs acutely (0-dpi) allows for cell engraftment, differentiation, and recovery. Currently, the literature suggests that shortening the delay between SCI and cell transplantation could impede the ability of neural cell populations to survive and differentiate into neurons and oligodendrocytes, and thus limit recovery (Okano 2002). However, as discussed above, numerous studies have shown that engrafted neural cells could also promote recovery by alternative mechanisms. We therefore hypothesized that acute HuCNS-SC transplantation after SCI could promote recovery via alternative mechanisms compared to the subacute paradigm, and investigated the consequence of the acute microenvironment on both the fate and migration of engrafted cells.

In contrast to our observations in the 9-dpi paradigm, immediate transplantation of HuCNS-SCs yielded no locomotor improvement in the transplanted versus control group. Histological analyses demonstrated survival and localization of engrafted human cells predominantly near the injury epicenter (Fig. 15.1A). We found successful engraftment in all of the HuCNS-SC transplanted animals. As in the case of the 9-dpi paradigm, engrafted cells transplanted at vertebral level T9 were able to migrate rostrally to T6 and caudally to T12, although at lower numbers than in the 9-dpi paradigm; migration past these levels was not investigated. Unbiased stereological quantification revealed an average of 210,000 HuCNS-SCs in the transplanted animals. In contrast to mice transplanted subacutely (9-dpi), a significant number of acutely transplanted HuCNS-SC (an average of approximately 94,000 cells per animal) migrated toward the lesion epicenter. Morphologically, human cells adjacent to the epicenter appeared astrocytic (data not shown). Cell fate was confirmed using a human-specific GFAP marker, which demonstrated that a majority of human cells near the lesion site differentiated into astrocytes; these findings are in contrast to the 9-dpi paradigm, in which only 3% of transplanted HuCNS-SCs differentiated into astrocytes. Notably, however, cells that migrated away from the SCI epicenter exhibited oligodendroglial and neuronal differentiation, as in the 9-dpi paradigm (Fig. 15.1B). These data suggest that environmental cues in the immediate injury niche affect cell fate (Hooshmand et al. 2007, 2008).

Presently, the implications of astrocytic differentiation following stem cell transplantation into the injured spinal cord are unclear. Scar formation has been shown to both facilitate recovery and impair regeneration after SCI. Reactive astrocytes could serve a beneficial role acutely after injury by mediating the repair of the blood–brain barrier (Faulkner et al. 2004; Sofroniew 2005). Chronically after SCI, however, the astroglial scar has been shown to function as both a physical and chemical barrier to axons (Davies et al. 1997; Fitch et al. 1999; Silver and Miller 2004) and could impede regeneration. However, stereological quantification for the total astroglial scar volume in our acute paradigm revealed no significant differences in transplanted versus control groups, suggesting that human GFAP+ cells did not contribute to the area of reactive glial scarring per se. Additionally, two studies transplanting murine-derived (Macias et al. 2006) and human-derived (Hofstetter et al. 2005) NSCs have raised concerns about a possible correlation between astrocyte differentiation and allodynia-like hypersensitivity to mechanical/thermal stimulation. However, in our acute paradigm, we found no evidence for increased mechanical allodynia in association with astrocytic cell fate.

Comparing the 0-dpi versus 9-dpi paradigms using identical cell populations suggests that local signals in the host microenvironment, defined here by the time of transplantation, affect cell fate and recovery of function. A potential candidate for regulating the fate and migration of HuCNS-SCs is the presence of myeloid cells, which begin infiltrating the site of injury starting immediately after trauma (Nguyen et al. 2008). Secretion of a variety of cytokines and soluble factors by inflammatory cells has been previously reported (Mantovani et al. 2004; Nguyen et al. 2007). Furthermore, the effects of signaling molecules and inflammatory cytokines on CNS cell fate have been shown both in vitro and in vivo (Barkho et al. 2006; Li and Grumet 2007; Nakanishi et al. 2007). Additionally, neural stem cell and CNS-resident microglia co-culture paradigms, as well as more direct experiments exposing NSCs to conditioned media from microglial cells, suggest the possibility that cells present within the CNS could release pro- and anti-inflammatory cytokines that would affect cell fate (Monje et al. 2003; Butovsky et al. 2006; Nakanishi et al. 2007; Jones and McTaggart 2008). The possibility that recruitment of myeloid cells into the injured environment immediately after SCI could influence the differentiation of transplanted cell populations remains unexplored, but it could partially explain our in vivo observations following acute transplantation.

CHRONIC TRANSPLANTATION OF HuCNS-SCs

Whereas most cell transplantation studies have focused on either the acute or subacute time frame, it is clinically important to investigate the effects of the chronic microenvironment on cell survival, fate, and functional recovery. Can the beneficial effects of HuCNS-SCs be extended beyond a 9-dpi subacute window?

Thus, we sought to assess cell survival, fate, locomotor recovery, and allodynia in NOD-scid mice receiving HuCNS-SCs 30-dpi (Salazar et al. 2006).

Similar to observations in animals in the 9-dpi paradigm, HuCNS-SC–transplanted animals in the 30-dpi paradigm performed significantly better on the BMS open field locomotor rating scale than vehicle-treated animals. HuCNS-SC–treated animals had improved recovery of coordination between the fore- and hindlimbs. CatWalk gait analysis revealed HuCNS-SC–treated mice had significantly improved stride length compared to vehicle-treated animals (Salazar et al. 2007). Furthermore, we assessed mechanical allodynia using von Frey hair testing and found that HuCNS-SC–treated mice did not exhibit evidence of increased sensitivity compared to controls.

We assessed survival and migration of transplanted HuCNS-SCs 16 weeks post-transplantation. We found successful engraftment in all of the HuCNS-SC transplanted animals. Unbiased stereological quantification estimated an average of 216,000 human cells per HuCNS-SC–transplanted animal. Additionally, we again found long-distance migration away from the transplant sites. As in the case of the 9-dpi and 0-dpi paradigms, engrafted cells transplanted at vertebral level T9 migrated rostrally to T6 and caudally to T12; migration past these levels was not investigated. Notably, as in the 9-dpi paradigm and in contrast to the 0-dpi paradigm, engrafted cells avoided the lesion and were concentrated in the spared tissue adjacent to the lesion and in the region 2mm rostral and 1mm caudal (Fig. 15.1E).

We also examined the fate and differentiation of the transplanted HuCNS-SCs by confocal double-immunofluorescent labeling. Similar to the 9-dpi paradigm, HuCNS-SCs rarely differentiated into astrocytes when transplanted 30-dpi, and of the cells that differentiated, the majority became oligodendrocytes with a smaller percentage of neurons; accordingly, human cell differentiation again exhibited white and gray matter specificity (Fig. 15.1F). Many studies transplanting either rat or mouse neural stem cells into injured spinal cord have reported that the differentiation of these cells is restricted to astrocytes. Few studies have examined chronic transplantation of NSCs into SCI models. One study found no survival of NSCs transplanted at 8 weeks post-injury (Karimi-Abdolrezaee et al. 2006), whereas another found differentiation restricted to astroglial and radial glial lineages (Pfeifer et al. 2006).

Lastly, we determined whether transplantation of HuCNS-SCs in the chronic model had an effect on lesion volume, spared tissue volume, or glial scar area, using unbiased stereological quantification. There were no significant differences between HuCNS-SC and control groups on any of these parameters, suggesting that the integration and differentiation of HuCNS-SCs are likely responsible for the improved locomotor recovery. It should be noted, however, that assessment of other possible host mechanisms remains to be completed and that the microenvironment of the chronic host has not been as thoroughly explored as in the subacute model (Salazar et al. 2008).

Currently, the mechanism of functional recovery observed in the chronic model is not known. The results of this study suggest that, as in the subacute model, HuCNS-SCs are capable of surviving and differentiating in an injured environment when transplantation is delayed 30-dpi. Overall these studies suggest that HuCNS-SCs have potential to treat SCI beyond the subacute phase, suggesting that HuCNS-SCs could be clinically relevant for SCI therapy.

THERAPEUTIC WINDOW FOR NSC TRANSPLANTATION

It has been suggested that there may be a narrow therapeutic time window for successful cell transplantation strategies following SCI (Okano 2002), because of a combination of acute toxicity in the SCI microenvironment and subsequent development of the glial scar. In our studies, acutely transplanted HuCNS-SCs exhibited successful engraftment, as did both subacute and chronically transplanted cells. Moreover, HuCNS-SC transplantation either 9-dpi or 30-dpi improved locomotor recovery in association with predominant differentiation to an oligodendroglial fate. Additionally, our data showed that survival of engrafted cells was required for maintenance of locomotor improvements, and that the contribution of host modifications was minimal, suggesting that the mechanism of action was via integration with the host CNS. Taken together, these data suggest that successful engraftment is possible in a wider window than previously suggested and support the working hypothesis that integration of transplanted HuCNS-SCs as oligodendrocytes is one mechanism for recovery of function.

We do not rule out the possibility of a contribution of neuronal integration— or the potential for a synergistic contribution of other host microenvironment modifications—to these observed effects. In this regard, future studies testing these hypotheses using fate-targeted selective ablation of human cells and further cell dose studies are necessary. However, focusing for the moment on remyelination, it is important to consider what aspects of the host microenvironment could affect the success of this cell therapeutic strategy, and what features of a therapeutic cell population contribute to the efficacy of this approach.

First, effective therapeutic remyelination after SCI may only be possible if the transplanted cell population is capable of extensive migration, enabling cells to reach demyelinated and/or dysmyelinated axons above and below the primary injury. We have shown the migration of engrafted HuCNS-SCs to multiple vertebral levels away from the transplantation site, suggesting that this population of NSCs is capable of navigating the injured microenvironment at multiple time points post-SCI.

Second, timing of transplantation within the post-SCI microenvironment must enable NSC differentiation along appropriate fate lineages. Whereas HuCNS-SCs were able to engraft and migrate extensively after acute transplantation, the majority of these cells were recruited toward the injury epicenter and failed to exhibit a predominant oligodendroglial fate, in contrast to the 9-dpi and 30-dpi paradigms.

Third, there must be functional spared host axons that remain demyelinated/ dysmyelinated at targeted transplantation times post-SCI. Mammalian SCI models have been reported to exhibit histological and electrophysiological evidence for chronic demyelination/dysmyelination in surviving axons (Blight 1989; Shi and Blight 1997; Shi et al. 1997; Karimi-Abdolrezaee et al. 2004), suggesting remyelination as a viable target. Few studies have examined demyelination in human pathological tissue following SCI, but in parallel to studies in animal models, these suggest that there are demyelinated and/or dysmyelinated fibers present in the chronic human spinal cord that could be a therapeutic target (Kakulas 1999; Norenberg et al. 2004; Guest et al. 2005). Again, timing post-SCI may be critical, as a significant number of demyelinated fibers were reported in clinical SCI cases within 1–2 years post-injury. Though the incidence declined over time post-injury, some evidence of demyelination was detected 10 years post-injury (Guest et al. 2005). Conversely, with regard to timing, myelination during critical phases in the subacute and early chronic stages post-SCI could enhance axon sparing (Blakemore 2000; Lasiene et al. 2008), resulting in further preservation of function or opportunities for host-mediated recovery and repair. In fact, the number of axons required for observable functional recovery may be quite small, perhaps 10% of pre-injury numbers (McDonald 1999). In contrast, other recent evidence has suggested that spared axons may undergo significant spontaneous host-mediated remyelination, resulting in few demyelinated axons 12 weeks after rat contusion injury (Lasiene et al. 2008). However, a delayed and secondary phase of demyelination beginning 4 months and continuing past 1 year in the chronic contusion-injured rat has recently been reported (Totoiu and Keirstead 2005), suggesting that the processes of demyelination and remyelination in the chronic SCI microenvironment are not completely understood. In sum, remyelination may be a viable transplantation target, but the viability of this strategy may depend on timing in the acute–chronic injury continuum and requires further exploration.

CONCLUSION

The microenvironment of the injured spinal cord is dynamic. It is clear that there is a progressive transition within the microenvironment from an acute to a chronic state over time. Thus, timing will alter the potential of transplanted cell populations to engraft and exert their intended therapeutic effects. We have identified multiple targets for therapeutic interventions focusing on cell transplantation approaches, discussed the application of multiple cells types in SCI models, and considered how cell-intrinsic properties as well as exogenous factors in the host microenvironment may influence the ability of various cell populations to survive, differentiate, and promote locomotor recovery following SCI. Finally, we described studies conducted in our own laboratory transplanting HuCNS-SCs at selected time points along the acute to chronic continuum, demonstrating that, depending on timing, HuCNS-SCs have the ability to promote locomotor recovery and that the microenvironment influences cell fate.

ACKNOWLEDGMENTS

We wish to thank our collaborators at StemCells, Inc. (Nobuko Uchida, Stanley Tamaki, Monika Dohse, Robert Tushinski, Ann Tsukamoto, and Dongping He), the Christopher & Dana Reeve Foundation (CDRF), and the CDRF SCI Core Facility technicians at UC Irvine (Rebecca Nishi, Hongli Liu, Chelsea Pagan, and Elizabeth Hoffman). This research was supported by the NIH grant R01NS049885 (AJA and BJC), by grant SBIR NS46975 (NU and AJA), and by the CDRF. D.L. Salazar was supported, in part, by a UC AGEP fellowship, NSF HRD0450366, and a CIRM Training Grant, TI-00008.

REFERENCES

Ackery, A., C. Tator and A. Krassioukov (2004). A global perspective on spinal cord injury epidemiology. *J Neurotrauma* 21(10):1355–70.

Anderson, A. J. (2002). Mechanisms and pathways of inflammatory responses in CNS trauma: spinal cord injury. *J Spinal Cord Med* 25(2):70–80.

Babu, H., G. Cheung, H. Kettenmann, T. D. Palmer and G. Kempermann (2007). Enriched monolayer precursor cell cultures from micro-dissected adult mouse dentate gyrus yield functional granule cell-like neurons. *PLoS ONE* 2(4):e388.

Bambakidis, N. C. and R. H. Miller (2004). Transplantation of oligodendrocyte precursors and sonic hedgehog results in improved function and white matter sparing in the spinal cords of adult rats after contusion. *Spine J* 4(1):16–26.

Baptiste, D. C. and M. G. Fehlings (2006). Pharmacological approaches to repair the injured spinal cord. *J Neurotrauma* 23(3–4):318–34.

Barkho, B. Z., H. Song, J. B. Aimone, R. D. Smrt, T. Kuwabara, K. Nakashima, F. H. Gage and X. Zhao (2006). Identification of astrocyte-expressed factors that modulate neural stem/progenitor cell differentiation. *Stem Cells Dev* 15(3):407–21.

Basso, D. M., M. S. Beattie and J. C. Bresnahan (1995). A sensitive and reliable locomotor rating scale for open field testing in rats. *J Neurotrauma* 12(1):1–21.

Basso, D. M., L. C. Fisher, A. J. Anderson, L. B. Jakeman, D. M. McTigue and P. G. Popovich (2006). Basso Mouse Scale for locomotion detects differences in recovery after spinal cord injury in five common mouse strains. *J Neurotrauma* 23(5): 635–59.

Belegu, V., M. Oudega, D. S. Gary and J. W. McDonald (2007). Restoring function after spinal cord injury: promoting spontaneous regeneration with stem cells and activity-based therapies. *Neurosurg Clin N Am* 18(1):143–68, xi.

Bethea, J. R., H. Nagashima, M. C. Acosta, C. Briceno, F. Gomez, A. E. Marcillo, K. Loor, J. Green and W. D. Dietrich (1999). Systemically administered interleukin-10 reduces tumor necrosis factor-alpha production and significantly improves functional recovery following traumatic spinal cord injury in rats. *J Neurotrauma* 16(10): 851–63.

Blakemore, W. F. (2000). Olfactory glia and CNS repair: a step in the road from proof of principle to clinical application. *Brain* 123(Pt 8):1543–4.

Blight, A. R. (1989). Effect of 4-aminopyridine on axonal conduction-block in chronic spinal cord injury. *Brain Res Bull* 22(1):47–52.

Bradbury, E. J., L. D. Moon, R. J. Popat, V. R. King, G. S. Bennett, P. N. Patel, J. W. Fawcett and S. B. McMahon (2002). Chondroitinase ABC promotes functional recovery after spinal cord injury. *Nature* 416(6881):636–40.

Brosamle, C., A. B. Huber, M. Fiedler, A. Skerra and M. E. Schwab (2000). Regeneration of lesioned corticospinal tract fibers in the adult rat induced by a recombinant, humanized IN-1 antibody fragment. *J Neurosci* 20(21):8061–8.

Brustle, O., K. Choudhary, K. Karram, A. Huttner, K. Murray, M. Dubois-Dalcq and R. D. McKay (1998). Chimeric brains generated by intraventricular transplantation of fetal human brain cells into embryonic rats. *Nat Biotechnol* 16(11):1040–4.

Butovsky, O., Y. Ziv, A. Schwartz, G. Landa, A. E. Talpalar, S. Pluchino, G. Martino and M. Schwartz (2006). Microglia activated by IL-4 or IFN-gamma differentially induce neurogenesis and oligodendrogenesis from adult stem/progenitor cells. *Mol Cell Neurosci* 31(1):149–60.

Cao, Q. L., R. M. Howard, J. B. Dennison and S. R. Whittemore (2002). Differentiation of engrafted neuronal-restricted precursor cells is inhibited in the traumatically injured spinal cord. *Exp Neurol* 177(2):349–59.

Cao, Q. L., Y. P. Zhang, R. M. Howard, W. M. Walters, P. Tsoulfas and S. R. Whittemore (2001). Pluripotent stem cells engrafted into the normal or lesioned adult rat spinal cord are restricted to a glial lineage. *Exp Neurol* 167(1):48–58.

Chaudhry, N. and M. T. Filbin (2007). Myelin-associated inhibitory signaling and strategies to overcome inhibition. *J Cereb Blood Flow Metab* 27(6):1096–107.

Chen, Z. J., Y. Ughrin and J. M. Levine (2002). Inhibition of axon growth by oligodendrocyte precursor cells. *Mol Cell Neurosci* 20(1):125–39.

Cheng, H., J. P. Wu and S. F. Tzeng (2002). Neuroprotection of glial cell line-derived neurotrophic factor in damaged spinal cords following contusive injury. *J Neurosci Res* 69(3):397–405.

Chow, S. Y., J. Moul, C. A. Tobias, B. T. Himes, Y. Liu, M. Obrocka, L. Hodge, A. Tessler and I. Fischer (2000). Characterization and intraspinal grafting of EGF/bFGF-dependent neurospheres derived from embryonic rat spinal cord. *Brain Res* 874(2):87–106.

Crowe, M. J., J. C. Bresnahan, S. L. Shuman, J. N. Masters and M. S. Beattie (1997). Apoptosis and delayed degeneration after spinal cord injury in rats and monkeys. *Nat Med* 3(1):73–6.

Cummings, B. J., C. Engesser-Cesar, G. Cadena and A. J. Anderson (2007). Adaptation of a ladder beam walking task to assess locomotor recovery in mice following spinal cord injury. *Behavioural Brain Research* 177(2):232–241.

Cummings, B. J., N. Uchida, S. J. Tamaki and A. J. Anderson (2006). Human neural stem cell differentiation following transplantation into spinal cord injured mice: association with recovery of locomotor function. *Neurological Research* 28(5):474–81.

Cummings, B. J., N. Uchida, S. J. Tamaki, D. L. Salazar, M. Hooshmand, R. Summers, F. H. Gage and A. J. Anderson (2005). Human neural stem cells differentiate and promote locomotor recovery in spinal cord-injured mice. *Proc Natl Acad Sci USA* 102 (39): 14069–74.

Daadi, M. M., A. L. Maag and G. K. Steinberg (2008). Adherent self-renewable human embryonic stem cell-derived neural stem cell line: functional engraftment in experimental stroke model. *PLoS ONE* 3(2):e1644.

Davies, J. E., C. Huang, C. Proschel, M. Noble, M. Mayer-Proschel and S. J. Davies (2006). Astrocytes derived from glial-restricted precursors promote spinal cord repair. *J Biol* 5(3):7.

Davies, S. J., M. T. Fitch, S. P. Memberg, A. K. Hall, G. Raisman and J. Silver (1997). Regeneration of adult axons in white matter tracts of the central nervous system. *Nature* 390(6661):680–3.

Einstein, O., N. Fainstein, I. Vaknin, R. Mizrachi-Kol, E. Reihartz, N. Grigoriadis, I. Lavon, M. Baniyash, H. Lassmann and T. Ben-Hur (2007). Neural precursors attenuate autoimmune encephalomyelitis by peripheral immunosuppression. *Ann Neurol* 61(3):209–18.

Engesser-Cesar, C., A. J. Anderson, D. M. Basso, V. R. Edgerton and C. W. Cotman (2005). Voluntary wheel running improves recovery from a moderate spinal cord injury. *J Neurotrauma* 22(1):157–71.

Faulkner, J. R., J. E. Herrmann, M. J. Woo, K. E. Tansey, N. B. Doan and M. V. Sofroniew (2004). Reactive astrocytes protect tissue and preserve function after spinal cord injury. *J Neurosci* 24(9):2143–55.

Fawcett, J. W. (2006). Overcoming inhibition in the damaged spinal cord. *J Neurotrauma* 23(3–4):371–83.

Fawcett, J. W. and R. A. Asher (1999). The glial scar and central nervous system repair. *Brain Res Bull* 49(6):377–91.

Fawcett, J. W., A. Curt, J. D. Steeves, W. P. Coleman, M. H. Tuszynski, D. Lammertse, P. F. Bartlett, A. R. Blight, V. Dietz, J. Ditunno, B. H. Dobkin, L. A. Havton, P. H. Ellaway, M. G. Fehlings, A. Privat, R. Grossman, J. D. Guest, N. Kleitman, M. Nakamura, M. Gaviria and D. Short (2007). Guidelines for the conduct of clinical trials for spinal cord injury as developed by the ICCP panel: spontaneous recovery after spinal cord injury and statistical power needed for therapeutic clinical trials. *Spinal Cord* 45(3):190–205.

Fitch, M. T., C. Doller, C. K. Combs, G. E. Landreth and J. Silver (1999). Cellular and molecular mechanisms of glial scarring and progressive cavitation: in vivo and in vitro analysis of inflammation-induced secondary injury after CNS trauma. *J Neurosci* 19(19):8182–98.

Flax, J. D., S. Aurora, C. Yang, C. Simonin, A. M. Wills, L. L. Billinghurst, M. Jendoubi, R. L. Sidman, J. H. Wolfe, S. U. Kim and E. Y. Snyder (1998). Engraftable human neural stem cells respond to developmental cues, replace neurons, and express foreign genes. *Nat Biotechnol* 16(11):1033–9.

Fleming, J. C., M. D. Norenberg, D. A. Ramsay, G. A. Dekaban, A. E. Marcillo, A. D. Saenz, M. Pasquale-Styles, W. D. Dietrich and L. C. Weaver (2006). The cellular inflammatory response in human spinal cords after injury. *Brain* 129(Pt 12):3249–69.

Foote, A. K. and W. F. Blakemore (2005a). Repopulation of oligodendrocyte progenitor cell-depleted tissue in a model of chronic demyelination. *Neuropathol Appl Neurobiol* 31(4):374–83.

Foote, A. K. and W. F. Blakemore (2005b). Inflammation stimulates remyelination in areas of chronic demyelination. *Brain* 128(Pt 3):528–39.

Fournier, A. E., B. T. Takizawa and S. M. Strittmatter (2003). Rho kinase inhibition enhances axonal regeneration in the injured CNS. *J Neurosci* 23(4):1416–23.

Fricker, R. A., M. K. Carpenter, C. Winkler, C. Greco, M. A. Gates and A. Bjorklund (1999). Site-specific migration and neuronal differentiation of human neural progenitor cells after transplantation in the adult rat brain. *J Neurosci* 19(14): 5990–6005.

Gage, F. H., J. Ray and L. J. Fisher (1995). Isolation, characterization, and use of stem cells from the CNS. *Ann Rev Neurosci* 18([issue?]):159–92.

Gerdoni, E., B. Gallo, S. Casazza, S. Musio, I. Bonanni, E. Pedemonte, R. Mantegazza, F. Frassoni, G. Mancardi, R. Pedotti and A. Uccelli (2007). Mesenchymal stem cells effectively modulate pathogenic immune response in experimental autoimmune encephalomyelitis. *Ann Neurol* 61(3):219–27.

Gimenez y Ribotta, M., D. Orsal, D. Feraboli-Lohnherr, A. Privat, J. Provencher and S. Rossignol (1998). Kinematic analysis of recovered locomotor movements of the hindlimbs in paraplegic rats transplanted with monoaminergic embryonic neurons. *Ann NY Acad Sci* 860:521–3.

Gonzenbach, R. R. and M. E. Schwab (2008). Disinhibition of neurite growth to repair the injured adult CNS: focusing on Nogo. *Cell Mol Life Sci* 65(1):161–76.

Greiner, D. L., R. A. Hesselton and L. D. Shultz (1998). SCID mouse models of human stem cell engraftment. *Stem Cells* 16(3):166–77.

Grill, R. J. (2005). User-defined variables that affect outcome in spinal cord contusion/compression models. *Exp Neurol* 196(1):1–5.

Guest, J. D., E. D. Hiester and R. P. Bunge (2005). Demyelination and Schwann cell responses adjacent to injury epicenter cavities following chronic human spinal cord injury. *Exp Neurol* 192(2):384–93.

Hamers, F. P., G. C. Koopmans and E. A. Joosten (2006). CatWalk-assisted gait analysis in the assessment of spinal cord injury. *J Neurotrauma* 23(3–4):537–48.

Heine, W., K. Conant, J. W. Griffin and A. Hoke (2004). Transplanted neural stem cells promote axonal regeneration through chronically denervated peripheral nerves. *Exp Neurol* 189(2):231–40.

Herrera, D. G., J. M. Garcia-Verdugo and A. Alvarez-Buylla (1999). Adult-derived neural precursors transplanted into multiple regions in the adult brain. *Ann Neurol* 46(6):867–77.

Hill, C. E., M. S. Beattie and J. C. Bresnahan (2001). Degeneration and sprouting of identified descending supraspinal axons after contusive spinal cord injury in the rat. *Exp Neurol* 171(1):153–69.

Hill, C. E., L. D. Moon, P. M. Wood and M. B. Bunge (2006). Labeled Schwann cell transplantation: cell loss, host Schwann cell replacement, and strategies to enhance survival. *Glia* 53(3):338–43.

Hill, C. E., C. Proschel, M. Noble, M. Mayer-Proschel, J. C. Gensel, M. S. Beattie and J. C. Bresnahan (2004). Acute transplantation of glial-restricted precursor cells into spinal cord contusion injuries: survival, differentiation, and effects on lesion environment and axonal regeneration. *Exp Neurol* 190(2):289–310.

Hofstetter, C. P., N. A. Holmstrom, J. A. Lilja, P. Schweinhardt, J. Hao, C. Spenger, Z. Wiesenfeld-Hallin, S. N. Kurpad, J. Frisen and L. Olson (2005). Allodynia limits the usefulness of intraspinal neural stem cell grafts; directed differentiation improves outcome. *Nat Neurosci* 8(3):346–53.

Hofstetter, C. P., E. J. Schwarz, D. Hess, J. Widenfalk, A. El Manira, D. J. Prockop and L. Olson (2002). Marrow stromal cells form guiding strands in the injured spinal cord and promote recovery. *Proc Natl Acad Sci USA* 99(4):2199–204.

Hooshmand, M. J., B. J. Cummings, D. L. Salazar, N. Uchida, S. J. Tamaki and A. J. Anderson (2007). Human neural stem cell fate is affected by the host microenvironment found at different times of transplantation after spinal cord injury. *Society for Neuroscience Abstracts* Poster #802.20.

Hooshmand, M. J., B. J. Cummings, C. J. Sontag, N. Uchida, S. J. Tamaki and A. J. Anderson (2008). Locomotor recovery in human CNS-stem cell-transplanted mice is not due to modification of the host environment. *Submitted.*

Hooshmand, M. J., B. J. Cummings, C. J. Sontag, N. Uchida, S. J. Tamaki, B. Tushinski, A. Tsukamoto and A. J. Anderson (2006). Locomotor recovery in human CNS-stem cell-transplanted mice is not due to modification of the host environment. *Society for Neuroscience Abstracts* Poster #475.19.

Hooshmand, M. J., B. J. Cummings, N. Uchida, S. J. Tamaki, C. J. Sontag, B. Tushinski, A. Tsukamoto and A. J. Anderson (2005). Human CNS-stem cell transplants survive, migrate, and promote functional recovery after spinal cord injury. *Society for Neuroscience Abstracts* Poster #438.5.

Hooshmand, M. J., H. X. Nguyen, B. J. Cummings, N. Uchida, S. J. Tamaki and A. J. Anderson (2008). Acute transplantation of human neural stem cells after spinal cord injury. *Society for Neuroscience Abstracts.*

Houle, J. D. and A. Tessler (2003). Repair of chronic spinal cord injury. *Exp Neurol* 182(2):247–60.

Ikegami, T., M. Nakamura, J. Yamane, H. Katoh, S. Okada, A. Iwanami, K. Watanabe, K. Ishii, F. Kato, H. Fujita, T. Takahashi, H. J. Okano, Y. Toyama and H. Okano (2005). Chondroitinase ABC combined with neural stem/progenitor cell transplantation enhances graft cell migration and outgrowth of growth-associated protein-43-positive fibers after rat spinal cord injury. *Eur J Neurosci* 22(12):3036–46.

Inman, D. M. and O. Steward (2003). Physical size does not determine the unique histopathological response seen in the injured mouse spinal cord. *J Neurotrauma* 20(1): 33–42.

Ishii, K., M. Nakamura, H. Dai, T. P. Finn, H. Okano, Y. Toyama and B. S. Bregman (2006). Neutralization of ciliary neurotrophic factor reduces astrocyte production from transplanted neural stem cells and promotes regeneration of corticospinal tract fibers in spinal cord injury. *J Neurosci Res* 84(8):1669–81.

Jakeman, L. B., Z. Guan, P. Wei, R. Ponnappan, R. Dzwonczyk, P. G. Popovich and B. T. Stokes (2000). Traumatic spinal cord injury produced by controlled contusion in mouse. *J Neurotrauma* 17(4):299–319.

Ji, B., M. Li, W. T. Wu, L. W. Yick, X. Lee, Z. Shao, J. Wang, K. F. So, J. M. McCoy, R. B. Pepinsky, S. Mi and J. K. Relton (2006). LINGO-1 antagonist promotes functional recovery and axonal sprouting after spinal cord injury. *Mol Cell Neurosci* 33(3): 311–20.

Jones, B. J. and S. J. McTaggart (2008). Immunosuppression by mesenchymal stromal cells: From culture to clinic. *Exp Hematol* 36(6):733–41.

Jones, T. B., E. E. McDaniel and P. G. Popovich (2005). Inflammatory-mediated injury and repair in the traumatically injured spinal cord. *Curr Pharm Des* 11(10): 1223–36.

Kakulas, B. A. (1999). A review of the neuropathology of human spinal cord injury with emphasis on special features. *J Spinal Cord Med* 22(2):119–24.

Kamei, N., N. Tanaka, Y. Oishi, T. Hamasaki, K. Nakanishi, N. Sakai and M. Ochi (2007). BDNF, NT-3, and NGF released from transplanted neural progenitor cells promote corticospinal axon growth in organotypic cocultures. *Spine* 32(12):1272–8.

Karimi-Abdolrezaee, S., E. Eftekharpour and M. G. Fehlings (2004). Temporal and spatial patterns of Kv1.1 and Kv1.2 protein and gene expression in spinal cord white matter after acute and chronic spinal cord injury in rats: implications for axonal patho-physiology after neurotrauma. *Eur J Neurosci* 19(3):577–89.

Karimi-Abdolrezaee, S., E. Eftekharpour, J. Wang, C. M. Morshead and M. G. Fehlings (2006). Delayed transplantation of adult neural precursor cells promotes remyelin-ation and functional neurological recovery after spinal cord injury. *J Neurosci* 26(13): 3377–89.

Keirstead, H. S., G. Nistor, G. Bernal, M. Totoiu, F. Cloutier, K. Sharp and O. Steward (2005). Human embryonic stem cell-derived oligodendrocyte progenitor cell trans-plants remyelinate and restore locomotion after spinal cord injury. *J Neurosci* 25(19): 4694–705.

Keyvan-Fouladi, N., G. Raisman and Y. Li (2003). Functional repair of the corticospinal tract by delayed transplantation of olfactory ensheathing cells in adult rats. *J Neurosci* 23(28):9428–34.

Kigerl, K. A., V. M. McGaughy and P. G. Popovich (2006). Comparative analysis of lesion development and intraspinal inflammation in four strains of mice following spi-nal contusion injury. *J Comp Neurol* 494(4):578–94.

Kim, B. G., H. N. Dai, J. V. Lynskey, M. McAtee and B. S. Bregman (2006). Degradation of chondroitin sulfate proteoglycans potentiates transplant-mediated axonal remodel-ing and functional recovery after spinal cord injury in adult rats. *J Comp Neurol* 497(2):182–98.

Kim, H. T., I. S. Kim, I. S. Lee, J. P. Lee, E. Y. Snyder and K. I. Park (2006). Human neu-rospheres derived from the fetal central nervous system are regionally and temporally specified but are not committed. *Exp Neurol* 199(1):222–35.

Kunkel-Bagden, E., H. N. Dai and B. S. Bregman (1993). Methods to assess the develop-ment and recovery of locomotor function after spinal cord injury in rats. *Exp Neurol* 119(2):153–64.

Lasiene, J., L. Shupe, S. Perlmutter and P. Horner (2008). No evidence for chronic demy-elination in spared axons after spinal cord injury in a mouse. *J Neurosci* 28(15): 3887–96.

Li, H. and M. Grumet (2007). BMP and LIF signaling coordinately regulate lineage restriction of radial glia in the developing forebrain. *Glia* 55(1):24–35.

Liu, S., Y. Qu, T. J. Stewart, M. J. Howard, S. Chakrabortty, T. F. Holekamp and J. W. McDon-ald (2000). Embryonic stem cells differentiate into oligodendrocytes and myelinate in culture and after spinal cord transplantation. *Proc Natl Acad Sci USA* 97(11):6126–31.

Liu, Y., B. T. Himes, M. Murray, A. Tessler and I. Fischer (2002). Grafts of BDNF-pro-ducing fibroblasts rescue axotomized rubrospinal neurons and prevent their atrophy. *Exp Neurol* 178(2):150–64.

Liu, Y., D. Kim, B. T. Himes, S. Y. Chow, T. Schallert, M. Murray, A. Tessler and I. Fischer (1999). Transplants of fibroblasts genetically modified to express BDNF pro-mote regeneration of adult rat rubrospinal axons and recovery of forelimb function. *J Neurosci* 19(11):4370–87.

Lu, J., F. Feron, A. Mackay-Sim and P. M. Waite (2002). Olfactory ensheathing cells pro-mote locomotor recovery after delayed transplantation into transected spinal cord. *Brain* 125(Pt 1):14–21.

Lu, P., L. L. Jones, E. Y. Snyder and M. H. Tuszynski (2003). Neural stem cells constitu-tively secrete neurotrophic factors and promote extensive host axonal growth after spinal cord injury. *Exp Neurol* 181(2):115–29.

Macias, M. Y., M. B. Syring, M. A. Pizzi, M. J. Crowe, A. R. Alexanian and S. N. Kurpad (2006). Pain with no gain: allodynia following neural stem cell transplantation in spi-nal cord injury. *Exp Neurol* 201(2):335–48.

Mantovani, A., A. Sica, S. Sozzani, P. Allavena, A. Vecchi and M. Locati (2004). The chemokine system in diverse forms of macrophage activation and polarization. *Trends
Immunol* 25(12):677–86.

McDonald, J. W. (1999). Repairing the damaged spinal cord. *Sci Am* 281(3):64–73.

McDonald, J. W., X. Z. Liu, Y. Qu, S. Liu, S. K. Mickey, D. Turetsky, D. I. Gottlieb and
D. W. Choi (1999). Transplanted embryonic stem cells survive, differentiate and promote recovery in injured rat spinal cord. *Nat Med* 5(12):1410–2.

Monje, M. L., H. Toda and T. D. Palmer (2003). Inflammatory blockade restores adult
hippocampal neurogenesis. *Science* 302(5651):1760–5.

Muir, G. D. and I. Q. Whishaw (1999). Complete locomotor recovery following corticospinal tract lesions: measurement of ground reaction forces during overground locomotion in rats. *Behav Brain Res* 103(1):45–53.

Murray, M., D. Kim, Y. Liu, C. Tobias, A. Tessler and I. Fischer (2002). Transplantation
of genetically modified cells contributes to repair and recovery from spinal injury.
Brain Res Brain Res Rev 40(1–3):292–300.

Nakanishi, M., T. Niidome, S. Matsuda, A. Akaike, T. Kihara and H. Sugimoto (2007).
Microglia-derived interleukin-6 and leukaemia inhibitory factor promote astrocytic
differentiation of neural stem/progenitor cells. *Eur J Neurosci* 25(3):649–58.

Namiki, J., A. Kojima and C. H. Tator (2000). Effect of brain-derived neurotrophic factor,
nerve growth factor, and neurotrophin-3 on functional recovery and regeneration after
spinal cord injury in adult rats. *J Neurotrauma* 17(12):1219–31.

Nguyen, H. X., K. D. Beck, M. D. Galvan, D. L. Salazar and A. J. Anderson (2008).
Quantative analysis of cellular inflammation after spinal cord injury: evidence for a
multiphasic inflammatory response in the acute to chronic envrionment. *Submitted.*

Nguyen, H. X., T. J. O'Barr and A. J. Anderson (2007). Polymorphonuclear leukocytes
promote neurotoxicity through release of matrix metalloproteinases, reactive oxygen
species, and TNF-alpha. *J Neurochem* 102(3):900–12.

Norenberg, M. D., J. Smith and A. Marcillo (2004). The pathology of human spinal cord
injury: defining the problems. *J Neurotrauma* 21(4):429–40.

Nothias, J. M., T. Mitsui, J. S. Shumsky, I. Fischer, M. D. Antonacci and M. Murray
(2005). Combined effects of neurotrophin secreting transplants, exercise, and serotonergic drug challenge improve function in spinal rats. *Neurorehabil Neural Repair*
19(4):296–312.

Okano, H. (2002). Stem cell biology of the central nervous system. *J Neurosci Res*
69(6):698–707.

Palmer, T. D., E. A. Markakis, A. R. Willhoite, F. Safar and F. H. Gage (1999). Fibroblast
growth factor-2 activates a latent neurogenic program in neural stem cells from diverse
regions of the adult CNS. *J Neurosci* 19(19):8487–97.

Pearse, D. D., F. C. Pereira, A. E. Marcillo, M. L. Bates, Y. A. Berrocal, M. T. Filbin and
M. B. Bunge (2004). cAMP and Schwann cells promote axonal growth and functional
recovery after spinal cord injury. *Nat Med* 10(6):610–6.

Pfeifer, K., M. Vroemen, A. Blesch and N. Weidner (2004). Adult neural progenitor cells
provide a permissive guiding substrate for corticospinal axon growth following spinal
cord injury. *Eur J Neurosci* 20(7):1695–704.

Pfeifer, K., M. Vroemen, M. Caioni, L. Aigner, U. Bogdahn and N. Weidner (2006).
Autologous adult rodent neural progenitor cell transplantation represents a feasible
strategy to promote structural repair in the chronically injured spinal cord. *Regen Med*
1(2):255–66.

Pluchino, S., L. Zanotti, B. Rossi, E. Brambilla, L. Ottoboni, G. Salani, M. Martinello, A.
Cattalini, A. Bergami, R. Furlan, G. Comi, G. Constantin and G. Martino (2005).

Neurosphere-derived multipotent precursors promote neuroprotection by an immuno-modulatory mechanism. *Nature* 436(7048):266–71.

Pollard, S. M., L. Conti, Y. Sun, D. Goffredo and A. Smith (2006). Adherent neural stem (NS) cells from fetal and adult forebrain. *Cereb Cortex* 16 (Suppl 1):i112–20.

Popovich, P. G. and T. B. Jones (2003). Manipulating neuroinflammatory reactions in the injured spinal cord: back to basics. *Trends Pharmacol Sci* 24(1):13–7.

Prakriya, M., P. M. McCabe and V. R. Holets (1993). A computerized grid walking system for evaluating the accuracy of locomotion in rats. *J Neurosci Methods* 48(1–2):15–25.

Ramer, L. M., E. Au, M. W. Richter, J. Liu, W. Tetzlaff and A. J. Roskams (2004). Peripheral olfactory ensheathing cells reduce scar and cavity formation and promote regeneration after spinal cord injury. *J Comp Neurol* 473(1):1–15.

Reynolds, B. A. and S. Weiss (1992). Generation of neurons and astrocytes from isolated cells of the adult mammalian central nervous system. *Science* 255(5052):1707–10.

Richards, L. J., T. J. Kilpatrick and P. F. Bartlett (1992). De novo generation of neuronal cells from the adult mouse brain. *Proc Natl Acad Sci USA* 89(18):8591–5.

Rivlin, A. S. and C. H. Tator (1977). Objective clinical assessment of motor function after experimental spinal cord injury in the rat. *J Neurosurg* 47(4):577–81.

Rus, H., C. Cudrici, F. Niculescu and M. L. Shin (2006). Complement activation in autoimmune demyelination: dual role in neuroinflammation and neuroprotection. *J Neuroimmunol* 180(1–2):9–16.

Salazar, D. L., B. J. Cummings, M. J. Hooshmand, N. Uchida, S. J. Tamaki, R. S. Tushinski, A. S. Tsukamoto and A. J. Anderson (2007). Delayed transplantation of human central nervous system stem cells into spinal cord injured NOD-SCID mice at 30 days post-injury results in functional recovery and increased engraftment compared to 9 day post-injury transplants. *ISSCR Annual Meeting* 287:234.

Salazar, D. L., B. J. Cummings, N. Uchida, S. J. Tamaki and A. J. Anderson (2008). Delayed transplantation of human neural stem cells promotes locomotor recovery in spinal cord injured mice. *Submitted*.

Salazar, D. L., B. J. Cummings, N. Uchida, S. J. Tamaki, R. S. Tushinski, A. S. Tsukamoto and A. J. Anderson (2006). Delayed transplantation of human central nervous system stem cells into a NOD/SCID mouse model of spinal cord injury. *2006 Neuroscience Meeting Planner. Atlanta, GA: Society for Neuroscience* Program No. 284.6.

Sasaki, M., B. C. Hains, K. L. Lankford, S. G. Waxman and J. D. Kocsis (2006). Protection of corticospinal tract neurons after dorsal spinal cord transection and engraftment of olfactory ensheathing cells. *Glia* 53(4):352–9.

Scheff, S. W., A. G. Rabchevsky, I. Fugaccia, J. A. Main and J. E. Lumpp, Jr. (2003). Experimental modeling of spinal cord injury: characterization of a force-defined injury device. *J Neurotrauma* 20(2):179–93.

Schwartz, M., O. Butovsky, W. Bruck and U. K. Hanisch (2006). Microglial phenotype: is the commitment reversible? *Trends Neurosci* 29(2):68–74.

Shi, R. and A. R. Blight (1997). Differential effects of low and high concentrations of 4-aminopyridine on axonal conduction in normal and injured spinal cord. *Neuroscience* 77(2):553–62.

Shi, R., T. M. Kelly and A. R. Blight (1997). Conduction block in acute and chronic spinal cord injury: different dose-response characteristics for reversal by 4-aminopyridine. *Exp Neurol* 148(2):495–501.

Shihabuddin, L. S., P. J. Horner, J. Ray and F. H. Gage (2000). Adult spinal cord stem cells generate neurons after transplantation in the adult dentate gyrus. *J Neurosci* 20(23):8727–35.

Silver, J. and J. H. Miller (2004). Regeneration beyond the glial scar. *Nat Rev Neurosci* 5(2):146–56.

Sipski, M. L. and D. D. Pearse (2006). Methylprednisolone and other confounders to spinal cord injury clinical trials. *Nat Clin Pract Neurol* 2(8):402–3.

Sofroniew, M. V. (2005). Reactive astrocytes in neural repair and protection. *Neuroscientist* 11(5):400–7.

Stokes, B. T. and L. B. Jakeman (2002). Experimental modelling of human spinal cord injury: a model that crosses the species barrier and mimics the spectrum of human cytopathology. *Spinal Cord* 40(3):101–9.

Swanger, S. A., B. Neuhuber, B. T. Himes, A. Bakshi and I. Fischer (2005). Analysis of allogeneic and syngeneic bone marrow stromal cell graft survival in the spinal cord. *Cell Transplant* 14(10):775–86.

Syed, Y. A., A. S. Baer, G. Lubec, H. Hoeger, G. Widhalm and M. R. Kotter (2008). Inhibition of oligodendrocyte precursor cell differentiation by myelin-associated proteins. *Neurosurg Focus* 24(3–4):E5.

Tarasenko, Y. I., J. Gao, L. Nie, K. M. Johnson, J. J. Grady, C. E. Hulsebosch, D. J. McAdoo and P. Wu (2007). Human fetal neural stem cells grafted into contusion-injured rat spinal cords improve behavior. *J Neurosci Res* 85(1):47–57.

Tator, C. H., E. G. Duncan, V. E. Edmonds, L. I. Lapczak and D. F. Andrews (1993). Changes in epidemiology of acute spinal cord injury from 1947 to 1981. *Surg Neurol* 40(3):207–15.

Teng, Y. D., E. B. Lavik, X. Qu, K. I. Park, J. Ourednik, D. Zurakowski, R. Langer and E. Y. Snyder (2002). Functional recovery following traumatic spinal cord injury mediated by a unique polymer scaffold seeded with neural stem cells. *Proc Natl Acad Sci USA* 99(5):3024–9.

Tobias, C. A., J. S. Shumsky, M. Shibata, M. H. Tuszynski, I. Fischer, A. Tessler and M. Murray (2003). Delayed grafting of BDNF and NT-3 producing fibroblasts into the injured spinal cord stimulates sprouting, partially rescues axotomized red nucleus neurons from loss and atrophy, and provides limited regeneration. *Exp Neurol* 184(1):97–113.

Totoiu, M. O. and H. S. Keirstead (2005). Spinal cord injury is accompanied by chronic progressive demyelination. *J Comp Neurol* 486(4):373–83.

Uchida, N., D. W. Buck, D. He, M. J. Reitsma, M. Masek, T. V. Phan, A. S. Tsukamoto, F. H. Gage and I. L. Weissman (2000). Direct isolation of human central nervous system stem cells. *Proc Natl Acad Sci USA* 97(26):14720–5.

Vroemen, M., L. Aigner, J. Winkler and N. Weidner (2003). Adult neural progenitor cell grafts survive after acute spinal cord injury and integrate along axonal pathways. *Eur J Neurosci* 18(4):743–51.

Wang, B., Z. Xiao, B. Chen, J. Han, Y. Gao, J. Zhang, W. Zhao, X. Wang and J. Dai (2008). Nogo-66 promotes the differentiation of neural progenitors into astroglial lineage cells through mTOR-STAT3 pathway. *PLoS ONE* 3(3):e1856.

Wells, J. E., R. J. Hurlbert, M. G. Fehlings and V. W. Yong (2003). Neuroprotection by minocycline facilitates significant recovery from spinal cord injury in mice. *Brain* 126(Pt 7):1628–37.

Yan, J., A. M. Welsh, S. H. Bora, E. Y. Snyder and V. E. Koliatsos (2004). Differentiation and tropic/trophic effects of exogenous neural precursors in the adult spinal cord. *J Comp Neurol* 480(1):101–14.

Yan, J., L. Xu, A. M. Welsh, G. Hatfield, T. Hazel, K. Johe and V. E. Koliatsos (2007). Extensive neuronal differentiation of human neural stem cell grafts in adult rat spinal cord. *PLoS Med* 4(2):e39.

Young, W. (2002). Spinal cord contusion models. *Prog Brain Res* 137:231–55.

Z'Graggen, W. J., G. A. Metz, G. L. Kartje, M. Thallmair and M. E. Schwab (1998). Functional recovery and enhanced corticofugal plasticity after unilateral pyramidal tract lesion and blockade of myelin-associated neurite growth inhibitors in adult rats. *J Neurosci* 18(12):4744–57.

Zhang, Y. W., J. Denham and R. S. Thies (2006). Oligodendrocyte progenitor cells derived from human embryonic stem cells express neurotrophic factors. *Stem Cells Dev* 15(6):943–52.

Zhao, X. H., W. L. Jin and G. Ju (2007). An in vitro study on the involvement of LINGO-1 and Rho GTPases in Nogo-A regulated differentiation of oligodendrocyte precursor cells. *Mol Cell Neurosci* 36(2):260–9.

Ziv, Y., H. Avidan, S. Pluchino, G. Martino and M. Schwartz (2006). Synergy between immune cells and adult neural stem/progenitor cells promotes functional recovery from spinal cord injury. *Proc Natl Acad Sci USA* 103(35):13174–9.

Chapter Sixteen

Spinal Cord Injury Pathology Differs with Injury Type, Age, and Exercise

Monica M. Siegenthaler and Hans S. Keirstead

Spinal cord injury (SCI) affects nearly 11,000 people a day in the United States alone. There is no cure for SCI, and very few therapies have been developed that better the pathological outcome and functional recovery following SCI. Elucidation of the pathology that occurs following SCI has proven useful in developing therapeutic strategies for neuroprotection and regeneration (Kwon et al. 2004). However, the field of SCI research is lacking in comprehensive studies that fully examine the pathogenesis of SCI. More importantly, dissection of each SCI type and examination of the demographical variables that may influence neural regeneration and plasticity following SCI are critical in identifying dissimilarities in pathological outcomes, which may suggest different therapeutic strategies.

SCI begins with a mechanical insult followed by immediate vasodilation, hyperemia, and petechial hemorrhage (Carlson et al. 1997a, 1997b; Hayes and Kakulas 1997). These immediate changes generate an environment that leads to a cascade of events that expands the primary lesion, resulting in further neurological deficits called secondary degeneration (Deumens et al. 2005; Injury 2005). These secondary events include edema, ischemia, excitotoxicicity, free-radical formation, and inflammation, which all eventually lead to cell death of neural and glial cell types (Schwab and Bartholdi 1996; Liu et al. 1997; Beattie et al. 2000). These secondary events often dictate the severity of SCI and are therefore important targets for the development of therapies with goals to: (1) provide neuroprotection,

(2) enhance axonal regeneration/plasticity, and (3) enhance remyelination (Kwon et al. 2004, 2005; Totoiu and Keirstead 2005; Tsai and Tator 2005).

Due to an increasing number of reports of widespread demyelination following trauma to the spinal cord, demyelination has been accepted as a therapeutic target (Keirstead et al. 2005; Klussmann and Martin-Villalba 2005; Totoiu and Keirstead 2005; Guest et al. 2006). In a recent series of studies from our laboratory, human embryonic stem cells (hESCs) were pre-differentiated into high-purity oligodendrocyte progenitor cells (OPCs)—the first demonstration that hESCs can be directed to differentiate into a high-purity neural population (Figure 16.1) (Nistor et al. 2005). This protocol has since been independently repeated and improved upon (Izrael et al. 2007). Transplantation of these cells into spinal cord–injured animals demonstrated pathotropism, cell survival and differentiation, enhanced remyelination, and significantly improved locomotor outcomes (Keirstead et al. 2005). Follow-up studies indicated that the procedure was safe, in that the transplant was not associated with tumor formation, scarring, tissue pathogenesis, or behavioral decline (Cloutier et al. 2006).

However, there is a degree of incongruence in human SCI cases with respect to injury type, age at time of injury, and general health conditions. For example, the average age at time of SCI has risen from 28.7 to 38 years of age since the 1970s, with more than half of the sustained cases occurring in the age range of 15–29 years of age (CDC 2006; NSCISC 2006). Additionally, the percentage of people over the age of 60 at time of SCI has increased since the 1970s from 4.7% to 11.5% (NSCISC 2006). Statistical data such as these indicate that there is a need to comparatively characterize the effects of variables such as injury type, age, and physical activity on SCI in animal models. Thorough characterization

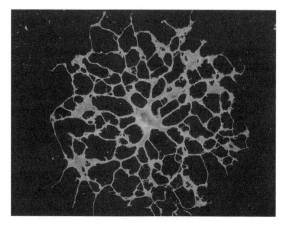

Figure 16.1 Photomicrograph of galactocerebroside-immunostained oligodendrocyte derived from human embryonic stem cell cultures. (See color Figure 16.1)

of demyelination and remyelination in different animal models of SCI that encompass demographical variables such as differing injury types, ages at time of injury, and levels of physical activity are key in elucidating the viability of demyelination as a therapeutic target in all cases of SCI. Additionally, these studies are of value in directing the future of SCI therapies.

MYELIN PATHOLOGY DIFFERS FOLLOWING CONTUSION AND LACERATION SPINAL CORD INJURY

The majority of spinal cord injuries are contusions, which are caused by a blunt force to the spinal cord resulting in bruising. Fewer cases are lacerations, which are caused by the penetration of a sharp object into the spinal cord (Liverman et al. 2005). Determining whether there are pathological differences between the injury types is necessary for developing therapies that specifically target pathology caused by the injury. Previous studies suggest that the time course and extent of damage within the spinal cord may differ between contusion and laceration SCI. For example, Dusart and Schwab (1994) describe a small, focal lesion site that corresponds to the region of primary mechanical damage one hour following transection of the adult rodent spinal cord. In contrast, the lesion size following contusion injury extends more than 8mm along the craniocaudal axis of the rat spinal cord within 15 minutes of injury (Grossman et al. 2001).

Morphometric and histopathological analyses of contused and hemisected rat spinal cords two months post-injury support the hypothesis that laceration and contusion SCI pathologies differ. Specifically, the extent of injured tissue, and the degree of tissue destruction within that region, is much greater in contused spinal cords. The area of pathology at 2mm and 4mm distal to the injury epicenter following a contusion injury is 7× and 8× greater, respectively, as compared to a laceration injury. This indicates that contusion SCI results in widespread pathology that is more extensive and greater than that of the localized pathology seen following laceration SCI (Siegenthaler et al. 2007).

Oligodendrocytes are sensitive to many components of the secondary degenerative cascade, which is primarily accountable for the enlargement of the initial injury area. Within the injury area are free radicals, inflammatory cells, and excess glutamate (Beattie 2004; Norenberg et al. 2004; Park et al. 2004; Klussmann and Martin-Villalba 2005). An examination of macrophage infiltration at early time points following injury indicates that contusion SCI produces a robust response, whereas laceration SCI produces a localized macrophage response (Dusart and Schwab 1994; Popovich and Hickey 2001; Byrnes et al. 2005; Siegenthaler et al. 2007). Interestingly, the extent of pathology and macrophage infiltration is similar to the extent and amount of apoptotic cells following contusion and laceration SCI. Cleaved caspase-3 and terminal dUTP nick end labeling (TUNEL) immunostaining reveal that contusion SCI results in more extensive and greater amounts of apoptotic mature oligodendrocytes as compared to laceration SCI. This differential loss of oligodendrocytes is reflected in a differing amount and extent of demyelination following contusion and laceration SCI, in which demyelination is greater and more extensive following contusion SCI (Siegenthaler et al. 2007).

Several clinical case studies have used imaging to demonstrate an extensive pathological region in human contusion SCI (Finnerup et al. 2003; Ellingson et al. 2006, 2008), supporting the notion that contusion SCI produces a greater amount of pathology. This suggests that the rat-contusion SCI model is a more appropriate model of human SCI compared to the rat-laceration SCI model. Most importantly, the studies outlined above indicate that demyelination may not be a suitable therapeutic target for laceration SCI, as it is for contusion SCI (Keirstead et al. 2005; Totoiu and Keirstead 2005).

AGE DETRIMENTALLY AFFECTS MYELIN PATHOLOGY AND FUNCTIONAL OUTCOME FOLLOWING SCI

Given that the average age at time of SCI has increased since the 1970s, it is important to understand how age may influence the pathology and recovery from SCI. The majority of rodent SCI studies utilize 2–3-month-old animals, which may not properly represent the average age at time of injury in humans. Although age comparisons between humans and rats are difficult to make, it can be estimated that rats of 2–3 months of age are equivalent to an adolescent human (Adams and Boice 1983; Quinn 2005). A rat that is 12 months of age is approximately equivalent to an adult human in his/her 30s, which is a better representation of the average age of humans at the time of SCI. Humans sustaining a SCI over the age of 60 are better represented by 24-month-old rats (Adams and Boice 1983; Quinn 2005).

Studies demonstrate a notable age-associated decline in neural maintenance, protection, repair, and recovery in the central nervous system (CNS). The aged CNS differs from a young CNS in many regards, including the amount of oxidative stress, mitochondrial damage, glial activation, circulating growth factors, and hormones (Hoffman et al. 1992; Hayashi et al. 1997; Genazzani et al. 1998; Morales et al. 1998; Keller et al. 2000; Kyrkanides et al. 2001; Navarro and Boveris 2007a, 2007b). These changes that occur with aging predispose the aged CNS to loss of integrity and functionality of neural systems, greatly affecting the intact white matter of the CNS as observed by compromised myelin integrity with age (Kullberg et al. 1998; Peters and Sethares 2003; Kovari et al. 2004; Raz et al. 2005; Raz and Rodrigue 2006).

With respect to the spinal cord in particular, 12-month-old rats remyelinate at a slower rate than 3-month-old rats following toxin-induced demyelination (Hinks and Franklin 2000), suggesting a slower recovery from injury with age. This age-related difference is attributed to a delay in growth factor gene expression, a decline in OPC colonization of OPC-depleted spinal cord tissue, and differences in early inflammatory responses (Hinks and Franklin 2000; Chari et al. 2003; Zhao et al. 2006). Moreover, 12-month-old rats exhibit slower locomotor behavioral recovery following transection SCI as compared to young (1.5- and 2-month-old) rats (Gwak et al. 2004). Similarly, clip compression of the spinal cord results in more extensive and severe pathology, leukocyte infiltration, and nitrotyrosine levels, accompanied by decreased behavioral recovery in 18-month-old rats as compared to 3-month-old rats (Genovese et al. 2006).

In the contusion SCI model, 12- and 24-month-old rats have delayed and lesser locomotor and bladder recovery as compared to 3-month-old rats following SCI. Contusion SCI also results in a greater area of pathology in 12- and 24-month-old rats as compared to 3-month-old rats. Similarly, contusion SCI results in greater demyelination and less remyelination in 12- and 24-month-old rats as compared to 3-month-old rats (Siegenthaler et al. 2008b). These data support and extend previous findings that neuroprotection is compromised with age (Hayashi et al. 1997; Azcoitia et al. 2003; Veiga et al. 2003, 2004; Ciriza et al. 2004a, 2004b; Genovese et al. 2006; Garcia-Segura et al. 2007).

EXERCISE ATTENUATES THE AGE-ASSOCIATED DEFICITS FOLLOWING SPINAL CORD INJURY

Vaynman and Gomez-Pinilla (2005) discuss several effects of exercise on the intact and injured CNS, including the ability of exercise to lessen the degree of damage by limiting the secondary degenerative response. Exercise prior to CNS injury is neuroprotective (Stummer et al. 1994; Ang et al. 2003; Ding et al. 2006b). The exercise-induced neuroprotection may be linked to the exercise-induced increase in neurotrophins and growth factors such as brain-derived neurotrophic factor (BDNF) and insulin-like growth factor 1 (IGF-1) (Schwarz et al. 1996; Trejo et al. 2001; Heinemeier et al. 2003; Ding et al. 2006a). Additionally, exercise attenuates the effects of oxidative stress, as indicated by a reduction in the level of membrane lipid peroxidation and oxidative damage to DNA and proteins (Radak et al. 2001a, 2001b; Vaynman and Gomez-Pinilla 2005).

Beneficial effects of exercise are well documented in young animals following SCI. Physical activity improves recovery of function following SCI in young rodents, perhaps due to the ability of exercise to alter the levels of neurotrophins, influencing growth and synaptic plasticity following SCI (Edgerton et al. 2001;

Multon et al. 2003; Van Meeteren et al. 2003; Engesser-Cesar et al. 2005, 2007; Ying et al. 2005; Erschbamer et al. 2006).

Similarly, there are beneficial effects of long-term exercise on recovery from contusion SCI in aged rats as well. Siegenthaler et al. (2008a) demonstrate that chronic voluntary wheel running improves locomotor recovery, lessens the amount of pathology and demyelination, and improves the efficiency of remyelination following contusion SCI in aged rats. These studies suggest that exercise decreases the age-associated loss in neuroprotection following SCI injury and increases the reparative mechanisms that are deficient in the aged rat following SCI.

AGE AND EXERCISE SPECIFICALLY AFFECT THE PROLIFERATION, PURITY, AND MIGRATION OF OPCs

The effect of age and exercise on the demyelination and remyelination that occurs following contusion SCI raises the question of how age and exercise affect endogenous OPC populations. In addition, what are the implications of the aging and exercise effects for cell replacement strategies? Specifically, how may the microenvironment of the injured spinal cord of aged and exercised animals influence transplanted hESC-derived OPCs?

Endogenous remyelination following SCI-induced demyelination begins with the recruitment of OPCs. Sources of OPCs include progenitors residing in the local gray and white matters, and early progenitors from the subventricular and subependymal regions within the spinal cord (Adrian and Walker 1962; Weiss et al. 1996; Horner et al. 2000; Becker et al. 2003). Once recruited to the site of demyelination, OPCs proliferate prior to differentiating into mature myelin-producing oligodendrocytes (McTigue et al. 1998, 2001; Watanabe et al. 2002; McDonald and Belegu 2006; Yang et al. 2006).

This multifaceted process of OPC recruitment, proliferation, and differentiation is in part orchestrated by the expression of specific growth factors. Motility of OPCs is induced by platelet-derived growth factor (PDGF) and basic fibroblast growth factor (bFGF) (Noble et al. 1988; McKay et al. 1997; Milner et al. 1997; Woodruff and Franklin 1999). Interestingly, the expression of PDGF and fibroblast growth factor 2 (FGF2) also inhibits the differentiation of OPCs into mature oligodendrocytes (Noble et al. 1988; Murtie et al. 2005; Wang et al. 2007), which is important in fully enabling recruitment because differentiating OPCs are limited in their migration and subsequent integration after injury (McDonald and Belegu 2006). Known mitogens of OPCs include PDGF, bFGF, IGF-1, and hepatocyte growth factor (Noble et al. 1988; Wolswijk et al. 1991; Wolswijk and Noble 1992; Engel and Wolswijk 1996; Cui and Almazan 2007; Ohya et al. 2007). Differentiation of OPCs is initiated by a decrease in PDGF and FGF2 expression coinciding with an increased expression of growth factors such as IGF-1 (McKay et al. 1997; Woodruff and Franklin 1999; Wilson et al. 2003).

There is evidence of dysregulation in the expression of these myelination-associated growth factors with age. The age-associated delay in remyelination following toxin-induced demyelination is suggested to be a result of delayed expression of PDGF and IGF-1, which in turn delays recruitment and differentiation of OPCs (Shields et al. 1999; Hinks and Franklin 2000; Franklin et al. 2002; Sim et al. 2002). Such age-associated dysregulation of growth factors implicated in remyelination following toxin-induced demyelination may also result in the age-associated differences in demyelination and remyelination following SCI (Siegenthaler et al. 2008b).

In vitro examination of the effects of proteins from 3-month-old rats, 12-month-old sedentary rats, and 12-month-old exercised rats 7 days post-SCI on the proliferation, purity, and migration of hESC-derived OPCs lends insight into the molecular mechanisms behind the age-associated deficits in neuroprotection and repair, and the exercise-induced attenuation of age-associated deficits following contusion SCI. These studies demonstrated that exercise attenuates the decrease in OPC colony area when exposed to SCI proteins from both 3-month-old and 12-month-old sedentary rats, indicating that exercise is neuroprotective. Additionally, exercise increases proliferation of OPCs, significantly enhances OPC motility, and attenuates the age-associated decrease in the percentage of cells expressing PDGF receptor alpha (PDGFRα), a marker for OPCs, in culture (Siegenthaler and Keirstead 2008).

Examination of growth factor levels expressed within one centimeter of the injury epicenter 7 days post-SCI in 3-month-old, 12-month-old sedentary, and 12-month-old exercised rats indicates that exercise elevates the expression of PDGF, IGF-1, and BDNF. Additionally, 12-month-old sedentary SCI rats express lower levels of BDNF as compared to 3-month-old SCI rats (Siegenthaler and Keirstead 2008).

Addition of PDGF at high and low concentrations to OPC cultures demonstrates that OPCs migrate and proliferate in response to PDGF in a dose-dependent fashion. Functional block of PDGF in cultures exposed to SCI proteins from 3-month-old rats significantly decreases migration and decreases the percentage of cells expressing PDGFRα in culture. This suggests that the elevated PDGF levels 7 days following SCI in 12-month-old exercised rats may cause increased recruitment, proliferation, and maintenance of the PDGFRα phenotype (Siegenthaler and Keirstead 2008).

BDNF is known to be elevated with physical activity in both the brain and spinal cord (Neeper et al. 1995, 1996; Perreau et al. 2005). BDNF is known to protect oligodendrocytes from apoptosis following SCI, possibly by increasing the expression of free radical scavengers (Ikeda et al. 2002; Koda et al. 2002). Comparison of BDNF levels 7 days following SCI demonstrates that there is an age-associated decline in BDNF expression that is attenuated by exercise (Siegenthaler and Keirstead 2008). These differing levels of BDNF may therefore account for the age-associated increase in demyelination that is attenuated by exercise.

Locomotor training can also increase expression of tyrosine receptor kinase B (TrkB), a receptor for BDNF, in OPCs (Skup et al. 2002). By doing so, locomotor training may enhance the actions of BDNF, which has been shown to induce OPC proliferation and myelination following SCI (McTigue et al. 1998). This activity-induced myelination may also indicate that the increased remyelination efficiency following SCI in 12-month-old exercised rats (Siegenthaler et al. 2008a) is mediated by BDNF.

Functional block of BDNF in cultures exposed to SCI proteins from 3-month-old rats significantly increases the percentage of OPCs expressing cleaved caspase-3, suggesting that apoptosis is increased (Siegenthaler and Keirstead 2008). This is the first indication that BDNF suppresses apoptosis in OPCs. BDNF is implicated in the survival of early neural progenitors derived from mesenchymal stem cells (Zhao et al. 2004). It is possible that the BDNF-mediated cell survival in these early neural cells and in mature cell populations, such as neurons and oligodendrocytes, is inducing cell survival through the TrkB receptor in OPCs. Interestingly, hESC-derived OPCs in culture express BDNF, exerting neuroprotection and neuroregeneration on neuronal populations (Zhang et al. 2006). Whether the BDNF secreted by the OPCs also affects their self-survival remains to be determined.

CONCLUSIONS

Taken together, it is apparent that type of injury, age at time of injury, and physical activity are variables that may dictate differing therapies for the treatment of SCI. Current therapies aimed at ameliorating demyelination following SCI may not be suitable for laceration SCI. In contrast, contusion SCI may benefit greatly from therapies targeting demyelination. However, therapies aimed at remyelinating axons may be complicated by age-associated loss in neuroprotection and regeneration. Importantly, these age-associated deficits may be negated or attenuated in patients with a history of chronic exercise, or may be attenuated with proper rehabilitation and/or mimicry of the molecular microenvironment produced by physical activity.

REFERENCES

Adams N, Boice R (1983) A longitudinal study of dominance in an outdoor colony of domestic rats. *J Comp Psychol* 97:24–33.

Adrian EK, Jr., Walker BE (1962) Incorporation of thymidine-H3 by cells in normal and injured mouse spinal cord. *J Neuropathol Exp Neurol* 21:597–609.

Ang ET, Wong PT, Moochhala S, Ng YK (2003) Neuroprotection associated with running: is it a result of increased endogenous neurotrophic factors? *Neuroscience* 118: 335–45.

Azcoitia I, Sierra A, Veiga S, Garcia-Segura LM (2003) Aromatase expression by reactive astroglia is neuroprotective. *Ann NY Acad Sci* 1007:298–305.

Beattie MS (2004) Inflammation and apoptosis: linked therapeutic targets in spinal cord injury. *Trends Mol Med* 10:580–3.

Beattie MS, Farooqui AA, Bresnahan JC (2000) Review of current evidence for apoptosis after spinal cord injury. *J Neurotrauma* 17:915–25.

Becker D, Sadowsky CL, McDonald JW (2003) Restoring function after spinal cord injury. *Neurologist* 9:1–15.

Byrnes KR, Waynant RW, Ilev IK, Wu X, Barna L, Smith K, Heckert R, Gerst H, Anders JJ (2005) Light promotes regeneration and functional recovery and alters the immune response after spinal cord injury. *Lasers Surg Med* 36:171–85.

Carlson GD, Minato Y, Okada A, Gorden CD, Warden KE, Barbeau JM, Biro CL, Bahnuik E, Bohlman HH, Lamanna JC (1997b) Early time-dependent decompression for spinal cord injury: vascular mechanisms of recovery. *J Neurotrauma* 14:951–62.

Carlson GD, Warden KE, Barbeau JM, Bahniuk E, Kutina-Nelson KL, Biro CL, Bohlman HH, LaManna JC (1997a) Viscoelastic relaxation and regional blood flow response to spinal cord compression and decompression. *Spine* 22:1285–91.

CDC (2006) Spinal Cord Injury (SCI): Fact Sheet. In Chari DM, Crang AJ, Blakemore WF (2003) Decline in rate of colonization of oligodendrocyte progenitor cell (OPC)-depleted tissue by adult OPCs with age. *J Neuropathol Exp Neurol* 62:908–16.

Ciriza I, Azcoitia I, Garcia-Segura LM (2004a) Reduced progesterone metabolites protect rat hippocampal neurones from kainic acid excitotoxicity in vivo. *J Neuroendocrinol* 16:58–63.

Ciriza I, Carrero P, Azcoitia I, Lundeen SG, Garcia-Segura LM (2004b) Selective estrogen receptor modulators protect hippocampal neurons from kainic acid excitotoxicity: differences with the effect of estradiol. *J Neurobiol* 61:209–21.

Cloutier F, Siegenthaler MM, Nistor G, Keirstead HS (2006) Transplantation of human embryonic stem cell-derived oligodendrocyte progenitors into rat spinal cord injuries does not cause harm. *Regen Med* 1:469–79.

Cui QL, Almazan G (2007) IGF-I-induced oligodendrocyte progenitor proliferation requires PI3K/Akt, MEK/ERK, and Src-like tyrosine kinases. *J Neurochem* 100: 1480–93.

Deumens R, Koopmans GC, Joosten EA (2005) Regeneration of descending axon tracts after spinal cord injury. *Prog Neurobiol* 77:57–89.

Ding Q, Vaynman S, Akhavan M, Ying Z, Gomez-Pinilla F (2006a) Insulin-like growth factor I interfaces with brain-derived neurotrophic factor-mediated synaptic plasticity to modulate aspects of exercise-induced cognitive function. *Neuroscience* 140: 823–33.

Ding YH, Mrizek M, Lai Q, Wu Y, Reyes R, Jr., Li J, Davis WW, Ding Y (2006b) Exercise preconditioning reduces brain damage and inhibits TNF-alpha receptor expression after hypoxia/reoxygenation: an in vivo and in vitro study. *Curr Neurovasc Res* 3:263–71.

Dusart I, Schwab ME (1994) Secondary cell death and the inflammatory reaction after dorsal hemisection of the rat spinal cord. *Eur J Neurosci* 6:712–24.

Edgerton VR, Leon RD, Harkema SJ, Hodgson JA, London N, Reinkensmeyer DJ, Roy RR, Talmadge RJ, Tillakaratne NJ, Timoszyk W, Tobin A (2001) Retraining the injured spinal cord. *J Physiol* 533:15–22.

Ellingson BM, Ulmer JL, Prost RW, Schmit BD (2006) Morphology and morphometry in chronic spinal cord injury assessed using diffusion tensor imaging and fuzzy logic. *Conf Proc IEEE Eng Med Biol Soc* 1:1885–8.

Ellingson BM, Ulmer JL, Schmit BD (2008) Morphology and morphometry of human chronic spinal cord injury using diffusion tensor imaging and fuzzy logic. *Ann Biomed Eng* 36:224–36.

Engel U, Wolswijk G (1996) Oligodendrocyte-type-2 astrocyte (O-2A) progenitor cells derived from adult rat spinal cord: in vitro characteristics and response to PDGF, bFGF and NT-3. *Glia* 16:16–26.

Engesser-Cesar C, Anderson AJ, Basso DM, Edgerton VR, Cotman CW (2005) Voluntary wheel running improves recovery from a moderate spinal cord injury. *J Neurotrauma* 22:157–71.

Engesser-Cesar C, Ichiyama RM, Nefas AL, Hill MA, Edgerton VR, Cotman CW, Anderson AJ (2007) Wheel running following spinal cord injury improves locomotor recovery and stimulates serotonergic fiber growth. *Eur J Neurosci* 25:1931–9.

Erschbamer MK, Pham TM, Zwart MC, Baumans V, Olson L (2006) Neither environmental enrichment nor voluntary wheel running enhances recovery from incomplete spinal cord injury in rats. *Exp Neurol* 201:154–64.

Finnerup NB, Gyldensted C, Nielsen E, Kristensen AD, Bach FW, Jensen TS (2003) MRI in chronic spinal cord injury patients with and without central pain. *Neurology* 61: 1569–75.

Franklin RJ, Zhao C, Sim FJ (2002) Ageing and CNS remyelination. *Neuroreport* 13: 923–8.

Garcia-Segura LM, Diz-Chaves Y, Perez-Martin M, Darnaudery M (2007) Estradiol, insulin-like growth factor-I and brain aging. *Psychoneuroendocrinology* 32(Suppl) 1: S57–61.

Genazzani AR, Petraglia F, Bernardi F, Casarosa E, Salvestroni C, Tonetti A, Nappi RE, Luisi S, Palumbo M, Purdy RH, Luisi M (1998) Circulating levels of allopregnanolone in humans: gender, age, and endocrine influences. *J Clin Endocrinol Metab* 83: 2099–103.

Genovese T, Mazzon E, Di Paola R, Crisafulli C, Muia C, Bramanti P, Cuzzocrea S (2006) Increased oxidative-related mechanisms in the spinal cord injury in old rats. *Neurosci Lett* 393:141–6.

Grossman SD, Rosenberg LJ, Wrathall JR (2001) Temporal-spatial pattern of acute neuronal and glial loss after spinal cord contusion. *Exp Neurol* 168:273–82.

Guest J, Herrera LP, Qian T (2006) Rapid recovery of segmental neurological function in a tetraplegic patient following transplantation of fetal olfactory bulb-derived cells. *Spinal Cord* 44:135–42.

Gwak YS, Hains BC, Johnson KM, Hulsebosch CE (2004) Effect of age at time of spinal cord injury on behavioral outcomes in rat. *J Neurotrauma* 21:983–93.

Hayashi M, Yamashita A, Shimizu K (1997) Somatostatin and brain-derived neurotrophic factor mRNA expression in the primate brain: decreased levels of mRNAs during aging. *Brain Res* 749:283–9.

Hayes KC, Kakulas BA (1997) Neuropathology of human spinal cord injury sustained in sports-related activities. *J Neurotrauma* 14:235–48.

Heinemeier K, Langberg H, Kjaer M (2003) Exercise-induced changes in circulating levels of transforming growth factor-beta-1 in humans: methodological considerations. *Eur J Appl Physiol* 90:171–7.

Hinks GL, Franklin RJ (2000) Delayed changes in growth factor gene expression during slow remyelination in the CNS of aged rats. *Mol Cell Neurosci* 16:542–56.

Hoffman AR, Lieberman SA, Ceda GP (1992) Growth hormone therapy in the elderly: implications for the aging brain. *Psychoneuroendocrinology* 17:327–33.

Horner PJ, Power AE, Kempermann G, Kuhn HG, Palmer TD, Winkler J, Thal LJ, Gage
    FH (2000) Proliferation and differentiation of progenitor cells throughout the intact
    adult rat spinal cord. *J Neurosci* 20:2218–28.
Ikeda O, Murakami M, Ino H, Yamazaki M, Koda M, Nakayama C, Moriya H (2002)
    Effects of brain-derived neurotrophic factor (BDNF) on compression-induced spinal
    cord injury: BDNF attenuates down-regulation of superoxide dismutase expression
    and promotes up-regulation of myelin basic protein expression. *J Neuropathol Exp
    Neurol* 61:142–53.
Izrael M, Zhang P, Kaufman R, Shinder V, Ella R, Amit M, Itskovitz-Eldor J, Chebath J,
    Revel M (2007) Human oligodendrocytes derived from embryonic stem cells: Effect
    of noggin on phenotypic differentiation in vitro and on myelination in vivo. *Mol Cell
    Neurosci* 34:310–23.
Keirstead HS, Nistor G, Bernal G, Totoiu M, Cloutier F, Sharp K, Steward O (2005)
    Human embryonic stem cell-derived oligodendrocyte progenitor cell transplants remy-
    elinate and restore locomotion after spinal cord injury. *J Neurosci* 25: 4694–705.
Keller JN, Huang FF, Markesbery WR (2000) Decreased levels of proteasome activity
    and proteasome expression in aging spinal cord. *Neuroscience* 98:149–56.
Klussmann S, Martin-Villalba A (2005) Molecular targets in spinal cord injury. *J Mol
    Med* 83:657–71.
Koda M, Murakami M, Ino H, Yoshinaga K, Ikeda O, Hashimoto M, Yamazaki M,
    Nakayama C, Moriya H (2002) Brain-derived neurotrophic factor suppresses delayed
    apoptosis of oligodendrocytes after spinal cord injury in rats. *J Neurotrauma*
    19:777–85.
Kovari E, Gold G, Herrmann FR, Canuto A, Hof PR, Michel JP, Bouras C, Giannakopou-
    los P (2004) Cortical microinfarcts and demyelination significantly affect cognition in
    brain aging. *Stroke* 35:410–4.
Kullberg S, Ramirez-Leon V, Johnson H, Ulfhake B (1998) Decreased axosomatic input
    to motoneurons and astrogliosis in the spinal cord of aged rats. *J Gerontol A Biol Sci
    Med Sci* 53:B369–79.
Kwon BK, Fisher CG, Dvorak MF, Tetzlaff W (2005) Strategies to promote neural repair
    and regeneration after spinal cord injury. *Spine* 30:S3–13.
Kwon BK, Tetzlaff W, Grauer JN, Beiner J, Vaccaro AR (2004) Pathophysiology and
    pharmacologic treatment of acute spinal cord injury. *Spine J* 4:451–64.
Kyrkanides S, O'Banion MK, Whiteley PE, Daeschner JC, Olschowka JA (2001)
    Enhanced glial activation and expression of specific CNS inflammation-related mole-
    cules in aged versus young rats following cortical stab injury. *J Neuroimmunol* 119:
    269–77.
Liu XZ, Xu XM, Hu R, Du C, Zhang SX, McDonald JW, Dong HX, Wu YJ, Fan GS,
    Jacquin MF, Hsu CY, Choi DW (1997) Neuronal and glial apoptosis after traumatic
    spinal cord injury. *J Neurosci* 17:5395–406.
Liverman CT, Altevogt BM, Joy JE, Johnson RT (2005) *Spinal cord injury: Progress,
    promise, and priorities*. Washington, DC: National Academies Press.
McDonald JW, Belegu V (2006) Demyelination and remyelination after spinal cord injury.
    J Neurotrauma 23:345–59.
McKay JS, Blakemore WF, Franklin RJ (1997) The effects of the growth factor-antago-
    nist, trapidil, on remyelination in the CNS. *Neuropathol Appl Neurobiol* 23:50–58.
McTigue DM, Horner PJ, Stokes BT, Gage FH (1998) Neurotrophin-3 and brain-derived
    neurotrophic factor induce oligodendrocyte proliferation and myelination of regener-
    ating axons in the contused adult rat spinal cord. *J Neurosci* 18:5354–65.

McTigue DM, Wei P, Stokes BT (2001) Proliferation of NG2-positive cells and altered oligodendrocyte numbers in the contused rat spinal cord. *J Neurosci* 21: 3392–400.

Milner R, Anderson HJ, Rippon RF, McKay JS, Franklin RJ, Marchionni MA, Reynolds R, Ffrench-Constant C (1997) Contrasting effects of mitogenic growth factors on oligodendrocyte precursor cell migration. *Glia* 19:85–90.

Morales AJ, Haubrich RH, Hwang JY, Asakura H, Yen SS (1998) The effect of six months treatment with a 100 mg daily dose of dehydroepiandrosterone (DHEA) on circulating sex steroids, body composition and muscle strength in age-advanced men and women. *Clin Endocrinol* (Oxf) 49:421–32.

Multon S, Franzen R, Poirrier AL, Scholtes F, Schoenen J (2003) The effect of treadmill training on motor recovery after a partial spinal cord compression-injury in the adult rat. *J Neurotrauma* 20:699–706.

Murtie JC, Zhou YX, Le TQ, Armstrong RC (2005) In vivo analysis of oligodendrocyte lineage development in postnatal FGF2 null mice. *Glia* 49:542–54.

Navarro A, Boveris A (2007a) The mitochondrial energy transduction system and the aging process. *Am J Physiol Cell Physiol* 292:C670–86.

Navarro A, Boveris A (2007b) Brain mitochondrial dysfunction in aging: conditions that improve survival, neurological performance and mitochondrial function. *Front Biosci* 12:1154–63.

Neeper SA, Gomez-Pinilla F, Choi J, Cotman C (1995) Exercise and brain neurotrophins. *Nature* 373:109.

Neeper SA, Gomez-Pinilla F, Choi J, Cotman CW (1996) Physical activity increases mRNA for brain-derived neurotrophic factor and nerve growth factor in rat brain. *Brain Res* 726:49–56.

Nistor GI, Totoiu MO, Haque N, Carpenter MK, Keirstead HS (2005) Human embryonic stem cells differentiate into oligodendrocytes in high purity and myelinate after spinal cord transplantation. *Glia* 49:385–96.

Noble M, Murray K, Stroobant P, Waterfield MD, Riddle P (1988) Platelet-derived growth factor promotes division and motility and inhibits premature differentiation of the oligodendrocyte/type-2 astrocyte progenitor cell. *Nature* 333:560–2.

Norenberg MD, Smith J, Marcillo A (2004) The pathology of human spinal cord injury: defining the problems. *J Neurotrauma* 21:429–40.

NSCISC (2006) Facts and Figures at a Glance. In Ohya W, Funakoshi H, Kurosawa T, Nakamura T (2007) Hepatocyte growth factor (HGF) promotes oligodendrocyte progenitor cell proliferation and inhibits its differentiation during postnatal development in the rat. *Brain Res* 1147:51–65.

Park E, Velumian AA, Fehlings MG (2004) The role of excitotoxicity in secondary mechanisms of spinal cord injury: a review with an emphasis on the implications for white matter degeneration. *J Neurotrauma* 21:754–74.

Perreau VM, Adlard PA, Anderson AJ, Cotman CW (2005) Exercise-induced gene expression changes in the rat spinal cord. *Gene Expr* 12:107–21.

Peters A, Sethares C (2003) Is there remyelination during aging of the primate central nervous system? *J Comp Neurol* 460:238–54.

Popovich PG, Hickey WF (2001) Bone marrow chimeric rats reveal the unique distribution of resident and recruited macrophages in the contused rat spinal cord. *J Neuropathol Exp Neurol* 60:676–85.

Quinn R (2005) Comparing rat's to human's age: how old is my rat in people years? *Nutrition* 21:775–7.

Radak Z, Kaneko T, Tahara S, Nakamoto H, Pucsok J, Sasvari M, Nyakas C, Goto S (2001b) Regular exercise improves cognitive function and decreases oxidative damage in rat brain. *Neurochem Int* 38:17–23.

Radak Z, Taylor AW, Ohno H, Goto S (2001a) Adaptation to exercise-induced oxidative stress: from muscle to brain. *Exerc Immunol Rev* 7:90–107.

Raz N, Lindenberger U, Rodrigue KM, Kennedy KM, Head D, Williamson A, Dahle C, Gerstorf D, Acker JD (2005) Regional brain changes in aging healthy adults: general trends, individual differences and modifiers. *Cereb Cortex* 15:1676–89.

Raz N, Rodrigue KM (2006) Differential aging of the brain: patterns, cognitive correlates and modifiers. *Neurosci Biobehav Rev* 30:730–48.

Schwab ME, Bartholdi D (1996) Degeneration and regeneration of axons in the lesioned spinal cord. *Physiol Rev* 76:319–70.

Schwarz AJ, Brasel JA, Hintz RL, Mohan S, Cooper DM (1996) Acute effect of brief low- and high-intensity exercise on circulating insulin-like growth factor (IGF) I, II, and IGF-binding protein-3 and its proteolysis in young healthy men. *J Clin Endocrinol Metab* 81:3492–7.

Shields SA, Gilson JM, Blakemore WF, Franklin RJ (1999) Remyelination occurs as extensively but more slowly in old rats compared to young rats following gliotoxin-induced CNS demyelination. *Glia* 28:77–83.

Siegenthaler MM, Ammon DL, Keirstead HS (2008b) Age-associated deficits following SCI. *Exp Neurol* doi: 10.1016/j.expneurol.2008.06.015.

Siegenthaler MM, Berchtold NC, Cotman CW, Keirstead HS (2007b) Voluntary running attenuates age-related deficits following SCI. *Exp Neurol* 210:207–16.

Siegenthaler MM, Keirstead H (2008) Age and exercise at time of SCI in rats affects the proliferation, survival, and migration of hESC-derived OPCs in vitro. Manuscript in Preparation.

Siegenthaler MM, Tu MK, Keirstead HS (2007a) The extent of myelin pathology differs following contusion and transection spinal cord injury. *J Neurotrauma* 24:1631–46.

Sim FJ, Zhao C, Penderis J, Franklin RJ (2002) The age-related decrease in CNS remyelination efficiency is attributable to an impairment of both oligodendrocyte progenitor recruitment and differentiation. *J Neurosci* 22:2451–9.

Skup M, Dwornik A, Macias M, Sulejczak D, Wiater M, Czarkowska-Bauch J (2002) Long-term locomotor training up-regulates TrkB(FL) receptor-like proteins, brain-derived neurotrophic factor, and neurotrophin 4 with different topographies of expression in oligodendroglia and neurons in the spinal cord. *Exp Neurol* 176:289–307.

Stummer W, Weber K, Tranmer B, Baethmann A, Kempski O (1994) Reduced mortality and brain damage after locomotor activity in gerbil forebrain ischemia. *Stroke* 25: 1862–9.

Totoiu MO, Keirstead HS (2005) Spinal cord injury is accompanied by chronic progressive demyelination. *J Comp Neurol* 486:373–83.

Trejo JL, Carro E, Torres-Aleman I (2001) Circulating insulin-like growth factor I mediates exercise-induced increases in the number of new neurons in the adult hippocampus. *J Neurosci* 21:1628–34.

Tsai EC, Tator CH (2005) Neuroprotection and regeneration strategies for spinal cord repair. *Curr Pharm Des* 11:1211–22.

Van Meeteren NL, Eggers R, Lankhorst AJ, Gispen WH, Hamers FP (2003) Locomotor recovery after spinal cord contusion injury in rats is improved by spontaneous exercise. *J Neurotrauma* 20:1029–37.

Vaynman S, Gomez-Pinilla F (2005) License to run: exercise impacts functional plasticity in the intact and injured central nervous system by using neurotrophins. *Neurorehabil Neural Repair* 19:283–95.

Veiga S, Garcia-Segura LM, Azcoitia I (2003) Neuroprotection by the steroids pregnenolone and dehydroepiandrosterone is mediated by the enzyme aromatase. *J Neurobiol* 56:398–406.

Veiga S, Melcangi RC, Doncarlos LL, Garcia-Segura LM, Azcoitia I (2004) Sex hormones and brain aging. *Exp Gerontol* 39:1623–31.

Wang Z, Colognato H, Ffrench-Constant C (2007) Contrasting effects of mitogenic growth factors on myelination in neuron-oligodendrocyte co-cultures. *Glia* 55: 537–45.

Watanabe M, Toyama Y, Nishiyama A (2002) Differentiation of proliferated NG2-positive glial progenitor cells in a remyelinating lesion. *J Neurosci Res* 69:826–36.

Weiss S, Dunne C, Hewson J, Wohl C, Wheatley M, Peterson AC, Reynolds BA (1996) Multipotent CNS stem cells are present in the adult mammalian spinal cord and ventricular neuroaxis. *J Neurosci* 16:7599–609.

Wilson HC, Onischke C, Raine CS (2003) Human oligodendrocyte precursor cells in vitro: phenotypic analysis and differential response to growth factors. *Glia* 44: 153–65.

Wolswijk G, Noble M (1992) Cooperation between PDGF and FGF converts slowly dividing O-2Aadult progenitor cells to rapidly dividing cells with characteristics of O-2Aperinatal progenitor cells. *J Cell Biol* 118:889–900.

Wolswijk G, Riddle PN, Noble M (1991) Platelet-derived growth factor is mitogenic for O-2Aadult progenitor cells. *Glia* 4:495–503.

Woodruff RH, Franklin RJ (1999) The expression of myelin protein mRNAs during remyelination of lysolecithin-induced demyelination. *Neuropathol Appl Neurobiol* 25: 226–35.

Yang H, Lu P, McKay HM, Bernot T, Keirstead H, Steward O, Gage FH, Edgerton VR, Tuszynski MH (2006) Endogenous neurogenesis replaces oligodendrocytes and astrocytes after primate spinal cord injury. *J Neurosci* 26:2157–66.

Ying Z, Roy RR, Edgerton VR, Gomez-Pinilla F (2005) Exercise restores levels of neurotrophins and synaptic plasticity following spinal cord injury. *Exp Neurol* 193:411–9.

Zhang YW, Denham J, Thies RS (2006) Oligodendrocyte progenitor cells derived from human embryonic stem cells express neurotrophic factors. *Stem Cells Dev* 15: 943–52.

Zhao C, Li WW, Franklin RJ (2006) Differences in the early inflammatory responses to toxin-induced demyelination are associated with the age-related decline in CNS remyelination. *Neurobiol Aging* 27:1298–307.

Zhao LX, Zhang J, Cao F, Meng L, Wang DM, Li YH, Nan X, Jiao WC, Zheng M, Xu XH, Pei XT (2004) Modification of the brain-derived neurotrophic factor gene: a portal to transform mesenchymal stem cells into advantageous engineering cells for neuroregeneration and neuroprotection. *Exp Neurol* 190:396–406.

INDEX

Note: Page numbers followed by *f* indicate figures; page numbers followed by *t* indicate tables.